Thank you ♡ for all your support!

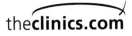

RHEUMATIC DISEASE CLINICS OF NORTH AMERICA

Scleroderma

GUEST EDITOR
Fredrick M. Wigley, MD

February 2008 • Volume 34 • Number 1

SAUNDERS

An Imprint of Elsevier, Inc.
PHILADELPHIA   LONDON   TORONTO   MONTREAL   SYDNEY   TOKYO

W.B. SAUNDERS COMPANY
A Division of Elsevier Inc.

1600 John F. Kennedy Boulevard • Suite 1800 • Philadelphia, Pennsylvania 19103-2899

http://www.theclinics.com

RHEUMATIC DISEASE
CLINICS OF NORTH AMERICA
February 2008
Editor: Rachel Glover

Volume 34, Number 1
ISSN 0889-857X
ISBN 13: 978-1-4160-5863-2
ISBN 10: 1-4160-5863-X

The ideas and opinions expressed in *Rheumatic Disease Clinics of North America* do not necessarily reflect those of the Publisher. The Publisher does not assume any responsibility for any injury and/or damage to persons or property arising out of or related to any use of the material contained in this periodical. The reader is advised to check the appropriate medical literature and the product information currently provided by the manufacturer of each drug to be administered to verify the dosage, the method and duration of administration, or contraindications. It is the responsibility of the treating physician or other health care professional, relying on independent experience and knowledge of the patient, to determine drug dosages and the best treatment of the patient. Mention of any product in this issue should not be construed as endorsement by the contributors, editors, or the Publisher of the product or manufacturers' claims.

Rheumatic Disease Clinics of North America (ISSN 0889-857X) is published quarterly by Elsevier Inc., 360 Park Avenue South, New York, NY 10010-1710. Months of issue are February, May, August, and November. Business and editorial offices: 1600 John F. Kennedy Boulevard, Suite 1800, Philadelphia, PA 19103-2899. Customer Service offices: 6277 Sea Harbor Drive, Orlando, FL 32887-4800. Periodicals postage paid at New York, NY and additional mailing offices. Subscription prices are USD 226 per year for US individuals, USD 370 per year for US institutions, USD 113 per year for US students and residents, USD 267 per year for Canadian individuals, USD 448 per year for Canadian institutions, USD 297 per year for international individuals, USD 448 per year for international institutions and USD 149 per year for Canadian and foreign students/residents. To receive student/resident rate, orders must be accompanied by name of affiliated institution, date of term, and the *signature* of program/residency coordinator on institution letterhead. Orders will be billed at individual rate until proof of status received. Foreign air speed delivery is included in all *Clinics* subscription prices. All prices are subject to change without notice. POSTMASTER: Send address changes to *Rheumatic Disease Clinics of North America*, Elsevier Journals Customer Service, 6277 Sea Harbor Drive, Orlando, FL 32887-4800. **Customer Service: 1-800-654-2452 (USA). From outside of the USA, call (+1) 407-563-6020. Fax: 1-407-363-9661. E-mail: JournalsCustomerService-usa@elsevier.com.**

Reprints. For copies of 100 or more of articles in this publication, please contact the Commercial Reprints Department, Elsevier Inc., 360 Park Avenue South, New York, 10010-1710; Tel.: (+1) 212-633-3813, Fax: (+1) 212-462-1935, and E-mail: reprints@elsevier.com.

Rheumatic Disease Clinics of North America is covered in *Index Medicus, Current Contents/Clinical Medicine, Science Citation Index, ISI/BIOMED,* and *EMBASE/Excerpta Medica.*

Printed in the United States of America.

GUEST EDITOR

FREDRICK M. WIGLEY, MD, Associate Director, Division of Rheumatology; and Director, Johns Hopkins Scleroderma Center, Johns Hopkins University, Baltimore, Maryland

CONTRIBUTORS

SANDEEP K. AGARWAL, MD, PhD, Division of Rheumatology, Department of Internal Medicine, The University of Texas Health Sciences Center at Houston, Houston, Texas

FRANK C. ARNETT, MD, Division of Rheumatology, Department of Internal Medicine, The University of Texas Health Sciences Center at Houston, Houston, Texas

FRANCESCO BOIN, MD, Instructor of Medicine, Division of Rheumatology, Johns Hopkins University School of Medicine, Baltimore, Maryland

HUNTER C. CHAMPION, MD, PhD, Assistant Professor of Medicine, Division of Cardiology, Department of Medicine, The Johns Hopkins Medical Institutions, Johns Hopkins University School of Medicine, Baltimore, Maryland

CHRISTOPHER P. DENTON, PhD, FRCP, Professor of Experimental Rheumatology, Centre for Rheumatology, Royal Free Hospital, London, United Kingdom

JÖRG DISTLER, MD, Department of Internal Medicine III; and Institute of Clinical Immunology, University Erlangen–Nuremberg, Erlangen, Germany

OLIVER DISTLER, MD, Department of Rheumatology, Center for Experimental Rheumatology, University Hospital Zurich, Zurich, Switzerland

NICHOLAS A. FLAVAHAN, PhD, Professor and Director of Research, Department of Anesthesiology and Critical Care Medicine, Johns Hopkins University, Baltimore, Maryland

JO NADINE FLEMING, MD, Department of Pathology, University of Washington, Seattle, Washington

ARIANE HERRICK, MD, FRCP, Reader in Rheumatology, University of Manchester; and Salford Royal NHS Foundation Trust, Salford, United Kingdom

LAURA K. HUMMERS, MD, Assistant Professor of Medicine, Division of Rheumatology; and Co-Director, Scleroderma Center, Johns Hopkins University School of Medicine, Baltimore, Maryland

BASHAR KAHALEH, MD, Professor and Chief, Division of Rheumatology and Immunology, University of Toledo Medical Center, Toledo, Ohio

MARY JO MULLIGAN-KEHOE, PhD, Research Associate Professor of Surgery, Angiogenesis Research Center; and Department of Surgery, Vascular Section, Dartmouth-Hitchcock Medical Center, Dartmouth Medical School, Lebanon, New Hampshire

SVETLANA I. NIHTYANOVA, MBBS, Centre for Rheumatology, Royal Free Hospital, London, United Kingdom

LEWIS J. RUBIN, MD, Professor of Medicine, University of California, San Diego School of Medicine, La Jolla, California

STEPHEN MARK SCHWARTZ, MD, PhD, Department of Pathology, University of Washington, Seattle, Washington

AMI A. SHAH, MD, Post-Doctoral Fellow, Division of Rheumatology, Johns Hopkins University, Baltimore, Maryland

MICHAEL SIMONS, MD, A.G. Huber Professor of Medicine, Angiogenesis Research Center; Department of Medicine, Cardiology Section; and Department of Pharmacology and Toxicology, Dartmouth-Hitchcock Medical Center, Dartmouth Medical College, Lebanon, New Hampshire

VIRGINIA D. STEEN, MD, Professor of Medicine, Department of Medicine, Georgetown University, Washington, DC

FILEMON K. TAN, MD, PhD, Division of Rheumatology, Department of Internal Medicine, The University of Texas Health Sciences Center at Houston, Houston, Texas

MARIA TROJANOWSKA, PhD, Division of Rheumatology, Medical University of South Carolina, Charleston, South Carolina

JOHN A. VARGA, MD, Division of Rheumatology, Northwestern University, Feinberg School of Medicine, Chicago, Illinois

FREDRICK M. WIGLEY, MD, Associate Director, Division of Rheumatology; and Director, Johns Hopkins Scleroderma Center, Johns Hopkins University, Baltimore, Maryland

FRANCISCO ZULIAN, MD, Professor, Department of Pediatrics, Rheumatology Unit, University of Padova, Padova, Italy

CONTENTS

trigger it. These findings have true translational implications, because modifiers of these key mediators and key mechanisms are often in clinical use in other disease indications, such as cancer. This article summarizes the clinical and preclinical evidence of examples of these novel antifibrotic treatment approaches in systemic sclerosis, including stem cell transplantation, modifiers of transforming growth factor-β1 signaling, intravenous immunoglobulins, tyrosine kinase inhibitors, and histone deacetylase inhibitors.

Skin sclerosis is a clinical hallmark of systemic sclerosis (SSc) and provides a means to classify and evaluate patients. In the diffuse cutaneous subset, skin involvement is often extensive and warrants direct therapy. Currently, broad spectrum immunosuppressive strategies are used, but more targeted specific approaches are now emerging. This article reviews the evidence for efficacy of current treatment approaches and future developments for managing skin disease in early diffuse cutaneous SSc.

The heart is one of the major organs involved in scleroderma, the involvement of which can be manifested by myocardial disease, conduction system abnormalities, arrhythmias, or pericardial disease. Additionally, scleroderma renal crisis and pulmonary hypertension lead to significant cardiac dysfunction secondary to damage in the kidney and lung. This article summarizes the types and mechanism of abnormalities in the heart in scleroderma. The concept of cardiac dysfunction in scleroderma and other rheumatologic conditions has received new interest with the advent of newer noninvasive imaging techniques, as well as the interest in detecting subclinical disease. With this increased interest in cardiac manifestations in scleroderma comes the realization that long-term studies are needed to better assess the appropriate screening and treatment in this patient population.

Although progress has been made in treatment of pulmonary arterial hypertension, serious challenges remain. This article provides an overview of the challenges faced in treatment of PAH caused by scleroderma. It also provides a glimpse into the future, based on recent developments in the field that hold promise for enhancing the treatment of this disease.

FORTHCOMING ISSUES

RECENT ISSUES

ELSEVIER
SAUNDERS

Rheum Dis Clin N Am
34 (2008) xi–xiii

RHEUMATIC
DISEASE CLINICS
OF NORTH AMERICA

Preface

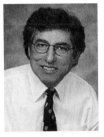

Fredrick M. Wigley, MD
Guest Editor

Systemic sclerosis (scleroderma) is unique among our rheumatic diseases, both in its clinical expression and its resistance to recovery when using our usual anti-inflammatory medications. The reason for this difference is now becoming apparent as the biology of the scleroderma process is better understood. It is now recognized that the disease expression is quite heterogeneous and that several different clinical but distinct phenotypes exist. Dr. Steen points out in her article that the different subtypes of scleroderma associate with specific autoantibodies that can be used to predict outcome and prognosis, thus providing the physician with a biologic footprint to help guide clinical decisions and management.

It is also now clear that scleroderma is a complex polygenetic disease. Understanding gene interactions, influences of environmental triggers, and epigenetic factors are allowing us to appreciate the reason that there is varied and a unique expression of scleroderma. Drs. Agarwal, Tan, and Arnett review past concepts and provide insight into how we need to use new technology to unravel the genetic influence on the biology of scleroderma.

While most agree that scleroderma is an autoimmune disease characterized by T-cell activation, auto-antibody production, and abnormal cytokine release, the pathologic features and biologic processes that make it unique are the presence of a diffuse microvascular injury and widespread activation of fibroblasts. Fibroblast activation leads to increased production of collagen, resulting in diffuse vascular damage and fibrosis of various organs including the heart, lungs, kidneys, and skin. The presence of Raynaud's phenomenon and the clear evidence of peripheral and microvascular disease

doi:10.1016/j.rdc.2008.01.002
rheumatic.theclinics.com

in the involved organ systems argue that the principle target of insult in scleroderma is the blood vessel. In this issue, the pathology, mechanism, and consequences of the vascular disease are reviewed by Drs. Fleming, Schwartz, Kahaleh, Mulligan-Kehoe, Simons, and Flavahan; Dr. Herrick then summarizes our current approach to methods to detect vascular changes and current approaches to manage this aspect of the disease. It is evident that understanding and directly managing the scleroderma vasculopathy is a major challenge for the future, and key to controlling and preventing disease progression.

At the same time, one must recognize that fibrosis is the pathologic hallmark of scleroderma and that it is this process in blood vessels, skin, and involved organs that ultimately causes organ failure and the associated morbidity and mortality. New understanding of the biologic processes that trigger and sustain tissue fibrosis is reviewed by Drs. Trojanowska and Varga.

Despite all the exciting discoveries that are happening in the research laboratory, we face many challenges in treating patients that we encounter with active and life threatening disease. Drs. Jorg and Oliver Distler provide a detailed discussion of current and novel therapeutic approaches to the treatment of inflammation and fibrosis, whereas Drs. Nihtyanova and Denton outline past therapy and their approach to early active diffuse scleroderma. The heart, lung, and pulmonary circulation are primary targets of the disease and the major cause for death among patients who have scleroderma. Current organ specific therapy is helpful, but Drs. Champion and Rubin point out that new insight into the biology of heart and lung disease is needed and novel approaches to the treatment of pulmonary hypertension are not only essential but approachable.

There are several disorders that mimic scleroderma. Drs. Boin and Hummers detail the current understanding of the pathogenesis of nephrogenic systemic fibrosis, eosinophilic fasciitis, scleromyxedema, and scleredema; these disorders are often referred to the rheumatologist who must be able to recognize and treat appropriately. In fact, therapy can be quite effective in controlling these disorders.

When dealing with patients who have scleroderma, we must recognize the varied expression of the disease and certainly manage the common manifestations, but we must not forget uncommon associated complications and manifestations that occur and need attention. Dr. Shah and I attempted to review several of these issues to make one aware and to suggest a treatment approach. Finally, we must not forget that though systemic sclerosis is usually a disease of adults, children are affected by both the systemic disease and, more commonly, localized scleroderma skin disease. Dr. Zulian reminds us of the manifestations of childhood scleroderma, the new insights into classification and clinical manifestations, and current efforts of management.

I thank all the authors for their brilliant and hard work, and hope this issue adds to the reader's knowledge. I acknowledge the Scleroderma

Research Foundation, and Nancy Bechtle and the Center's other Board members for their support of the Johns Hopkins Scleroderma Center. It is an exciting time to be working in the scleroderma field because of the burst of new work bringing us closer to understanding the disease process, the impressive number of new therapeutic options, and the intense interest supported by new technology to allow us to tackle the challenges of managing this complex human disease we call scleroderma.

Fredrick M. Wigley, MD
Johns Hopkins Scleroderma Center
John Hopkins University
5200 Eastern Avenue, Suite 4100
Mason F. Lord Building, Center Tower
Baltimore, MD 21224, USA

E-mail address: fwig@jhmi.edu

ELSEVIER
SAUNDERS

Rheum Dis Clin N Am
34 (2008) 1–15

RHEUMATIC
DISEASE CLINICS
OF NORTH AMERICA

The Many Faces of Scleroderma

Virginia D. Steen, MD

Department of Medicine, Georgetown University, 3800 Reservoir Road,
LL Gorman, Washington, DC 20007, USA

Scleroderma was first described in 1842 [1]. At that time the classic description of the disease was one of diffuse skin thickening and multisystem organ involvement. A subgroup of patients with calcinosis, Raynaud's, sclerodactyly, and telangiectasias (CRST) was identified as a milder form of the disease that was not felt to have internal organ involvement. When it was clear that these patients had significant esophageal dysmotility, Velayos and colleagues added an E and thus, the classic CREST syndrome was defined [2,3]. This syndrome was felt to have a much-improved survival compared with those patients with progressive systemic sclerosis. In the late 1970s an American Rheumatism Association subcommittee developed criteria for systemic sclerosis [4]. Patients entered into the study must have had the diagnosis of scleroderma for less than 2 years. Thus, since most CREST patients have Raynaud's phenomenon for many years before they develop other scleroderma symptoms, they were less likely included in this study. The primary criterion for systemic sclerosis was skin thickening proximal to the metacarpalphalangeal joints (MCPs). This automatically excluded most of the CREST syndrome patients who only have skin thickening of the fingers. The secondary criteria were two of the following: sclerodactyly, digital pitting scars, and interstitial fibrosis. This covered about 50% of "CREST" syndrome patients, but did not include a large number of patients who have sclerodactyly and severe gastrointestinal dysmotility. During that time there were "camps" who felt that CREST syndrome was really just the same as systemic sclerosis and others who felt that is was a distinct milder disease.

Autoantibodies were first identified in systemic sclerosis in the 1960s [5]. In the early 1980s several important observations showed that the two subsets were similar but that CREST was not a benign disease. Pulmonary arterial hypertension, which was seen almost exclusively in CREST patients, was shown to be a deadly complication of scleroderma, negating the

---

E-mail address: steenv@georgetown.edu

0889-857X/08/$ - see front matter © 2008 Elsevier Inc. All rights reserved.
doi:10.1016/j.rdc.2007.12.001   *rheumatic.theclinics.com*

impression that this was a milder disease [6]. Also, patients with CREST syndrome were identified with severe small intestinal involvement. About the same time, scleroderma-specific autoantibodies were identified that were closely associated with these two subsets of patients. Anti-Scl 70 antibody [7], an antibody to the enzyme topoisomerase I, was clinically associated with classic diffuse scleroderma. And anticentromere antibody, an antibody to the centromere of the nucleus, was associated with the classic CREST syndrome [8]. This confirmed that there were two distinct subsets within scleroderma but that the CREST syndrome was not benign and had many features that were almost identical to the diffuse form of the disease. Thus, both "camps" were right [2,9,10].

In 1988, we compared patients with positive anticentromere antibody (ACA) to those with anti-Scl 70 antibody (TOPO) [2]. This study showed that there were major differences between the subsets, including pulmonary arterial hypertension (PAH) occurring almost exclusively in ACA and renal crisis occurring almost exclusively in the TOPO group. We also showed that there were distinct genetic factors, HLA-DR 1 was associated with ACA and HLA DR 5 in TOPO. None of our patients had both antibodies and this has only rarely been reported [11]. At the same time, it was shown that the frequency and type of gastrointestinal manifestations were almost identical in the two subsets [12]. One interpretation of these data was that they were two completely different diseases; however, I tended to be a "lumper" and did not encourage this conclusion.

Over the next 10 years, various observations led to blurring of the differences between the subsets, both clinically and prognostically: PAH was seen in diffuse scleroderma [13], renal crisis was reported in CREST syndrome patients [14], "CREST" syndrome was reported in diffuse scleroderma patients with calcinosis and telangiectasias [12], CREST syndrome patients had skin thickening proximal to the MCPs [15], and pulmonary fibrosis was seen in "CREST" syndrome patients [16]. This led the scleroderma thought leaders to publish an editorial that defined limited cutaneous and diffuse cutaneous in more descriptive terms trying not to focus on only on the "CREST" manifestations [9].

In the 1990s, additional scleroderma-specific autoantibodies were identified that were associated with different clinical subsets of patients [17–20]. Although these antibody subsets tend to be associated with limited or diffuse cutaneous disease, the pattern of internal organ involvement was more variable, particularly in terms of lung involvement. Within the limited and diffuse subsets, the autoantibodies were associated with significant differences in the frequency and specific of organ involvement. Also, genetic studies show that the genetic associations were closely correlated with the specific autoantibodies and not just with limited and diffuse cutaneous subsets [21–25]. Patients with a specific genetic makeup may respond in a certain way to an antigen resulting in a specific set of disease manifestations and a specific antibody. Reproducible genetic associations have been identified with most of the antibodies [23]; however, only 1.6% of patients have a first-degree relative with scleroderma [26]. Recent twin studies did not show an increase in frequency of scleroderma in identical twins compared with fraternal twins although a positive antinuclear antibody was seen more frequently in the nonaffected twin in the identical twins [27].

Clinical features and the frequency of scleroderma subsets and antibodies are different in different countries and ethnicities supporting the importance of genetic background in the pathogenesis of systemic sclerosis [28]. In England, the ratio of limited to diffuse scleroderma is 4.7:1; in the United States it is closer to 1.5:1 [29,30]. French patients have more TOPO patients and fewer anti-RNA polymerase III (POL 3) patients than US patients [31]. Italian patients have a high percentage of anti-TOPO [32,33], but only 8% of Italian patients have POL 3 compared with 25% to 33% of patients from other countries [20,34]. In Thailand, where 100% of patients had diffuse scleroderma, anti-TOPO was present in 76% and many of the others had a nucleolar pattern [35]. This is in contrast to Australians where most patients have limited scleroderma (6:1) and 50% have ACA [35].

There is a marked increase in the prevalence of scleroderma in the Choctaw Indians who have TOPO, which has led to intensive studies looking for the gene related to scleroderma in this population [36]. Tan and colleagues [37], using microsatellite arrays, have demonstrated and hypothesized that the fibrillin 1 gene or one nearby on chromosome 15q gives an increased susceptibility in the Choctaw Indians with TOPO. This all supports that genetics play a major role in the different features of the disease within the autoantibody subsets.

Antibodies in scleroderma are not yet known to have a distinct role in the pathogenesis of the disease but appear primarily to be markers of clinical, genetic, and possibly etiologic patient subsets. The targets of the antibodies are specific components of the cell including kinetochore proteins, ribonuclear proteins, topoisomerase, and RNA polymerase enzymes. Theories include that they may be biologic markers of tissue injury, or they could cause epitope spreading [38] or could be a receptor that mediates contractions in mouse muscles [39]. None of these theories have adequate data to account for the entire disease process and most importantly they have little to no correlation with the clinical manifestations of the disease [40]. There have been several studies that suggest that the level of anti-topoisomerase antibodies may reflect the degree of activity or severity of the disease process [41–43]. Although there is no known relationship of these cellular components to the disease pathogenesis, in the future, research may show that each of these antibodies reflects specific unique pathogenic pathways. Genetic studies should specifically be looking at the antibody subsets to have a better understanding of the pathogenesis of the disease [44].

There are several "new" non-nuclear autoantibodies that have been identified in scleroderma patients. These "new" autoantibodies may actually have a role in vascular damage and in tissue fibrosis [45]. Anti-endothelial cell antibodies [46], anti-fibrillin-1 antibodies [47], anti-matrix metalloproteinases [48], and antiplatelet-derived growth factor receptor antibodies [49] have all recently been shown to be associated with specific pathogenic features in scleroderma. None of these, though, have been associated with clinical or genetic subsets, so how do these "new" antibodies relate to the other nuclear antibodies. It seems unlikely that these four (or more) very different autoantibodies are all needed for the development of the vascular and fibrotic changes seen in scleroderma. However, it would be very exciting if we could identify such an antibody that we could focus on very early in the disease process rather than the end organ process. With a better understanding of the genetics and the antibodies, we may be able to determine what role they have in developing different aspects of the disease.

Antinuclear antibodies are the hallmark of autoimmune diseases. In systemic sclerosis, autoantibodies are seen in more than 95% of patients. At this point there are seven scleroderma-specific ones that have been described with distinct subsets. Additional antibodies are being identified that may prove to be even more specific for the manifestations within an antibody subset. Others are less frequent and less specific, and there are still some that are yet to be identified with unknown clinical significance. The scleroderma-specific ones are infrequently seen in other connective tissues diseases and are even less common in non–immune mediated processes. These antibodies are usually present at the onset of symptoms and do not switch from one antibody to a different one during the course of the disease. Patients rarely have multiple antibodies [50]. Autoantibodies have been noted before any manifestations of the disease, are present at the time of diagnosis of scleroderma, and remain throughout the course of the disease [51]. Antibodies, as in this study, are usually mutually exclusive and do not change from one antibody to a different antibody during the illness [52–54].

Clinical studies have shown that the use of limited cutaneous and diffuse cutaneous scleroderma does not adequately predict the prognosis in many patients. Perhaps systemic sclerosis should be used as a generic term such as "cancer" or "heart disease" and then use the autoantibody subset as a distinct form of the disease. Treatment is still focused on individual organ systems and different antibody subsets have different frequency and severity of organ involvement. Thus, the antibody subsets still need to be lumped under the umbrella of systemic sclerosis. At this point, it seems prudent to put more emphasis on the autoantibody subsets. Although pulmonary fibrosis appears similar in all groups of patients, it may be that the pathogenesis of fibrosis in the topoisomerase patient is quite different from that seen in patients with the Th/To or U3 RNP autoantibody. It is highly likely that the distinct clinical patterns and the distinct genetic correlations with these autoantibodies represent unique syndromes within the overall disease of systemic sclerosis. This chapter will focus on the clinical differences within these antibody subsets but other recent reviews have discussed the immunology and genetics in much greater detail. It will explain the importance of using them for monitoring patients, making decisions about therapy, and for prognosis factors. It hopefully will convince the reader that the differences in the frequency and severity of the vascular, fibrotic, and inflammatory manifestations in these different autoantibody subsets reflect that the pathogenesis of the disease varies significantly within these different autoantibody subsets of patients. It is time to consider scleroderma as seven or more distinct "diseases."

Limited scleroderma

Traditionally, systemic sclerosis has been divided into limited and diffuse scleroderma because of the major differences in the extent of cutaneous disease and the type of organ systems that are involved in these subsets. However, this was based on the classic old terms "CREST" and "progressive systemic sclerosis." Patients with limited scleroderma can have one of four of the scleroderma-specific antibodies. Table 1 describes some of the major differences between these autoantibody subsets.

Table 1
Features of patients with limited scleroderma-specific autoantibodies

Antibody	ACA	Th/To	Pm/Scl	U1-RNP
No. of patients	291	72	36	71
Male sex, %*	**8**	19	19	21
African African, %*	3	4	3	**13**
Age of onset*	42	40	38	**33**
Diffuse SSc, %*	5	7	22	20
Disease duration				
At diagnosis*	**8.7**	**7.9**	3.2	3.2
Joints, %*	60	60	75	**94**
Digital ulcers, %*	**61**	29	47	49
Gangrene, %*	**18**	5	5	11
Digital tuft	**27**	7	**32**	17
Resorption* (x-ray numbers actually performed)	(41/151)	(2/28)	(7/22)	(5/29)
Calcinosis, %*	**46**	**22**	**39**	14
Muscle inflammation, %*	1	6	**58**	**27**
Any GI, %	57	33	39	39
Severe GI, %*	8	**13**	0	14
Any lung, %	45	62	58	53
Number with PFTs	(184)	(49)	(22)	(49)
Severe fibrosis, %*	6	**16**	**27**	**22**
Lowest FVC,* % predicted	87	**70**	74	75
Isolated PAH*	**19**	**32**	3	14
Severe heart, %*	4	7	6	11
Renal crisis, %*	1	4	4	7
Survival, % cumulative survival from diagnosis				
5 y, 10 y	85,75	**78,65**	95,72	**78,65**

Major differences in bold.

Abbreviations: ACA, anticentromere antibody; FVC, forced vital capacity; GI, gastrointestinal; PFT, pulmonary function test; PAH, pulmonary arterial hypertension; SSc, systemic sclerosis.

* $P < .001$ by analysis of variance.

Anticentromere antibody

Anticentromere antibody (ACA) patients are older, and have a high percentage of women and a low frequency in African American patients. The natural history is one of long-standing Raynaud's phenomenon followed by puffy fingers. At some point, patients will develop persistent swelling of fingers, reflux, heartburn, or digital ulcers. When the physician obtains laboratory studies and finds an anticentromere antibody, the diagnosis of scleroderma is made. Patients with this antibody have limited cutaneous disease and rarely have skin thickening above the distal forearms. They have facial changes of mouth furrowing and telangiectasias on face, tongue, and fingers. They frequently have digital ulcers, gangrene, and digital tip loss both from chronic ulcers as well acroosteolysis with shortening of the fingers. After many years of disease, they develop calcinosis, which most frequently occurs on the fingertips, forearms, and shins. Gastrointestinal involvement is almost always present with esophageal dysmotility. Since patients do not die early of kidney, lung, or pulmonary fibrosis, they usually have more severe esophageal, small intestine involvement with malabsorption and pseudo obstruction, and severe colon hypomotility late in their course.

Severe interstitial fibrosis and renal crisis almost never occurs, but PAH occurs in about 20% of ACA patients. Half of ACA patients who die of scleroderma will die of PAH [55–57]. The major risk factor of PAH in these patients is a low-diffusing capacity for carbon monoxide [57–59]. An increase in the pulmonary artery systolic pressure on echocardiogram may be present before definite diagnosis of PAH, but it is not yet clear whether this is a risk factor. Cardiac involvement is probably more common than realized but cardiac deaths, which are distinct from other causes of cardiac diseases, are uncommon in ACA patients. Supraventricular arrhythmias, conduction defects, and pericardial effusions are more common than severe cardiomyopathies in these patients.

Anti-Th/To antibodies

A nucleolar pattern for antinuclear antibodies in connective tissue diseases is fairly specific for scleroderma [60–62], although it is seen in liver disease, hepatocellular cancer, and other malignancies [63,64]. One of the three nucleolar antibodies seen in scleroderma, anti-Th/To, occurs in limited scleroderma patients [18,65]. This antibody has a nucleolar pattern on immunofluorescent antibody testing, but is usually not identified with the enzyme-linked immunosorbent assay (ELISA) antinuclear antibody (ANA) method (thus, a negative ANA). The assay to identify the anti-Th/To antibody is an immunoprecipitation assay, which is difficult to do and is not likely to be easily available in the near future. Thus, we can only use the presence of a nucleolar pattern to help determine whether this antibody is present. Like the ACA patients, the Th/To patients are Caucasian but more males have this antibody than ACA (19% versus 8%). These patients tend to have a shorter duration of Raynaud's before other symptoms and get more swelling of their entire hands compared with the ACA patients [18,66]. Although the closer proximity of the onset of swollen hands to Raynaud's suggests diffuse scleroderma, Th/To patients do not get diffuse cutaneous disease and only rarely get renal crisis [18]. Digital ulcers and gangrene are less common but telangiectasias and calcinosis occur after many years of disease. Th/To patients had less esophageal involvement [66] but had more frequent severe small bowel involvement [18].

The major difference between the two limited scleroderma patient groups, ACA and the nucleolar antibody, Th/To, is that Th/To patients get both interstitial and vascular pulmonary disease [66,67]. Unlike ACA patients, Th/To patients can get significant interstitial fibrosis, which occurs early in the disease (similar to the TOPO patients). Even though they have fibrosis, they also develop a vasculopathic pulmonary hypertension. Since some of these patients do not have severe fibrosis or chronic hypoxemia, it is not thought to be a secondary pulmonary hypertension [67]. The degree of pulmonary hypertension is "out of proportion" to the degree of fibrosis. However, the overall disease duration at the time of PAH is significantly shorter than in the ACA patients (10.4 years versus 13 years). This increased frequency and severity of lung disease results in a decreased survival compared with other limited scleroderma patients [68].

Pm/Scl

Another nucleolar antibody, Pm/Scl, is the least common of these seven scleroderma autoantibodies, but these patients are very easily recognized [17]. It is less common in African Americans, and most patients present with the acute onset of inflammatory muscle disease. Along with the inflammatory muscle disease, they often have dermatomyositis cutaneous skin changes. However, they also have typical Raynaud's and scleroderma skin changes. About 20% actually develop diffuse cutaneous changes. They frequently get digital tip ulcerations and interestingly have a high frequency of acro-osteolysis. Calcinosis is common and often is similar in distribution to the linear calcinosis in the muscle seen in patients with myositis. Surprisingly, they do not seem to have severe gastrointestinal or cardiac muscle disease, but like other myositis patients they often have severe interstitial fibrosis.

U1-RNP

The other major overlap syndrome in scleroderma is associated with anti-U1-RNP, a high-titered speckled ANA. This antibody is associated with the classic mixed connective tissue disease (MCTD) [69]. Disease onset in these patients is early, there is a high frequency of African Americans, and it is the main antibody associated with limited scleroderma in African Americans. Patients have a high frequency of inflammatory muscle (27%) and joint problems (94%), which represent the myositis and lupus parts of the mixed connective tissue disease. Patients usually present with these inflammatory problems, which tend to quiet down over time. Raynaud's and puffy fingers occur early in the disease, but later these patients develop other more severe manifestations of scleroderma. Most of them have limited cutaneous disease [70], although 20% get diffuse cutaneous disease. Although they get all manifestations of scleroderma, the most serious complications are less common. PAH is the most common cause of death, but they can also get pulmonary fibrosis [71]. They can get scleroderma renal crisis but they also get lupus nephritis, so it is particularly important that one knows the autoantibody to be able to make this distinction.

Limited scleroderma patients with anti-Scl 70 antibody and U3 RNP

There are some limited scleroderma patients who have autoantibodies that are most typically seen in diffuse scleroderma patients. Almost 30% of the anti-topoisomerase patients and 25% of the U3 RNP patients will never develop diffuse cutaneous disease. Other than rarely developing renal crisis [72] and not developing diffuse cutaneous changes, they have the same frequency and severity of organ involvement as patients with the same antibody who have diffuse cutaneous scleroderma.

Diffuse cutaneous scleroderma

Anti-topoisomerase antibody

The autoantibodies in patients with diffuse cutaneous scleroderma are associated with distinctive and discriminating features (Table 2). The antinuclear pattern is either speckled or homogeneous. Occasionally it may be speckled. Patients with anti-TOPO have classic "diffuse" scleroderma. Thirty percent of African Americans with scleroderma have this autoantibody. Raynaud's is usually the first symptom and there is a variable time range before the onset of other symptoms. Most develop hand swelling within the first 2 years but sometimes they have Raynaud's for longer before developing diffuse cutaneous changes, making it somewhat unpredictable when and whether they will develop diffuse cutaneous scleroderma. Digital tip ulcers, gangrene, and acroosteolysis occur more frequently in anti-TOPO patients than in other diffuse scleroderma patients. Like all diffuse scleroderma patients, they have lots of joint and tendon involvement, particularly early in the disease. Most patients have diffuse cutaneous disease although about 30% will have slowly progressive cutaneous skin changes and about half of these will not get diffuse skin thickening. Generally, progression of

Table 2
Features of patients with diffuse scleroderma specific autoantibodies present

Antibody	TOPO	POL 3	U3 RNP
No. of patients	318	120	55
Male sex, %*	27	**19**	29
African African, %*	**17**	3	**29**
Age of onset*	43	44	**35**
Diffuse SSc, %*	71	**85**	64
Disease duration			
At diagnosis	2.2	1.5	2.9
Joints, %	**86**	**88**	**89**
Carpal tunnel, %*	28	**43**	27
Tendon rubs, %	**50**	**61**	**42**
Digital ulcers, %*	63	42	**58**
Gangrene, %*	**13**	3	9
Digital tuft	**28**	5	9
Resorption* (x-ray numbers actually performed)	49/173	3/54	2/22
Calcinosis, %*	17	14	**22**
Muscle inflammation, %*	9	4	**18**
Any GI, %	56	37	59
Severe GI, %*	8	5	**25**
Any lung %	73	49	67
Number with PFTs	(235)	(74)	(37)
Severe fibrosis, %*	**23**	7	**24**
Lowest FVC,* % predicted	67	81	68
Isolated PAH	2	6	24
Severe heart, %*	**16**	**7**	**18**
Renal crisis, %*	**10**	**28**	7
Survival, % cumulative survival from diagnosis			
5 y, 10 y	78,65	**90,75**	80,61

Major differences in bold.

Abbreviations: FVC, forced vital capacity; GI, gastrointestinal; PFT, pulmonary function test; PAH, pulmonary arterial hypertension; SSc, systemic sclerosis.

* $P < .001$ by analysis of variance.

the skin thickening occurs early in the disease, but in some it may not occur for 3 or 4 years [73]. Cardiac involvement and renal crisis occur most often early in those with rapid progression to diffuse cutaneous disease.

Severe lung disease is the hallmark of anti-TOPO patients, although fortunately not all patients get severe disease [74]. Alveolitis occurs early in the disease, so careful monitoring is particularly important in the first 3 to 4 years from the very first disease symptom [74]. At the time of diagnosis, patients with anti-TOPO should have pulmonary function tests and high resolution CT scans performed every 3 to 6 months until they are stable. Importantly, during this time patients may not have any or may only have mild respiratory symptoms, but this is when the disease is most active. Although most of the active disease occurs early, with time there is progression of disease from persistent low-level activity and/or complications from reflux or infection. Patients die of lung-related problems an average of 10 years after onset of scleroderma symptoms but have only had symptoms of their lung disease for 5 years

[74]. Most TOPO patients have chronic, stable, moderate fibrosis and function quite normally.

RNA polymerase III

Diffuse scleroderma patients with anti-RNA polymerase III (POL3) have the most severe skin disease and the highest frequency of renal crisis but they do NOT get severe interstitial fibrosis [20,75]. They present the earliest because of a high frequency of carpal tunnel syndrome, inflammatory joint symptoms, swollen hands, or swollen legs, often in the absence of Raynaud's [68]. Raynaud's phenomenon is not present at the time of diagnosis in 15% of patients. In spite of all the tendon and joint involvement, actual muscle inflammation is uncommon. Although an ELISA method of identifying the POL3 antibody is now clinically available, patients with this antibody can be recognized by the following combination of features: a speckled antibody (with or without a nucleolar pattern, but rarely nucleolar alone) [76], a negative anti-TOPO antibody, presentation to the physician very early in their disease with prominent skin and tendon involvement, and a forced vital capacity that is close to normal in spite of the severe skin disease. As soon as the diagnosis of scleroderma is made, these patients need *aggressive* physical and occupational therapy. They are at high risk for severe contractures related to the extent and rapidity of their skin disease. In many patients the diffuse skin disease will regress over time, but severe contractures are very difficult to improve. Severe peripheral vascular disease (and acroosteolysis) is uncommon, but these patients often have very difficult to manage ulcers on the dorsum of the finger joints primarily from the taut skin and repeated trauma.

Severe gastrointestinal disease is uncommon, and the POL 3 patients infrequently have severe lung disease. Less than 10% will have severe fibrosis (3%) or pulmonary hypertension (6%) [67]. They often will have completely normal PFTs in spite of the rapidly progressive cutaneous disease. Aggressive treatment of lung disease is generally not necessary and conservative treatment of the lung is prudent in spite of severe cutaneous disease. Pulmonary vascular disease is also uncommon and has been seen in a few patients with prior renal crisis [77]. POL3 patients have the highest risk for renal crisis; 25% to 33% will get renal crisis. Early studies suggested that rapidly progressive skin disease was a risk factor for renal crisis [15], and later it was found that this is because both severe skin and renal crisis were associated with the POL 3 antibody [20,34]. These patients should take their blood pressure regularly and when they have any symptoms and know what their normal pressure is. They must be educated to contact their physician if there is ever an elevation. Treatment with angiotensin converting enzyme (ACE) inhibitors has become life saving. Less than 10% of scleroderma-related deaths are from renal crisis now compared with 40% before ACE inhibitors [78]. Survival in patients with RNA-POL 3 is actually better than those with anti-TOPO since renal crisis is now more easily treated than pulmonary fibrosis [68]. More recent studies suggest that management continues to be challenging and that prophylactic ACE inhibitors may potentially be associated with worse outcomes [79,80]. These well-established outcomes should be considered in future therapeutic trials. Clinical management focusing on these differences could be life saving.

U3-RNP

Patients with the nucleolar antibody, U3-RNP, also have classic diffuse scleroderma with multiorgan involvement. This antibody is the most frequent in African Americans [19]. The mean age of onset is only 35, which is the youngest of the diffuse scleroderma patients. Most patients have diffuse scleroderma with areas of hypo- and hyperpigmentation, which is very difficult for them to deal with emotionally. They have fewer tendon and joint problems but more inflammatory and fibrotic muscle disease. Thus, they have milder hand contractures but more severe larger joint contractures.

These patients have the worst prognosis because of severe internal organ involvement. In addition to severe interstitial lung disease similar to the TOPO patients, they also can develop pulmonary hypertension similar to that seen in the other nucleolar antibody subset, anti-Th/To. The presence of a nucleolar antibody in either diffuse or limited cutaneous disease is often associated with severe lung disease and is the primary cause of scleroderma-related deaths in these patients. With similar type of lung disease as the nucleolar antibody, Th/To can use that pattern to anticipate the problems these patients will have. They need to be monitored early for alveolitis and development of fibrosis, and later, one must consider the development of a severe vascular pulmonary hypertension. This often has an acute onset and is out of proportion to the severity of fibrosis. Diagnosis is very important since treatment approaches are very different. Since African Americans also commonly have anti-TOPO, all African Americans should be aggressively monitored and treated for pulmonary fibrosis early in the disease. Severe small bowel involvement with pseudo obstruction and malabsorption occurs disproportionately in these patients. Some patients have had symptomatic peripheral neuropathies, which are uncommon in other scleroderma subsets.

In summary, scleroderma-specific autoantibodies are strongly associated with meaningful clinical manifestations. These antibodies can be helpful in determining prognosis, and monitoring and treating patients. They should be used in performing clinical trials and in doing genetic and basic research. Hopefully, these scleroderma antibodies will lead to a better understanding of the pathogenesis of scleroderma.

References

[1] Benedek TG, Rodnan GP. The early history and nomenclature of scleroderma and of its differentiation from sclerema neonatorum and scleroedema. Semin Arthritis Rheum 1982;12:52–67.

12   STEEN

[2] Steen VD, Powell DL, Medsger TA Jr. Clinical correlations and prognosis based on serum autoantibodies in patients with systemic sclerosis. Arthritis Rheum 1988;31:196–203.

[3] Velayos EE, Masi AT, Stevens MB, et al. The 'CREST' syndrome. Comparison with systemic sclerosis (scleroderma). Arch Intern Med 1979;139:1240–4.

[4] Masi AT, Rodman G, Medsger T, et al. Preliminary criteria for the classification of systemic sclerosis (scleroderma). Arthritis Rheum 1980;23:581–90.

[5] Rothfield NF, Rodnan GP. Serum antinuclear antibodies in progressive systemic sclerosis (scleroderma). Arthritis Rheum 1968;11:607–17.

[6] Salerni R, Rodnan GP, Leon DF, et al. Pulmonary hypertension in the CREST syndrome variant of progressive systemic sclerosis (scleroderma). Ann Intern Med 1977;86:394–9.

[7] Douvas AS, Achten M, Tan EM. Identification of a nuclear protein (Scl-70) as a unique target of human antinuclear antibodies in scleroderma. J Biol Chem 1979;254:10514–22.

[8] Moroi Y, Peebles C, Fritzler MJ, et al. Autoantibody to centromere (kinetochore) in scleroderma sera. Proc Natl Acad Sci U S A 1980;77:1627–31.

[9] Leroy EC, Black C, Fleischmajer R, et al. Scleroderma (systemic sclerosis): classification, subsets and pathogenesis. J Rheumatol 1988;15:202–5.

[10] Tan EM, Rodnan GP, Garcia I, et al. Diversity of antinuclear antibodies in progressive systemic sclerosis. Anti-centromere antibody and its relationship to CREST syndrome. Arthritis Rheum 1980;23:617–25.

[11] Kikuchi M, Inagaki T. Bibliographical study of the concurrent existence of anticentromere and antitopoisomerase I antibodies. Clin Rheumatol 2000;19:435–41.

[12] Furst DE, Clements PJ, Saab M, et al. Clinical and serological comparison of 17 chronic progressive systemic sclerosis (PSS) and 17 CREST syndrome patients matched for sex, age, and disease duration. Ann Rheum Dis 1984;43:794–801.

[13] Sacks DG, Okano Y, Steen VD, et al. Isolated pulmonary hypertension in systemic sclerosis with diffuse cutaneous involvement: association with serum anti-U3RNP antibody. J Rheumatol 1996;23:639–42.

[14] Sugimoto T, Soumura M, Danno K, et al. Scleroderma renal crisis in a patient with anticentromere antibody-positive limited cutaneous systemic sclerosis. Mod Rheumatol 2006;16:309–11.

[15] Steen VD, Medsger TA Jr, Osial TA Jr, et al. Factors predicting development of renal involvement in progressive systemic sclerosis. Am J Med 1984;76:779–86.

[16] Steen VD, Owens GR, Fino GJ, et al. Pulmonary involvement in systemic sclerosis (scleroderma). Arthritis Rheum 1985;28:759–67.

[17] Oddis CV, Okano Y, Rudert WA, et al. Serum autoantibody to the nucleolar antigen PM-Scl. Clinical and immunogenetic associations. Arthritis Rheum 1992;35:1211–7.

[18] Okano Y, Medsger TA Jr. Autoantibody to Th ribonucleoprotein (nucleolar 7-2 RNA protein particle) in patients with systemic sclerosis. Arthritis Rheum 1990;33:1822–8.

[19] Okano Y, Steen VD, Medsger TA Jr. Autoantibody to U3 nucleolar ribonucleoprotein (fibrillarin) in patients with systemic sclerosis. Arthritis Rheum 1992;35:95–100.

[20] Okano Y, Steen VD, Medsger TA Jr. Autoantibody reactive with RNA polymerase III in systemic sclerosis. Ann Intern Med 1993;119:1005–13.

[21] Falkner D, Wilson J, Fertig N, et al. Studies of HLA-DR and DQ alleles in systemic sclerosis patients with autoantibodies to RNA polymerases and U3-RNP (fibrillarin). J Rheumatol 2000;27:1196–202.

[22] Falkner D, Wilson J, Medsger TA Jr, et al. HLA and clinical associations in systemic sclerosis patients with anti- Th/To antibodies. Arthritis Rheum 1998;41:74–80.

[23] Johnson RW, Tew MB, Arnett FC. The genetics of systemic sclerosis. Curr Rheumatol Rep 2002;4:99–107.

[24] Morel PA, Chang HJ, Wilson JW, et al. HLA and ethnic associations among systemic sclerosis patients with anticentromere antibodies. Hum Immunol 1995;42:35–42.

[25] Morel PA, Chang HJ, Wilson JW, et al. Severe systemic sclerosis with anti-topoisomerase I antibodies is associated with an HLA-DRw11 allele. Hum Immunol 1994;40:101–10.

[26] Assassi S, Arnett FC, Reveille JD, et al. Clinical, immunologic, and genetic features of familial systemic sclerosis. Arthritis Rheum 2007;56:2031–7.

[27] Feghali-Bostwick C, Medsger TA Jr, Wright TM. Analysis of systemic sclerosis in twins reveals low concordance for disease and high concordance for the presence of antinuclear antibodies. Arthritis Rheum 2003;48:1956–63.

[28] Kuwana M, Kaburaki J, Arnett FC, et al. Influence of ethnic background on clinical and serologic features in patients with systemic sclerosis and anti-DNA topoisomerase I antibody. Arthritis Rheum 1999;42:465–74.

[29] Allcock RJ, Forrest I, Corris PA, et al. A study of the prevalence of systemic sclerosis in northeast England. Rheumatology (Oxford) 2004;43:596–602.

[30] Mayes MD, Lacey JV Jr, Beebe-Dimmer J, et al. Prevalence, incidence, survival, and disease characteristics of systemic sclerosis in a large US population. Arthritis Rheum 2003;48:2246–55.

[31] Meyer OC, Fertig N, Lucas M, et al. Disease subsets, antinuclear antibody profile, and clinical features in 127 French and 247 US adult patients with systemic sclerosis. J Rheumatol 2007;34:104–9.

[32] Ferri C, Valentini G, Cozzi F, et al. Systemic sclerosis: demographic, clinical, and serologic features and survival in 1,012 Italian patients. Medicine (Baltimore) 2002;81:139–53.

[33] Picillo U, Migliaresi S, Marcialis MR, et al. Clinical setting of patients with systemic sclerosis by serum autoantibodies. Clin Rheumatol 1997;16:378–83.

[34] Bunn CC, Denton CP, Shi-wen X, et al. Anti-RNA polymerases and other autoantibody specificities in systemic sclerosis. Br J Rheumatol 1998;37:15–20.

[35] McNeilage LJ, Youngchaiyud U, Whittingham S. Racial differences in antinuclear antibody patterns and clinical manifestations of scleroderma. Arthritis Rheum 1989;32:54–60.

[36] Zhou X, Tan FK, Wang N, et al. Genome-wide association study for regions of systemic sclerosis susceptibility in a Choctaw Indian population with high disease prevalence. Arthritis Rheum 2003;48:2585–92.

[37] Tan FK, Wang N, Kuwana M, et al. Association of fibrillin 1 single-nucleotide polymorphism haplotypes with systemic sclerosis in Choctaw and Japanese populations. Arthritis Rheum 2001;44:893–901.

[38] Brouwer R, Vree Egberts WT, Hengstman GJ, et al. Autoantibodies directed to novel components of the PM/Scl complex, the human exosome. Arthritis Res 2002;4:134–8.

[39] Goldblatt F, Gordon TP, Waterman SA. Antibody-mediated gastrointestinal dysmotility in scleroderma. Gastroenterology 2002;123:1144–50.

[40] Harris ML, Rosen A. Autoimmunity in scleroderma: the origin, pathogenetic role, and clinical significance of autoantibodies. Curr Opin Rheumatol 2003;15:778–84.

[41] Hu PQ, Fertig N, Medsger TA Jr, et al. Correlation of serum anti-DNA topoisomerase I antibody levels with disease severity and activity in systemic sclerosis. Arthritis Rheum 2003;48:1363–73.

[42] Kuwana M, Kaburaki J, Mimori T, et al. Longitudinal analysis of autoantibody response to topoisomerase I in systemic sclerosis. Arthritis Rheum 2000;43:1074–84.

[43] Sato S, Hamaguchi Y, Hasegawa M, et al. Clinical significance of anti-topoisomerase I antibody levels determined by ELISA in systemic sclerosis. Rheumatology (Oxford) 2001;40:1135–40.

[44] Okano Y. Antinuclear antibody in systemic sclerosis (scleroderma). Rheum Dis Clin North Am 1996;22:709–35.

[45] Arnett FC. Is scleroderma an autoantibody mediated disease? Curr Opin Rheumatol 2006;18:579–81.

[46] Ahmed SS, Tan FK, Arnett FC, et al. Induction of apoptosis and fibrillin 1 expression in human dermal endothelial cells by scleroderma sera containing anti-endothelial cell antibodies. Arthritis Rheum 2006;54:2250–62.

[47] Tan FK, Arnett FC, Reveille JD, et al. Autoantibodies to fibrillin 1 in systemic sclerosis: ethnic differences in antigen recognition and lack of correlation with specific clinical features or HLA alleles [in process citation]. Arthritis Rheum 2000;43:2464–71.

[48] Sato S, Hayakawa I, Hasegawa M, et al. Function blocking autoantibodies against matrix metalloproteinase-1 in patients with systemic sclerosis. J Invest Dermatol 2003;120:542–7.

[49] Baroni SS, Santillo M, Bevilacqua F, et al. Stimulatory autoantibodies to the PDGF receptor in systemic sclerosis. N Engl J Med 2006;354:2667–76.

[50] Ho KT, Reveille JD. The clinical relevance of autoantibodies in scleroderma. Arthritis Res Ther 2003;5:80–93.

[51] Tramposch HD, Smith CD, Senecal JL, et al. A long-term longitudinal study of anticentromere antibodies. Arthritis Rheum 1984;27:121–4.

[52] Dick T, Mierau R, Bartz-Bazzanella P, et al. Coexistence of antitopoisomerase I and anticentromere antibodies in patients with systemic sclerosis. Ann Rheum Dis 2002;61:121–7.

[53] Hildebrandt S, Jackh G, Weber S, et al. A long-term longitudinal isotypic study of antitopoisomerase I autoantibodies. Rheumatol Int 1993;12:231–4.

[54] Ruffatti A, Calligaro A, Ferri C, et al. Association of anti-centromere and anti-Scl 70 antibodies in scleroderma. Report of two cases. J Clin Lab Immunol 1985;16:227–9.

[55] Kane GC, Varga J, Conant EF, et al. Lung involvement in systemic sclerosis (scleroderma): relation to classification based on extent of skin involvement or autoantibody status. Respir Med 1996;90:223–30.

[56] Morelli S, Barbieri C, Sgreccia A, et al. Relationship between cutaneous and pulmonary involvement in systemic sclerosis. J Rheumatol 1997;24:81–5.

[57] Steen V, Medsger TA Jr. Predictors of isolated pulmonary hypertension in patients with systemic sclerosis and limited cutaneous involvement. Arthritis Rheum 2003;48:516–22.

[58] Freundlich B, Jimenez SA, Steen VD, et al. Treatment of systemic sclerosis with recombinant interferon-gamma. A phase I/II clinical trial. Arthritis Rheum 1992;35:1134–42.

[59] Macgregor AJ, Canavan R, Knight C, et al. Pulmonary hypertension in systemic sclerosis: risk factors for progression and consequences for survival. Rheumatology (Oxford) 2001; 40:453–9.

[60] Harvey G, Black C, Maddison P, et al. Characterization of antinucleolar antibody reactivity in patients with systemic sclerosis and their relatives. J Rheumatol 1997;24:477–84.

[61] Van Eenennaam H, Vogelzangs JH, Bisschops L, et al. Autoantibodies against small nucleolar ribonucleoprotein complexes and their clinical associations. Clin Exp Immunol 2002; 130:532–40.

[62] Van Eenennaam H, Vogelzangs JH, Lugtenberg D, et al. Identity of the RNase MRP- and RNase P-associated Th/To autoantigen. Arthritis Rheum 2002;46:3266–72.

[63] Imai H, Ochs RL, Kiyosawa K, et al. Nucleolar antigens and autoantibodies in hepatocellular carcinoma and other malignancies. Am J Pathol 1992;140:859–70.

[64] Strassburg CP, Manns MP. Antinuclear antibody (ANA) patterns in hepatic and extrahepatic autoimmune disease. J Hepatol 1999;31:751.

[65] Kipnis RJ, Craft J, Hardin JA. The analysis of antinuclear and antinucleolar autoantibodies of scleroderma by radioimmunoprecipitation assays. Arthritis Rheum 1990;33:1431–7.

[66] Mitri GM, Lucas M, Fertig N, et al. A comparison between anti-Th/To- and anticentromere antibody-positive systemic sclerosis patients with limited cutaneous involvement. Arthritis Rheum 2003;48:203–9.

[67] Steen VD, Lusas M, Fertig N, et al. Pulmonary arterial hypertension and severe pulmonary fibrosis in systemic sclerosis patients with a nuclear antibody. J Rheumatol 2007;34(11): 2230–5.

[68] Steen VD. Autoantibodies in systemic sclerosis. Semin Arthritis Rheum 2005;35(1):35–42.

[69] Aringer M, Steiner G, Smolen JS. Does mixed connective tissue disease exist? Yes. Rheum Dis Clin North Am 2005;31:411–20.

[70] Maddison PJ. Autoantibodies and clinical subsets: relevance to scleroderma [editorial] [in process citation]. Wien Klin Wochenschr 2000;112:684–6.

[71] Lundberg I, Antohi S, Takeuki K, et al. Kinetics of anti-fibrillin-1 autoantibodies in MCTD and CREST syndrome. J Autoimmun 2000;14:267–74.

[72] Steen VD, Medsger TA Jr. Epidemiology and natural history of systemic sclerosis. Rheum Dis Clin North Am 1990;16:1–10.

[73] Perera A, Fertig N, Lucas M, et al. Clinical subsets, skin thickness progression rate, and serum antibody levels in systemic sclerosis patients with anti-topoisomerase I antibody. Arthritis Rheum 2007;56:2740–6.

[74] Steen VD, Conte C, Owens GR, et al. Severe restrictive lung disease in systemic sclerosis. Arthritis Rheum 1994;37:1283–9.

[75] Santiago M, Baron M, Hudson M, et al. Antibodies to RNA polymerase III in systemic sclerosis detected by ELISA. J.Rheumatol 2007;34:1528–34.

[76] Kuwana M, Okano Y, Pandey JP, et al. Enzyme-linked immunosorbent assay for detection of anti-RNA polymerase III antibody: analytical accuracy and clinical associations in systemic sclerosis. Arthritis Rheum 2005;52:2425–32.

[77] Gunduz OH, Fertig N, Lucas M, et al. Systemic sclerosis with renal crisis and pulmonary hypertension: a report of eleven cases. Arthritis Rheum 2001;44:1663–6.

[78] Steen VD, Medsger TA Jr. Changes in causes of death in systemic sclerosis. Ann Rheum Dis 2007;34:2230–5.

[79] Penn H, Howie AJ, Kingdon EJ, et al. Scleroderma renal crisis: patient characteristics and long-term outcomes. QJM 2007;100:485–94.

[80] Teixeira L, Mahr A, Berezne A, et al. Scleroderma renal crisis, still a life-threatening complication. Ann N Y Acad Sci 2007;1108:249–58.

ELSEVIER
SAUNDERS

Rheum Dis Clin N Am
34 (2008) 17–40

RHEUMATIC
DISEASE CLINICS
OF NORTH AMERICA

Genetics and Genomic Studies in Scleroderma (Systemic Sclerosis)

Sandeep K. Agarwal, MD, PhD*,
Filemon K. Tan, MD, PhD,
Frank C. Arnett, MD

Division of Rheumatology, Department of Internal Medicine, The University of Texas Health Science Center at Houston, 6431 Fannin, MSB 5.270, Houston, TX 77030, USA

Scleroderma or systemic sclerosis is an autoimmune connective tissue disease clinically characterized by fibrosis of the skin and internal organs and obliterative vasculopathy. The complexities of scleroderma are evident from the variability in its clinical manifestations, which probably reflects the diverse mechanisms that underlie the development of disease subtypes. Despite recent advances in the understanding of some of the molecular pathways involved in scleroderma, the etiopathogenesis remains unknown. Although fibrosis and endothelial dysfunction are hallmarks of the disease, autoimmunity is probably the root cause. Autoimmunity and inflammation currently are best exemplified by the multiple but not overlapping patterns of specific autoantibodies in patients who have scleroderma. In fact, each of these autoantibodies tends to mark a distinct clinical subset of disease [1]. The presence of inflammatory infiltrates in the dermis early in the disease and increased circulating levels of cytokines and chemokines in patients who have scleroderma further implicate inflammation in the pathogenesis of scleroderma. It remains unknown how these autoimmune responses lead to certain patterns of organ damage that vary among different clinical subsets of scleroderma.

It currently is believed that scleroderma is a complex polygenic disease that occurs in genetically predisposed individuals who have encountered specific environment exposures and/or other stochastic factors. The nature of these genetic determinants and how they interact with environmental factors are areas of active investigation. This article discusses the evidence that

---

* Corresponding author.
E-mail address: sandeep.k.agarwal@uth.tmc.edu (S.K. Agarwal).

0889-857X/08/$ - see front matter © 2008 Elsevier Inc. All rights reserved.
doi:10.1016/j.rdc.2007.10.001

supports a strong genetic link to scleroderma. Also reviewed are the family and twin studies that suggest a genetic component in scleroderma, and recent genetic-association studies implicating specific genes in the pathogenetic triad of autoimmunity, endothelial dysfunction, and fibroblast activation. Last, this article highlights recent studies in scleroderma that use gene-expression microarray profiles seeking to identify pathogenetic pathways in scleroderma. Together these studies implicate potential pathogenetic mechanisms involved in scleroderma, which, it is hoped, may translate into clinical utility, including determination of disease risk, diagnosis, prognosis, and novel therapeutics.

Familial aggregation and twin studies

Determining that a disease occurs more commonly in families than in the general population is a first step in implicating potential genetic contributions. Robust estimates of prevalence and incidence rates of scleroderma, which are essential in determining familial aggregation, have varied widely in the general population, ranging from 3.1 to 20.8 per 100,000 and from 0.4 to 1.2 per 100,000, respectively [2–5]. A recent, well-conducted study estimated the prevalence of scleroderma to be 24.2 per 100,000 adults with an annual incidence of 1.93 per 100,000 adults [6]. Initial reports suggested that familial clustering was uncommon, but only recently has it been quantitated [7]. Ten cases of scleroderma in first-degree relatives among 710 proband cases were reported in the Sydney, Australia population, conferring a familial risk conservatively estimated at 11 (95% confidence interval [CI], 2.7–19.3) [8]. It was demonstrated subsequently that scleroderma recurred in 1.6% of families of scleroderma cases in three separate cohorts that had an estimated population risk of only 0.026% [9]. Although this absolute risk of familial scleroderma was relatively low, the familial relative risk was approximately 15-fold higher for siblings and 13-fold higher for first-degree relatives. A recent study suggested that the affected members within multicase scleroderma families tend to have concordant scleroderma-specific autoantibodies, further supporting the concept of a genetic predisposition [10]. Based on these studies, a positive family history of scleroderma confers the strongest known relative risk for disease.

The investigation of monozygotic twins is an important approach for assessing and quantifying the role of genetic versus environmental factors in specific diseases. Case reports have described concordance for scleroderma in twins [11,12]. Examination of 42 monozygotic and dizygotic twins collected from across the United States demonstrated similar scleroderma concordance rates (~5%), thus implying no genetic susceptibility [13]. The concordance rate of antinuclear antibodies was significantly higher in monozygotic twins (90%) than in dizygotic twins (40%), however [13]. A subsequent study compared gene-expression microarray profiles of cultured fibroblasts from 15 discordant mono- and dizygotic twin pairs [14].

Unsupervised hierarchical clustering segregated cultured fibroblasts into two distinct groups. Fibroblast lines from unaffected monozygotic, but not dizygotic, twins tended to group with cultured fibroblast cell lines from affected scleroderma patients rather than with normal controls. Together, as summarized in Table 1, these data suggest that genetic factors may play a significant role in susceptibility to scleroderma with regards to the production of autoantibodies and in vitro fibroblast activation. Although these data may partially explain the clustering of autoimmune diseases observed in some families, it is necessary to define the genetic factors that underlie scleroderma susceptibility.

Ethnic factors

It is apparent that ethnicity influences the susceptibility to autoimmune diseases, including scleroderma. African Americans have been reported to have a higher incidence of scleroderma (22.5 cases per million per year) than white women (12.8 cases per million per year) [15]. Furthermore, African American women have been reported likely to have more severe disease, earlier age of onset, and worse survival rates [15]. Reveille and colleagues [16] demonstrated in a prospective cohort that Hispanics and African Americans were more likely than whites to have diffuse skin involvement, digital ulcerations, and pulmonary hypertension.

Among the more intriguing observations with regards to ethnicity and scleroderma were those made in the Oklahoma Choctaw Indians [17]. The prevalence in full-blooded Choctaws was estimated at 469 cases per 100,000 over a 4-year period. This prevalence was significantly higher than that seen in non–full-blooded Choctaws, other Native Americans in Oklahoma, and whites. Furthermore, a majority of the Choctaw scleroderma cases had diffuse scleroderma, pulmonary fibrosis, and circulating anti-topoisomerase I antibodies and could be traced genealogically to a common founding family in the late 1700s. No environmental factors were identified in the Oklahoma environment, and the strongest risk factor was a nearly unique Amerindian HLA class II haplotype (*DRB1*1602, DQA1*0501, DQB1*0301*). Investigators using microsatellite markers in

Table 1
Estimates of scleroderma occurrence and risk in families

Population	Frequency (%)
General population (prevalence)	0.026
First-degree relatives of persons who have scleroderma (prevalence)	1.60
Siblings of persons who have scleroderma (prevalence)	0.40
Monozygotic twins of persons who have scleroderma (concordance)	5.00
Monozygotic twins with antinuclear antibody–positive concordance	90
Monozygotic twins with fibroblast gene profile concordance	50

three candidate regions found a shared haplotype on chromosome 15q containing the fibrillin-1 (*FBN1*) gene, an important structural protein and regulator of transforming growth factor-beta (TGF-β) within the extracellular matrix, to be significantly overrepresented in Choctaw scleroderma cases [18]. Similar studies of single-nucleotide polymorphisms (SNPs) supported a role for *FBN1* in Choctaw and Japanese scleroderma cases but did not show associations in whites [19]. Interestingly, a mouse model of scleroderma, the tight skin mouse (tsk-1), is caused by a genomic duplication of fibrillin-1 [20].

These studies demonstrate the influence of ethnicity on scleroderma susceptibility. Although multiple factors including socioeconomic factors, access to health care, and even environmental exposures may help explain these difference in scleroderma susceptibility or even clinical expression, genetic differences among ethnic groups probably are key determinants as well.

Genetic factors

HLA associations

The major histocompatibility complex (MHC) or HLA region is the most polymorphic region of the genome. Polymorphisms in HLA have been linked to a number of autoimmune diseases including rheumatoid arthritis, ankylosing spondylitis, systemic lupus erythematosus, and many others [1,21–23]. Scleroderma also has been associated with HLA polymorphisms, and these associations have been reviewed previously [24,25]. The associations of HLA polymorphisms with scleroderma susceptibility itself are modest but, more importantly, are consistent and are reproducible across different populations; these include associations with the HLA-DR5/11 and DR3 haplotypes in white patients and with HLA-DR2 haplotypes in Japanese and Choctaw Indian patients. Of particular interest is a finding of a significantly higher frequency of *HLA-DQA1*0501* in male patients who have scleroderma [26].

Stronger associations with HLA haplotypes exist for specific autoantibody subsets of scleroderma, including HLA *DRB1*1104* and, independently, *DPB1*1301* in whites, *DQB1*0301* and *DPB1*1301* in African Americans, and DR2 haplotypes in Japanese (*DRB1*1502, DQB1*0601, DPB1*090*) and Choctaws (*DRB1*1602, DQB1*0301, DPB1*1301*) with anti-topoisomerase antibody [27–32]. Furthermore, HLA *DQB1*0501* and other DQB1 alleles encoding nonpolar amino acids in position 26 are associated with anti-centromere antibody [27,33]. An association of HLA *DRB1*1302, DQB1*0604/0605* haplotypes has been found with anti-fibrillarin (anti-U3-RNP)–positive patients, who are more often male African Americans, and the HLA *DRB1*0301* haplotype has been shown to be associated with anti-PM-Scl antibody positivity in patients who tend to be nearly exclusively white [34,35]. Finally, an association was observed with

HLA *DQB1*0201* in patients who have anti-RNA polymerase I, II, and/or III antibodies, but this association has not been observed in other studies [32,36,37].

Non-HLA candidate-gene associations

Genetic-association studies seek to determine genetic variants associated with disease states or specific traits. As more studies have been undertaken in different complex diseases, it has become clear that the contribution of individual genes to the genetic risk for disease may be quite modest (relative risk, ∼ 1.5–2.0) and that multiple loci are involved. In this light, interpretation of genetic-association studies in an uncommon and phenotypically heterogeneous disease, such as scleroderma, must be performed using strict guidelines. Such studies often are limited by lack of sufficient statistical power to generate reliable and reproducible results because of small sample sizes in cases and controls, genetic heterogeneity, and the extent and degree of linkage disequilibrium among genetic markers that vary among populations [38,39]. Population stratification, differences in phenotype of complex diseases, and quality control also complicate the interpretation of genetic-association studies. The inability to replicate data across study cohorts, however, may represent real biologic differences in populations that originate from different genetic backgrounds, as has been shown recently in rheumatoid arthritis [40–45]. Nonetheless, it is necessary to replicate the findings of association studies in additional appropriately designed cohorts. Furthermore, candidate genes identified in genetic-association studies must be followed by functional studies, usually done in vitro, that demonstrate that these associations are, in fact, causal or at least biologically plausible.

Choosing which targets to investigate is based largely on current paradigms of pathogenesis from human and/or animal studies or, in some instances, on associations with other autoimmune diseases. Thus, selection of these candidate genes is colored by publication bias and incomplete scientific knowledge. The candidate genes for scleroderma that have been investigated have been related largely to autoimmunity/inflammation, vascular function, and fibrosis or extracellular matrix production.

Autoimmunity/Inflammation

Interleukin-1 alpha and beta

Interleukin-1 alpha (IL-1α) and interleukin-1 beta (IL-1β) are proinflammatory cytokines involved in a number of autoimmune diseases. Patients who have scleroderma have increased circulating levels of IL-1α and IL-β, and IL-1α is a potent stimulatory factor of cultured dermal scleroderma fibroblast behavior in vitro [46–48]. In a study comparing 86 Japanese patients who had scleroderma with 70 healthy controls, the CTG haplotype at positions −889, +4729, and +4845 of the *IL1A* gene was associated with scleroderma susceptibility as well as the presence of interstitial lung disease [49]. Attempts to confirm this association have not been successful. The −889C allele of *IL1A*, which is part of this haplotype, was not found to be associated with scleroderma in cohorts of Slovak and Italian patients [50,51]. In contradiction to the initial observation, the −889T allele of *IL1A* was found to be associated with scleroderma in Slovak patients [50]. These studies must be interpreted cautiously because of the small sample sizes. Alternatively, the conflicting results may be caused by differences in linkage disequilibrium within the *IL1* gene cluster among these populations.

Genetic associations with *IL1B* also have been investigated in patients who have scleroderma. Mattuzzi and colleagues [52] recently demonstrated significant associations of the *IL1B-31-C* and *IL1B-511-T* alleles with susceptibility to scleroderma. Given the potential importance of IL-1β in scleroderma, it will be interesting to see if these genetic associations are replicated. Furthermore, additional genes involved in the IL-1α and IL-1β pathways may be involved in scleroderma susceptibility and should be considered for future studies.

Allograft inflammatory factor-1

Allograft inflammatory factor-1 (AIF-1) is a newly identified protein identified in rat cardiac allografts undergoing chronic rejection [53]. The function and regulation of AIF-1 expression has not been characterized thoroughly. AIF-1 is expressed by macrophages and neutrophils, and immunohistochemical analyses of scleroderma biopsies have demonstrated increased AIF-1 expression in the infiltrating cells within lesions [54–56]. A recent study demonstrated that AIF-1 promoted T-cell infiltration and induced the expression types I and III collagen and cytokines by normal dermal fibroblasts, providing additional evidence for a role of AIF-1 in scleroderma [57]. A comparison of 140 patients who had scleroderma with 97 controls demonstrated an association of the *AIF1* +889A allele with scleroderma [58]. This polymorphism, which is located in exon 3 of AIF-1, generates a nonsynonymous change (tryptophan to arginine). Investigators using the relatively large cohort of 548 patients who had scleroderma in the Scleroderma Family Registry and DNA Repository and an additional 467 patients from the Genetics versus Environment in Scleroderma Outcomes Study noted a modest association with this AIF-1 polymorphism, but only with the anti-centromere antibody (ACA)–positive subset of scleroderma [59]. Although the *AIF1* gene maps within the MHC class II region, the association of *AIF1* with ACA-positive scleroderma was not explained completely by linkage disequilibrium, suggesting an independent association of *AIF1* with ACA-positive scleroderma [59]. Additional studies are needed to confirm these associations and to advance the understanding of the functional importance of AIF-1 in the pathogenesis of scleroderma.

Protein tyrosine phosphatase non-receptor 22

Protein tyrosine phosphatase non-receptor 22 (PTPN22) is a class I cysteine-based tyrosine phosphatase expressed in hematopoietic cells. In functional studies, PTPN22 exerts a negative regulatory function of T-cell receptor signaling [60,61]. The *PTPN22 R620W* mutation has been shown to increase this negative regulatory effect on T-cell receptor signaling [62]. The *PTPN22 R620W* mutation has been associated with several diseases, including type I diabetes mellitus, systemic lupus erythematosus, and rheumatoid arthritis, but not ankylosing spondylitis, Crohn's disease, or primary Sjögren's syndrome [43,45,63–67]. Two initial reports with small sample sizes failed to show an association of *PTPN22* and scleroderma [68,69]. This finding is not surprising, given the modest genetic risk conferred by *PTPN22* for diseases such as rheumatoid arthritis (odds ratio [OR], ~1.5) [43,45]. In contrast, a study combining three different cohorts, totaling 1120 patients who had scleroderma and 816 control subjects, found an association between the *PTPN22 R620W* SNP and both anti-topoisomerase-I (OR, 2.14; 95% CI, 1.4–3.2) and ACA-positive scleroderma (OR, 1.67; 95% CI, 1.2–2.4) [70]. This large study cohort provides strong evidence that inherent immunoregulatory defects common to some, but not all, autoimmune diseases also may play a role in scleroderma.

Macrophage migration inhibitory factor

Macrophage migration inhibitory factor (MIF) is a proinflammatory cytokine that is released from activated T cells and macrophages [71,72]. MIF promotes production of tumor necrosis factor-alpha and other cytokines by macrophages and T cells [71,72]. MIF expression is increased in patients who have rheumatoid arthritis and recently has been shown to be increased in scleroderma as well [73,74]. *MIF* polymorphisms were characterized in a cohort of 486 patients who had scleroderma and 254 healthy subjects [75]. The −173C *MIF* promoter polymorphism and the associated haplotype containing −173C and −794 7-CATT (C7) were found to be underrepresented in patients who had limited scleroderma compared with patients who had diffuse scleroderma or healthy controls. The genetic-association study was followed up by complementary functional studies of the effects of the polymorphisms that emphasize its potential relevance in disease pathogenesis. Fibroblasts from patients with this haplotype produced increased levels of MIF in vitro, consistent with a functional role of the C7 *MIF* haplotype in limited scleroderma but not diffuse scleroderma [75].

Chemokines

Multiple chemokines are involved in the pathogenesis of scleroderma where they mediate chemoattraction of inflammatory cells to the site of dermal fibrosis as well as influence cellular activation, angiogenesis, and fibrosis. Specifically, chemokines including CCL-2 (monocyte chemoattractant protein-1, MCP-1), CCL-5 (regulated on activation, normal T-cell expressed and secreted, RANTES), CCL-3 (microphage inflammatory protein alpha-1, MIP-α1), and CXCL-8 (interleukin 8, IL-8) have been shown to be involved in scleroderma [76–79]. For example, lesional and nonlesional scleroderma skin biopsies show increased expression of CCL-2 protein and mRNA, and murine studies have confirmed an important role for CCL-2 in dermal fibrosis [78,80–82].

A small study of 18 patients who had scleroderma investigated *CCL-2* polymorphisms and identified an association of the −2518 GG genotype of *CCL-2* with scleroderma [83]. This polymorphism is within the promoter region and was further demonstrated to be associated with increased CCL-2 production in vitro [83]. Another recent report in 99 patients who had scleroderma enrolled at Seoul National University Hospital failed to show any significant associations of scleroderma with polymorphisms in CCL-2, CXCL-8, CCL-5, CCL-3, and multiple chemokine receptors [84]. A significant and interesting interaction between polymorphisms of CCL-5 and CXCL-8 and susceptibility to scleroderma was noted using two different statistical approaches, however. These data are intriguing and point to the importance of potential gene–gene interactions in complex diseases such as scleroderma.

Other candidate genes in autoimmunity/inflammation

Many additional genetic-association studies of genes involved in autoimmunity and inflammation have been conducted in scleroderma. These reports often have studied small cohorts from different ethnic backgrounds, with conflicting results. These reports are briefly summarized in Table 2 and have been discussed previously in review articles [99,100]. These studies have shown associations of scleroderma with polymorphisms in genes encoding tumor necrosis factor-alpha, cytotoxic T-lymphocyte-associated antigen 4, killer cell immunoglobulin-like receptors, and CD19 receptor, along with others listed in Table 2 [58,88,90,97,98,101,102]. Additional studies are needed to replicate these studies using larger cohorts.

Vascular function

Nitric oxide synthase

Nitric oxide, a potent vasodilator and critical regulator of vascular tone, is synthesized from L-arginine by nitric oxide synthase (NOS). Three isoforms of NOS are known: NOS_1 (neural NOS, nNOS), NOS_2 (inducible NOS, iNOS), and NOS_3 (endothelial NOS, eNOS). Multiple studies have shown dysregulation of nitric oxide production (summarized in Ref. [103]). Because of the complexities of nitric oxide functions, it remains unclear if nitric oxide plays a beneficial or pathologic role in scleroderma [103]. Given the importance of nitric oxide in the regulation of vascular tone and vascular endothelial dysfunction in scleroderma, the nitric oxide pathway is an intriguing candidate to consider for genetic-association studies.

Table 2
Candidate genes in inflammation and scleroderma susceptibility

Candidate gene	Number of patients	Association	Reference
AIF-1	144	A-allele of rs2269475 associated with SSc	[58]
	1015	T-allele of rs2269475 associated with ACA+ SSc	[59]
CD19	134	−499T allele associated with SSc	[85]
CD22	126	c.2304 A/A genotype associated with limited SSc	[86]
CD86	221	−3479G allele associated with SSc	[87]
CTLA-4	137	+49 AG heterozygotes associated with SSc in African Americans	[88]
	62	+49A associated with RNP+ SSc only	[89]
	83	−1722C, −1661G and −318T (not +49A) associated with SSc	[90]
	43	−318T and +49A not associated with SSc	[91]
CCL-2	18	−2518 GG genotype was associated with SSc	[83]
CCL-5	99	No association with SSc alone, but a gene–gene interaction with CXCL-8 and SSc was observed	[84]
CXCL-8	99	No association with SSc alone, but a gene–gene interaction with CCL-5 and SSc was observed	[84]
CXCR-2	128	+785 CC and 1208 TT homozygotes associated with SSc	[92]
IL-1α	86	CTG haplotype association with SSc	[49]
	46	IL-1a −889T allele associated with SSc	[50]
	204	No association with SSc	[51]
IL-1β	204	No association with SSc	[51]
	78	IL-1B31-C and IL-1B-511-T associated with SSc	[52]
IL-2	78	IL-2-384G associated with SSc	[52]
IL-10	140	GCC haplotype underrepresented in SSc	[93]
	161	GCC haplotype associated with SCL70+ SSc	[94]
IL-13	174	rs18000925 C/T genotype and rs2243204T allele associated with SSc	[95]
IL-13RA2	97	rs638376 G allele associated with diffuse SSc	[96]
MIF	486	C7 haplotype associated with limited SSc	[75]
PTPN22	121	No association with SSc	[69]
	54	No association with SSc	[68]
	1120	R620W associated with anti-topo and ACA+ SSc	[70]
TNF-α	214	−1031C and −863A alleles associated with ACA+ SSc	[97]
	114	−238A allele and +489 AG genotype associated with SSc	[98]
	144	−1031T/T and −237G/G genotypes associated with SSc	[58]

Abbreviations: CTLA, cytotoxic T-lymphocyte antigen; *IL-13RA2,* interleukin 13 receptor alpha 2; *TNF-α,* tumor necrosing factor alpha.

Although an initial study in Italians failed to show an association of *NOS* polymorphisms, a subsequent study of 73 Italian patients who had scleroderma demonstrated that the *eNOS 894T* allele was associated with disease [104,105]. The *eNOS 849T* allele subsequently was demonstrated to be associated with altered blood-flow profiles in patients who had scleroderma [106]. Additional studies, however, have failed to demonstrate a consistent association of this polymorphism with scleroderma susceptibility [107,108]. Two polymorphisms and a pentanucleotide repeat in *iNOS* were found to be associated with pulmonary arterial hypertension in a cohort of 78 Japanese patients who had scleroderma, but it was not associated with the risk of scleroderma [109]. Consistent with the hypothesis that *iNOS* is decreased in scleroderma, in vitro experiments demonstrated that the pentanucleotide repeat was associated with less *iNOS* transcription [109]. No additional genetic-association studies with *iNOS* polymorphisms have been reported.

Angiotensin-converting enzyme

Angiotensin-converting enzyme (ACE) catalyzes the conversion of angiotensin I into angiotensin II, which is vasoactive, stimulates aldosterone, and inactivates the vasodilator bradykinin. An insertion/deletion polymorphism of the *ACE* gene is associated with higher tissue and plasma ACE levels (D-allele) [110]. In a study of 73 Italian patients who had scleroderma, the D-allele was associated with scleroderma [105], but this association was not confirmed in a study of 164 American patients who had scleroderma [107].

Vascular endothelial growth factor

Vascular endothelial growth factor (VEGF) is a major angiogenic factor and prime endothelial cell growth factor. Despite defects in angiogenesis, patients who have scleroderma have high levels of circulating VEGF [111,112]. *VEGF* polymorphisms have been associated with alterations in VEGF levels and with other diseases, including giant cell arteritis [113,114]. In a genetic-association study of 416 patients who had scleroderma and 249 controls, no differences in allele and genotype frequencies were observed [115].

Endothelin-1

Endothelin-1 (ET-1) is a potent vasoconstrictive peptide that plays a crucial role in vascular damage. Through interaction with its receptors (ET_A and ET_B), ET-1 also regulates tissue remodeling and fibrosing by promoting fibroblast activation and proliferation [116]. Serum and bronchoalveolar lavage fluid from patients who have scleroderma have increased levels of ET-1 that correlate with severity [117,118]. A recent report evaluated the distribution of polymorphisms in ET-1 (*EDN1*), ET_A receptor (*EDNRA*), and ET_B receptor (*EDNRB*) [119]. No differences were observed between patients who had scleroderma with controls. Patients who had diffuse scleroderma, however, had an increased frequency of the *EDNRB-1A, EDNRB-2A,* and *EDNRB-3G* alleles. Furthermore, the presence of anti-RNA polymerase antibodies in patients who had scleroderma was associated with the *EDNRA* alleles H323H/C and E335E/A [119].

Fibrosis and extracellular matrix production

Transforming growth factor beta-1

The importance of TGF-β in scleroderma pathogenesis has been demonstrated and reviewed extensively in the past [120,121]. TGF-β, its receptor, and downstream signaling molecules (eg, Smad3) are expressed at increased levels in affected organs. TGF-β activates dermal fibroblasts leading to increased production of extracellular matrix. Given the importance of TGF-β in scleroderma, it has been hypothesized that polymorphisms in TGF-β may contribute to scleroderma susceptibility. Supporting this hypothesis is a study of 152 patients who had scleroderma that demonstrated an association of the *TGFβ +889 C* allele with both limited and diffuse scleroderma [122]. These data, however, were not replicated in a subsequent study [123]. More studies with large cohorts as well as studies investigating polymorphisms in the TGF-β receptor, Smad proteins, and non-canonical TGB-β signaling pathways may provide important insight into the role of TGF-β in scleroderma.

Connective tissue growth factor

Connective tissue growth factor (CTGF), also known as CCN2, is a heparin-binding 38-kD polypeptide that induces proliferation, extracellular matrix production, and chemotaxis of mesenchymal cells [124–126]. These processes are central to the development of fibrosis of skin and internal organs observed in scleroderma. The production of CTGF is increased in scleroderma skin biopsies and in fibroblasts cultured from patients who have scleroderma [14,127–129]. These observations led to interest in determining if polymorphisms in *CTGF* were associated with susceptibility to scleroderma [130]. In a cohort of 200 patients who had scleroderma and 188 controls, an association of scleroderma with homozygosity for the G-allele at position −945 of *CTGF* was observed. Furthermore, this association was replicated in a second cohort of 300 patients who had scleroderma and 312 controls. The odds ratio for the GG genotype using the combination of both cohorts was 2.2 (95% CI, 1.5–3.2). Furthermore, homozygosity for the G-allele was associated with the presence of fibrosing alveolitis and the presence of anti-topoisomerase I antibodies. These data point to an association between the G-945C polymorphism in *CTGF* and scleroderma susceptibility.

In the same report, the authors extended the initial genetic association using in vitro studies to demonstrate a potential functional relevance of the *CTGF* G-945C polymorphism in scleroderma [130]. Because this polymorphism occurs in the promoter region of *CTGF*, the approach focused on the transcription of CTGF. DNA from the *CTGF* promoter region of five patients who had the CC genotype and five patients who had the GG genotype was cloned into luciferase promoter-reporter constructs. The GG genotype had higher rates of transcription in vitro than the CC genotype. Additional studies demonstrated that Sp1 (an activator of transcription) bound less efficiently to the CTGF promoter with the GG genotype than with the CC genotype. In contrast, Sp3 (a repressor of transcription) had increased binding to the CTGF promoter with the GG genotype. The shift in the balance of Sp1 binding toward Sp3 binding is consistent with an increase in transcription of the *CTGF* gene. The combination of the genetic association of the G-945C *CTGF* promoter polymorphism with scleroderma in two cohorts and the functional data strongly support an important role for CTGF in scleroderma.

Secreted protein, acidic and rich in cysteine

Secreted protein, acidic and rich in cysteine (SPARC) is a matricellular protein in the extracellular matrix that is overexpressed by scleroderma fibroblasts [131]. SPARC regulates cell-to-cell and cell-to-matrix interactions and also is involved in the production of extracellular matrix by scleroderma fibroblasts [132,133]. In a cohort of 20 Choctaw patients who had scleroderma and 178 patients from the GENOSIS cohort, the C allele at +998 position of *SPARC* was found to be associated with scleroderma across four ethnic populations [131]. Furthermore, fibroblasts isolated from patients homozygous for the +998C allele had more stable expression of SPARC mRNA than fibroblasts from heterozygotes, confirming a functional relevance for the polymorphism that is consistent with the role of SPARC in the pathogenesis of scleroderma [131]. Despite the potential functional importance of this polymorphism in *SPARC*, a subsequent study was unable to confirm a genetic association with susceptibility to scleroderma [134].

Genome-wide studies

Genome-wide association studies have been a powerful approach to the identification of genetic susceptibility loci in complex genetic disorders such as rheumatoid arthritis, inflammatory bowel disease, and coronary artery disease [135–138]. Genome-wide association studies allow the investigator to identify new mechanisms and pathways without predefined assumptions or biases. Such studies rely on large cohorts of patients who have well-defined disease phenotypes. The only genome-wide association study in scleroderma was performed in the Choctaw Indians, who have the highest known prevalence of scleroderma [139]. This study used 400 microsatellite markers to identify 17 chromosome regions associated with susceptibility to scleroderma, including the HLA region and regions near the *SPARC*, *FBN1*, and topoisomerase I (*TOPOI*) genes. These data must be replicated in other populations, and better resolution of the genes within these chromosomal regions is needed. With recent technological advances, high-density genotyping experiments using SNP arrays to study DNA variations are increasingly reported. Current platforms are able to interrogate more than 1 million SNPs on a single microarray. These high-density, large, genome-wide association studies in patients who have scleroderma are currently underway and will be important in defining the future direction of disease association as well as mechanistic research in scleroderma.

Microarray studies

Several technologies that have emerged since the sequencing of the human genome are particularly useful in dissecting the molecular mechanisms of complex biologic processes. Gene-expression profiling using whole-genome microarrays is one such powerful technique that allows simultaneous analysis of thousands of mRNA transcripts. The investigator can learn about multiple pathways involved in diseases and discover completely novel pathways that previously would not have been hypothesized to be involved. This approach also enables the investigation of complex biologic processes in a relatively unbiased manner. These studies, however, must use rigid statistical approaches and must use alternative methodologies to confirm the results. With these requirements in mind, several studies have used microarray expression profiling in scleroderma, and the data that are emerging certainly will guide the direction of future research.

Patterns of gene expression were determined in biopsies of lesional and nonlesional skin from four patients who had scleroderma and four healthy controls [140]. Initial analyses demonstrated that expression of 2776 genes varied by more than twofold, and unsupervised hierarchical clustering grouped all but one of the scleroderma samples into a single group. This group included both lesional and nonlesional skin biopsies from patients who had scleroderma. Clusters of genes that differed among patients who had scleroderma and healthy controls were groups of genes expressed in endothelial cells, smooth muscle cells, T lymphocytes, and B lymphocytes, as well as genes involved in extracellular matrix. No differences in gene-expression profiles were seen in the small number of cultured normal or scleroderma fibroblasts studied [140,141].

A more recent study compared the gene-expression profiles of skin biopsies and corresponding cultured fibroblasts from nine patients who had scleroderma and nine controls [142]. Unsupervised clustering of all skin biopsy samples demonstrated that the scleroderma phenotype was the dominant influence on the expression profile. Expression profiles of scleroderma and control biopsies differed in 1839 genes ($P < .01$). Alterations in TGF-β and Wnt pathways, extracellular matrix proteins, and the CCN family were notable in scleroderma skin biopsies. A key finding of these data is that scleroderma in the skin has a distinct and complex gene-expression profile that is reflected only partially in matched explanted fibroblasts cultured under standard conditions. Despite the large numbers of genes differentially expressed in scleroderma skin biopsies, the expression profile from the cultured fibroblasts differed only in the expression of 223 genes ($P < .01$). These data emphasize the importance of studying skin biopsies and also suggest a significant unmet need to develop better in vitro systems for the study of the complex molecular mechanisms of scleroderma. One such model has been reported recently in which normal dermal fibroblasts are transfected with adenovirus vector expressing TGF-β receptor-1 [143,144]. The overexpression of TGF-β receptor-1 in dermal fibroblasts causes alterations in the gene-expression profile that are similar to those of scleroderma fibroblasts [143,144].

Dysregulation of the immune system is central to the pathogenesis of scleroderma. Prior investigations of circulating immune cells have focused largely on individual populations of cells, such as T lymphocytes. These studies are critical to advancing the understanding but are limited in that they are unable to capture changes that may be observed when multiple populations of cells are allowed to interact with each other. To obtain a global view of the differences in gene-expression profile in early scleroderma, total RNA harvested from peripheral blood cells (PBCs) from 18 patients who had untreated, diffuse scleroderma with recent disease onset and 18 matched controls was analyzed using transcriptional profiling [145]. Global analyses demonstrated an increase in the expression of 244 genes and decreased expression of 138 genes in scleroderma PBCs compared with controls. These studies demonstrated differential expression of 18 interferon-α–inducible genes, including six genes that also are altered in lupus peripheral blood mononuclear cells. Recently, this interferon signature has been confirmed in another microarray study of scleroderma peripheral blood mononuclear cells [146]. Furthermore, this report demonstrated that activation of interferon-regulated genes was dependent on the Toll-like receptors, TLR-7 and TLR-9 [146]. In addition to interferon-regulated genes, microarray analyses of PBCs from patients who had scleroderma demonstrated increased expression of AIF-1 and cellular adhesion molecules including selectin and integrin family members [145]. In total, 13 biologic pathways were differentially regulated in scleroderma PBCs, including GATA-3, a key transcription factor involved in T-helper cell type 2 differentiation [145]. These data are available for review online at http://www. uth.tmc.edu/scleroderma. Taken together these reports demonstrate that transcriptional profiling can discriminate reliably between scleroderma and control PBCs and will be useful in the identification of hitherto unrecognized disease subsets and in the discovery of molecular pathways involved in scleroderma.

Summary and future directions

The evidence for a strong genetic contribution to scleroderma pathogenesis continues to mount. Epidemiologic studies suggest that a family history is the strongest risk factor, but ethnicity also contributes. The candidate-gene association studies presented in this article identify several individual genes that may be involved in scleroderma. Biologic pathways do not act in isolation, however. More often than not, any given pathway will have significant crosstalk with a multitude of other pathways through common intracellular signal transduction molecules and transcription factors. Indeed the whole-genome microarray expression studies of skin biopsies and peripheral blood cells from patients who have scleroderma, as described in previous sections, supports the involvement of multiple pathways in the development of scleroderma. The end result is a complex regulatory network of genes and pathways that, because of limitations in knowledge, initially may appear counterintuitive. Future studies need to foster the understanding of the genes and proteins involved in these pathways and how they interact with one another to lead ultimately to the development of scleroderma.

Although the gene-association studies reviewed provide insight into the development of scleroderma, they have significant limitations that can be addressed in future studies. Many candidate-gene association studies used small cohorts of patients who had scleroderma and controls. Population stratification and differences in linkage disequilibrium make interpretation of the data from these studies difficult. To help address these limitations, it is imperative that future studies be performed in large cohorts of patients to help determine the genetic effects that are involved in scleroderma. Because of the low prevalence of scleroderma, extensive multi-institutional collaborations will be necessary to develop these large cohorts. These collaborations also will enable the formation of cohorts for replication studies, a critical step in confirming initial observations.

The clinical heterogeneity of scleroderma is a substantial obstacle to the design and interpretation of studies. Although large sample sizes are essential, future cohorts also must be able to characterize the patients carefully according to demographics, clinical phenotype, autoantibody profiles, and clinical course. Associations between distinct scleroderma autoantibody profiles and clinical manifestations may allow better definition of scleroderma disease subsets. Indeed, as discussed previously, stratification of patients based on autoantibody profiles demonstrates stronger associations with HLA polymorphisms and with other candidate genes (Table 3).

Another significant limitation of the candidate-gene approach that has been used to date is the inability to investigate large numbers of genes concomitantly. The completion of the human genome, advances in the understanding of the genome, and progress in the development of high-throughput molecular and genetic technologies have facilitated the use of genome-wide association studies to study genetic determinants of complex diseases. Although these studies require large cohorts and sophisticated statistical analyses, they can be performed without bias in terms of the genes that are considered for analysis. In addition, genome-wide approaches will make possible the identification of completely novel genes involved in scleroderma susceptibility that would not have been considered using the traditional candidate-gene approach. This approach now is being used

Table 3
Genetic associations based on autoantibody subsets in scleroderma

Autoantibody	Clinical characteristics	HLA associations	Candidat-gene associations

Anti-topoisomerase I	Diffuse skin involvement
	Pulmonary fibrosis
		Whites: *DRB1*1104, DPB1*1301*
		African Americans: *DQB1*0301, DPB1*1301*
		Japanese: *DRB1*1502, DQB1*0601,*
		  DPB1*0901
		Choctaw: *DRB1*1602, DQB1*0301,*
		  DPB1*1301
			PTPN22 R620W
			CTGF G-945C

Anti-centromere	LSSc	*DQB1*0501* and other *DQB1* alleles having polar amino acids in position 26	*AIF-1* +899T
	Pulmonary hypertension; digital ulcers		*PTPN22* R620W
Anti-RNA polymerase	Renal crisis Rapid progressive skin fibrosis	*DQB1*0201*	*EDNRA* H323H/C and E335E/A
Anti-PM-Scl	Overlap myositis Young age of onset	*DRB1*0301*	
Anti-U3RNP (fibrillarin)	African Americans and males	*DRB1*1302, DQB1*0604/0605*	

Abbreviation: LSSc, limited scleroderma.

extensively and already has provided significant insight into diseases such as rheumatoid arthritis and systemic lupus erythematosus [135,136].

Following the identification of individual genetic determinants of scleroderma susceptibility, it will be necessary to increase the understanding of how these genetic polymorphisms relate to the development of scleroderma. Central to this understanding will be defining complex gene–gene and gene–environment interactions. In addition, biologic confirmation of these genetic alterations into functional studies is essential to determine whether these associations are, in fact, causal. Such studies will depend on the availability of model systems for scleroderma that are amenable to experimental manipulation and accurately reflect the disease phenotype. Last, efforts also should focus on translating these findings into the care of the patient who has scleroderma. Ultimately, these genetic factors may have great importance in the diagnosis, prognosis, and perhaps treatment of patients who have scleroderma.

References

[1] Arnett FC. HLA and autoimmunity in scleroderma (systemic sclerosis). Int Rev Immunol 1995;12(2–4):107–28.

[2] Medsger TA Jr. Epidemiology of systemic sclerosis. Clin Dermatol 1994;12(2):207–16.

[3] Medsger TA Jr, Masi AT. Epidemiology of systemic sclerosis (scleroderma). Ann Intern Med 1971;74(5):714–21.

[4] Steen VD, Oddis CV, Conte CG, et al. Incidence of systemic sclerosis in Allegheny County, Pennsylvania. A twenty-year study of hospital-diagnosed cases, 1963–1982. Arthritis Rheum 1997;40(3):441–5.

[5] Michet CJ Jr, McKenna CH, Elveback LR, et al. Epidemiology of systemic lupus erythematosus and other connective tissue diseases in Rochester, Minnesota, 1950 through 1979. Mayo Clin Proc 1985;60(2):105–13.

[6] Mayes MD, Lacey JV Jr, Beebe-Dimmer J, et al. Prevalence, incidence, survival, and disease characteristics of systemic sclerosis in a large US population. Arthritis Rheum 2003; 48(8):2246–55.

[7] McGregor AR, Watson A, Yunis E, et al. Familial clustering of scleroderma spectrum disease. Am J Med 1988;84(6):1023–32.

[8] Englert H, Small-McMahon J, Chambers P, et al. Familial risk estimation in systemic sclerosis. Aust N Z J Med 1999;29(1):36–41.

[9] Arnett FC, Cho M, Chatterjee S, et al. Familial occurrence frequencies and relative risks for systemic sclerosis (scleroderma) in three United States cohorts. Arthritis Rheum 2001; 44(6):1359–62.

[10] Assassi S, Arnett FC, Reveille JD, et al. Clinical, immunologic, and genetic features of familial systemic sclerosis. Arthritis Rheum 2007;56(6):2031–7.

[11] Cook NJ, Silman AJ, Propert J, et al. Features of systemic sclerosis (scleroderma) in an identical twin pair. Br J Rheumatol 1993;32(10):926–8.

[12] De Keyser F, Peene I, Joos R, et al. Occurrence of scleroderma in monozygotic twins. J Rheumatol 2000;27(9):2267–9.

[13] Feghali-Bostwick C, Medsger TA Jr, Wright TM. Analysis of systemic sclerosis in twins reveals low concordance for disease and high concordance for the presence of antinuclear antibodies. Arthritis Rheum 2003;48(7):1956–63.

[14] Zhou X, Tan FK, Xiong M, et al. Monozygotic twins clinically discordant for scleroderma show concordance for fibroblast gene expression profiles. Arthritis Rheum 2005;52(10): 3305–14.

[15] Laing TJ, Gillespie BW, Toth MB, et al. Racial differences in scleroderma among women in Michigan. Arthritis Rheum 1997;40(4):734–42.

[16] Reveille JD, Fischbach M, McNearney T, et al. Systemic sclerosis in 3 US ethnic groups: a comparison of clinical, sociodemographic, serologic, and immunogenetic determinants. Semin Arthritis Rheum 2001;30(5):332–46.

[17] Arnett FC, Howard RF, Tan F, et al. Increased prevalence of systemic sclerosis in a Native American tribe in Oklahoma. Association with an Amerindian HLA haplotype. Arthritis Rheum 1996;39(8):1362–70.

[18] Tan FK, Stivers DN, Foster MW, et al. Association of microsatellite markers near the fibrillin 1 gene on human chromosome 15q with scleroderma in a Native American population. Arthritis Rheum 1998;41(10):1729–37.

[19] Tan FK, Wang N, Kuwana M, et al. Association of fibrillin 1 single-nucleotide polymorphism haplotypes with systemic sclerosis in Choctaw and Japanese populations. Arthritis Rheum 2001;44(4):893–901.

[20] Siracusa LD, McGrath R, Ma Q, et al. A tandem duplication within the fibrillin 1 gene is associated with the mouse tight skin mutation. Genome Res 1996;6(4):300–13.

[21] Arnett FC, Bias WB, Reveille JD. Genetic studies in Sjogren's syndrome and systemic lupus erythematosus. J Autoimmun 1989;2(4):403–13.

[22] Schlosstein L, Terasaki PI, Bluestone R, et al. High association of an HL-A antigen, W27, with ankylosing spondylitis. N Engl J Med 1973;288(14):704–6.

[23] Nepom GT, Seyfried CE, Holbeck SL, et al. Identification of HLA-Dw14 genes in DR4+ rheumatoid arthritis. Lancet 1986;2(8514):1002–5.

[24] Tan FK, Arnett FC. Genetic factors in the etiology of systemic sclerosis and Raynaud phenomenon. Curr Opin Rheumatol 2000;12(6):511–9.

[25] Tan FK. Systemic sclerosis: the susceptible host (genetics and environment). Rheum Dis Clin North Am 2003;29(2):211–37.

[26] Lambert NC, Distler O, Muller-Ladner U, et al. HLA-DQA1*0501 is associated with diffuse systemic sclerosis in Caucasian men. Arthritis Rheum 2000;43(9):2005–10.

[27] Reveille JD, Durban E, MacLeod-St Clair MJ, et al. Association of amino acid sequences in the HLA-DQB1 first domain with antitopoisomerase I autoantibody response in scleroderma (progressive systemic sclerosis). J Clin Invest 1992;90(3):973–80.

[28] Tan FK, Stivers DN, Arnett FC, et al. HLA haplotypes and microsatellite polymorphisms in and around the major histocompatibility complex region in a Native American population with a high prevalence of scleroderma (systemic sclerosis). Tissue Antigens 1999;53(1): 74–80.

[29] Kuwana M, Kaburaki J, Okano Y, et al. The HLA-DR and DQ genes control the autoimmune response to DNA topoisomerase I in systemic sclerosis (scleroderma). J Clin Invest 1993;92(3):1296–301.

[30] Kuwana M, Medsger TA Jr, Wright TM. T cell proliferative response induced by DNA topoisomerase I in patients with systemic sclerosis and healthy donors. J Clin Invest 1995;96(1): 586–96.

[31] Morel PA, Chang HJ, Wilson JW, et al. Severe systemic sclerosis with anti-topoisomerase I antibodies is associated with an HLA-DRw11 allele. Hum Immunol 1994;40(2):101–10.

[32] Gilchrist FC, Bunn C, Foley PJ, et al. Class II HLA associations with autoantibodies in scleroderma: a highly significant role for HLA-DP. Genes Immun 2001;2(2):76–81.

[33] Morel PA, Chang HJ, Wilson JW, et al. HLA and ethnic associations among systemic sclerosis patients with anticentromere antibodies. Hum Immunol 1995;42(1):35–42.

[34] Arnett FC, Reveille JD, Goldstein R, et al. Autoantibodies to fibrillarin in systemic sclerosis (scleroderma). An immunogenetic, serologic, and clinical analysis. Arthritis Rheum 1996; 39(7):1151–60.

[35] Marguerie C, Bunn CC, Copier J, et al. The clinical and immunogenetic features of patients with autoantibodies to the nucleolar antigen PM-Scl. Medicine (Baltimore) 1992;71(6): 327–36.

[36] Fanning GC, Welsh KI, Bunn C, et al. HLA associations in three mutually exclusive auto-antibody subgroups in UK systemic sclerosis patients. Br J Rheumatol 1998;37(2):201–7.

[37] Falkner D, Wilson J, Fertig N, et al. Studies of HLA-DR and DQ alleles in systemic sclerosis patients with autoantibodies to RNA polymerases and U3-RNP (fibrillarin). J Rheumatol 2000;27(5):1196–202.

[38] Campbell H, Rudan I. Interpretation of genetic association studies in complex disease. Pharmacogenomics J 2002;2(6):349–60.

[39] Lohmueller KE, Pearce CL, Pike M, et al. Meta-analysis of genetic association studies supports a contribution of common variants to susceptibility to common disease. Nat Genet 2003;33(2):177–82.

[40] Caponi L, Petit-Teixeira E, Sebbag M, et al. A family based study shows no association between rheumatoid arthritis and the PADI4 gene in a white French population. Ann Rheum Dis 2005;64(4):587–93.

[41] Kang CP, Lee HS, Ju H, et al. A functional haplotype of the PADI4 gene associated with increased rheumatoid arthritis susceptibility in Koreans. Arthritis Rheum 2006;54(1):90–6.

[42] Martinez A, Valdivia A, Pascual-Salcedo D, et al. PADI4 polymorphisms are not associated with rheumatoid arthritis in the Spanish population. Rheumatology (Oxford) 2005;44(10):1263–6.

[43] Plenge RM, Padyukov L, Remmers EF, et al. Replication of putative candidate-gene associations with rheumatoid arthritis in >4,000 samples from North America and Sweden: association of susceptibility with PTPN22, CTLA4, and PADI4. Am J Hum Genet 2005;77(6):1044–60.

[44] Suzuki A, Yamada R, Chang X, et al. Functional haplotypes of PADI4, encoding citrullinating enzyme peptidylarginine deiminase 4, are associated with rheumatoid arthritis. Nat Genet 2003;34(4):395–402.

[45] Begovich AB, Carlton VE, Honigberg LA, et al. A missense single-nucleotide polymorphism in a gene encoding a protein tyrosine phosphatase (PTPN22) is associated with rheumatoid arthritis. Am J Hum Genet 2004;75(2):330–7.

[46] Kanangat S, Postlethwaite AE, Higgins GC, et al. Novel functions of intracellular IL-1ra in human dermal fibroblasts: implications in the pathogenesis of fibrosis. J Invest Dermatol 2006;126(4):756–65.

[47] Kawaguchi Y, Hara M, Wright TM. Endogenous IL-1alpha from systemic sclerosis fibroblasts induces IL-6 and PDGF-A. J Clin Invest 1999;103(9):1253–60.

[48] Kawaguchi Y, McCarthy SA, Watkins SC, et al. Autocrine activation by interleukin 1alpha induces the fibrogenic phenotype of systemic sclerosis fibroblasts. J Rheumatol 2004;31(10):1946–54.

[49] Kawaguchi Y, Tochimoto A, Ichikawa N, et al. Association of IL1A gene polymorphisms with susceptibility to and severity of systemic sclerosis in the Japanese population. Arthritis Rheum 2003;48(1):186–92.

[50] Hutyrova B, Lukac J, Bosak V, et al. Interleukin 1alpha single-nucleotide polymorphism associated with systemic sclerosis. J Rheumatol 2004;31(1):81–4.

[51] Beretta L, Bertolotti F, Cappiello F, et al. Interleukin-1 gene complex polymorphisms in systemic sclerosis patients with severe restrictive lung physiology. Hum Immunol 2007;68(7):603–9.

[52] Mattuzzi S, Barbi S, Carletto A, et al. Association of polymorphisms in the IL1B and IL2 genes with susceptibility and severity of systemic sclerosis. J Rheumatol 2007;34(5):997–1004.

[53] Utans U, Arceci RJ, Yamashita Y, et al. Cloning and characterization of allograft inflammatory factor-1: a novel macrophage factor identified in rat cardiac allografts with chronic rejection. J Clin Invest 1995;95(6):2954–62.

[54] Del Galdo F, Maul GG, Jimenez SA, et al. Expression of allograft inflammatory factor 1 in tissues from patients with systemic sclerosis and in vitro differential expression of its

isoforms in response to transforming growth factor beta. Arthritis Rheum 2006;54(8): 2616–25.

[55] Utans U, Quist WC, McManus BM, et al. Allograft inflammatory factory-1. A cytokine-responsive macrophage molecule expressed in transplanted human hearts. Transplantation 1996;61(9):1387–92.

[56] Del Galdo F, Artlett CM, Jimenez SA. The role of allograft inflammatory factor 1 in systemic sclerosis. Curr Opin Rheumatol 2006;18(6):588–93.

[57] Galdo FD, Jimenez SA. T cells expressing allograft inflammatory factor 1 display increased chemotaxis and induce a profibrotic phenotype in normal fibroblasts in vitro. Arthritis Rheum 2007;56(10):3478–88.

[58] Otieno FG, Lopez AM, Jimenez SA, et al. Allograft inflammatory factor-1 and tumor necrosis factor single nucleotide polymorphisms in systemic sclerosis. Tissue Antigens 2007;69(6):583–91.

[59] Alkassab F, Gourh P, Tan FK, et al. An allograft inflammatory factor 1 (AIF1) single nucleotide polymorphism (SNP) is associated with anticentromere antibody positive systemic sclerosis. Rheumatology (Oxford) 2007;46(8):1248–51.

[60] Bottini N, Musumeci L, Alonso A, et al. A functional variant of lymphoid tyrosine phosphatase is associated with type I diabetes. Nat Genet 2004;36(4):337–8.

[61] Rieck M, Arechiga A, Onengut-Gumuscu S, et al. Genetic variation in PTPN22 corresponds to altered function of T and B lymphocytes. J Immunol 2007;179(7):4704–10.

[62] Vang T, Congia M, Macis MD, et al. Autoimmune-associated lymphoid tyrosine phosphatase is a gain-of-function variant. Nat Genet 2005;37(12):1317–9.

[63] Onengut-Gumuscu S, Ewens KG, Spielman RS, et al. A functional polymorphism (1858C/T) in the PTPN22 gene is linked and associated with type I diabetes in multiplex families. Genes Immun 2004;5(8):678–80.

[64] Orozco G, Sanchez E, Gonzalez-Gay MA, et al. Association of a functional single-nucleotide polymorphism of PTPN22, encoding lymphoid protein phosphatase, with rheumatoid arthritis and systemic lupus erythematosus. Arthritis Rheum 2005;52(1):219–24.

[65] Orozco G, Garcia-Porrua C, Lopez-Nevot MA, et al. Lack of association between ankylosing spondylitis and a functional polymorphism of PTPN22 proposed as a general susceptibility marker for autoimmunity. Ann Rheum Dis 2006;65(5):687–8.

[66] van Oene M, Wintle RF, Liu X, et al. Association of the lymphoid tyrosine phosphatase R620W variant with rheumatoid arthritis, but not Crohn's disease, in Canadian populations. Arthritis Rheum 2005;52(7):1993–8.

[67] Ittah M, Gottenberg JE, Proust A, et al. No evidence for association between 1858 C/T single-nucleotide polymorphism of PTPN22 gene and primary Sjogren's syndrome. Genes Immun 2005;6(5):457–8.

[68] Balada E, Simeon-Aznar CP, Serrano-Acedo S, et al. Lack of association of the PTPN22 gene polymorphism R620W with systemic sclerosis. Clin Exp Rheumatol 2006;24(3): 321–4.

[69] Wipff J, Allanore Y, Kahan A, et al. Lack of association between the protein tyrosine phosphatase non-receptor 22 (PTPN22)*620W allele and systemic sclerosis in the French Caucasian population. Ann Rheum Dis 2006;65(9):1230–2.

[70] Gourh P, Tan FK, Assassi S, et al. Association of the PTPN22 R620W polymorphism with anti-topoisomerase I- and anticentromere antibody-positive systemic sclerosis. Arthritis Rheum 2006;54(12):3945–53.

[71] Bacher M, Meinhardt A, Lan HY, et al. Migration inhibitory factor expression in experimentally induced endotoxemia. Am J Pathol 1997;150(1):235–46.

[72] Calandra T, Bernhagen J, Mitchell RA, et al. The macrophage is an important and previously unrecognized source of macrophage migration inhibitory factor. J Exp Med 1994; 179(6):1895–902.

[73] Morand EF, Leech M, Weedon H, et al. Macrophage migration inhibitory factor in rheumatoid arthritis: clinical correlations. Rheumatology (Oxford) 2002;41(5):558–62.

[74] Selvi E, Tripodi SA, Catenaccio M, et al. Expression of macrophage migration inhibitory factor in diffuse systemic sclerosis. Ann Rheum Dis 2003;62(5):460–4.

[75] Wu SP, Leng L, Feng Z, et al. Macrophage migration inhibitory factor promoter polymorphisms and the clinical expression of scleroderma. Arthritis Rheum 2006;54(11):3661–9.

[76] Kadono T, Kikuchi K, Ihn H, et al. Increased production of interleukin 6 and interleukin 8 in scleroderma fibroblasts. J Rheumatol 1998;25(2):296–301.

[77] Distler O, Rinkes B, Hohenleutner U, et al. Expression of RANTES in biopsies of skin and upper gastrointestinal tract from patients with systemic sclerosis. Rheumatol Int 1999; 19(1–2):39–46.

[78] Kimura M, Kawahito Y, Hamaguchi M, et al. SKL-2841, a dual antagonist of MCP-1 and MIP-1 beta, prevents bleomycin-induced skin sclerosis in mice. Biomed Pharmacother 2007;61(4):222–8.

[79] Yamamoto T, Eckes B, Krieg T. High expression and autoinduction of monocyte chemoattractant protein-1 in scleroderma fibroblasts. Eur J Immunol 2001;31(10):2936–41.

[80] Yamamoto T, Eckes B, Hartmann K, et al. Expression of monocyte chemoattractant protein-1 in the lesional skin of systemic sclerosis. J Dermatol Sci 2001;26(2):133–9.

[81] Distler O, Pap T, Kowal-Bielecka O, et al. Overexpression of monocyte chemoattractant protein 1 in systemic sclerosis: role of platelet-derived growth factor and effects on monocyte chemotaxis and collagen synthesis. Arthritis Rheum 2001;44(11):2665–78.

[82] Ferreira AM, Takagawa S, Fresco R, et al. Diminished induction of skin fibrosis in mice with MCP-1 deficiency. J Invest Dermatol 2006;126(8):1900–8.

[83] Karrer S, Bosserhoff AK, Weiderer P, et al. The −2518 promotor polymorphism in the MCP-1 gene is associated with systemic sclerosis. J Invest Dermatol 2005;124(1):92–8.

[84] Lee EB, Zhao J, Kim JY, et al. Evidence of potential interaction of chemokine genes in susceptibility to systemic sclerosis. Arthritis Rheum 2007;56(7):2443–8.

[85] Tsuchiya N, Kuroki K, Fujimoto M, et al. Association of a functional CD19 polymorphism with susceptibility to systemic sclerosis. Arthritis Rheum 2004;50(12):4002–7.

[86] Hitomi Y, Tsuchiya N, Hasegawa M, et al. Association of CD22 gene polymorphism with susceptibility to limited cutaneous systemic sclerosis. Tissue Antigens 2007;69(3): 242–9.

[87] Abdallah AM, Renzoni EA, Anevlavis S, et al. A polymorphism in the promoter region of the CD86 (B7.2) gene is associated with systemic sclerosis. Int J Immunogenet 2006;33(3): 155–61.

[88] Hudson LL, Silver RM, Pandey JP. Ethnic differences in cytotoxic T lymphocyte associated antigen 4 genotype associations with systemic sclerosis. J Rheumatol 2004;31(1):85–7.

[89] Takeuchi F, Kawasugi K, Nabeta H, et al. Association of CTLA-4 with systemic sclerosis in Japanese patients. Clin Exp Rheumatol 2002;20(6):823–8.

[90] Almasi S, Erfani N, Mojtahedi Z, et al. Association of CTLA-4 gene promoter polymorphisms with systemic sclerosis in Iranian population. Genes Immun 2006;7(5):401–6.

[91] Balbi G, Ferrera F, Rizzi M, et al. Association of −318 C/T and +49 A/G cytotoxic T lymphocyte antigen-4 (CTLA-4) gene polymorphisms with a clinical subset of Italian patients with systemic sclerosis. Clin Exp Immunol 2007;149(1):40–7.

[92] Renzoni E, Lympany P, Sestini P, et al. Distribution of novel polymorphisms of the interleukin-8 and CXC receptor 1 and 2 genes in systemic sclerosis and cryptogenic fibrosing alveolitis. Arthritis Rheum 2000;43(7):1633–40.

[93] Crilly A, Hamilton J, Clark CJ, et al. Analysis of the 5' flanking region of the interleukin 10 gene in patients with systemic sclerosis. Rheumatology (Oxford) 2003;42(11):1295–8.

[94] Beretta L, Cappiello F, Barili M, et al. Proximal interleukin-10 gene polymorphisms in Italian patients with systemic sclerosis. Tissue Antigens 2007;69(4):305–12.

[95] Granel B, Chevillard C, Allanore Y, et al. Evaluation of interleukin 13 polymorphisms in systemic sclerosis. Immunogenetics 2006;58(8):693–9.

[96] Granel B, Allanore Y, Chevillard C, et al. IL13RA2 gene polymorphisms are associated with systemic sclerosis. J Rheumatol 2006;33(10):2015–9.

[97] Sato H, Lagan AL, Alexopoulou C, et al. The TNF-863A allele strongly associates with anticentromere antibody positivity in scleroderma. Arthritis Rheum 2004;50(2): 558–64.

[98] Tolusso B, Fabris M, Caporali R, et al. −238 and +489 TNF-alpha along with TNF-RII gene polymorphisms associate with the diffuse phenotype in patients with systemic sclerosis. Immunol Lett 2005;96(1):103–8.

[99] Assassi S, Tan FK. Genetics of scleroderma: update on single nucleotide polymorphism analysis and microarrays. Curr Opin Rheumatol 2005;17(6):761–7.

[100] Herrick AL, Worthington J. Genetic epidemiology: systemic sclerosis. Arthritis Res 2002; 4(3):165–8.

[101] Pandey JP, Takeuchi F. TNF-alpha and TNF-beta gene polymorphisms in systemic sclerosis. Hum Immunol 1999;60(11):1128–30.

[102] Momot T, Koch S, Hunzelmann N, et al. Association of killer cell immunoglobulin-like receptors with scleroderma. Arthritis Rheum 2004;50(5):1561–5.

[103] Matucci Cerinic M, Kahaleh MB. Beauty and the beast. The nitric oxide paradox in systemic sclerosis. Rheumatology (Oxford) 2002;41(8):843–7.

[104] Biondi ML, Marasini B, Leviti S, et al. Genotyping method for point mutation detection in the endothelial nitric oxide synthase exon 7 using fluorescent probes. Clinical validation in systemic sclerosis patients. Clin Chem Lab Med 2001;39(3):281–2.

[105] Fatini C, Gensini F, Sticchi E, et al. High prevalence of polymorphisms of angiotensin-converting enzyme (I/D) and endothelial nitric oxide synthase (Glu298Asp) in patients with systemic sclerosis. Am J Med 2002;112(7):540–4.

[106] Fatini C, Mannini L, Sticchi E, et al. Hemorheologic profile in systemic sclerosis: role of NOS3 −786T > C and 894G > T polymorphisms in modulating both the hemorheologic parameters and the susceptibility to the disease. Arthritis Rheum 2006;54(7):2263–70.

[107] Assassi S, Mayes MD, McNearney T, et al. Polymorphisms of endothelial nitric oxide synthase and angiotensin-converting enzyme in systemic sclerosis. Am J Med 2005;118(8): 907–11.

[108] Tikly M, Gulumian M, Marshall S. Lack of association of eNOS(G894T) and p22phox NADPH oxidase submit (C242T) polymorphisms with systemic sclerosis in a cohort of French Caucasian patients. Clin Chim Acta 2005;358(1–2):196–7.

[109] Kawaguchi Y, Tochimoto A, Hara M, et al. NOS2 polymorphisms associated with the susceptibility to pulmonary arterial hypertension with systemic sclerosis: contribution to the transcriptional activity. Arthritis Res Ther 2006;8(4):R104.

[110] Rigat B, Hubert C, Alhenc-Gelas F, et al. An insertion/deletion polymorphism in the angiotensin I-converting enzyme gene accounting for half the variance of serum enzyme levels. J Clin Invest 1990;86(4):1343–6.

[111] Distler O, Del Rosso A, Giacomelli R, et al. Angiogenic and angiostatic factors in systemic sclerosis: increased levels of vascular endothelial growth factor are a feature of the earliest disease stages and are associated with the absence of fingertip ulcers. Arthritis Res 2002; 4(6):R11.

[112] Distler O, Distler JH, Scheid A, et al. Uncontrolled expression of vascular endothelial growth factor and its receptors leads to insufficient skin angiogenesis in patients with systemic sclerosis. Circ Res 2004;95(1):109–16.

[113] Watson CJ, Webb NJ, Bottomley MJ, et al. Identification of polymorphisms within the vascular endothelial growth factor (VEGF) gene: correlation with variation in VEGF protein production. Cytokine 2000;12(8):1232–5.

[114] Rueda B, Lopez-Nevot MA, Lopez-Diaz MJ, et al. A functional variant of vascular endothelial growth factor is associated with severe ischemic complications in giant cell arteritis. J Rheumatol 2005;32(9):1737–41.

[115] Allanore Y, Borderie D, Airo P, et al. Lack of association between three vascular endothelial growth factor gene polymorphisms and systemic sclerosis: results from a multicenter EUSTAR study of European Caucasian patients. Ann Rheum Dis 2007;66(2):257–9.

[116] Herrick AL. Vascular function in systemic sclerosis. Curr Opin Rheumatol 2000;12(6): 527–33.

[117] Cambrey AD, Harrison NK, Dawes KE, et al. Increased levels of endothelin-1 in bronchoalveolar lavage fluid from patients with systemic sclerosis contribute to fibroblast mitogenic activity in vitro. Am J Respir Cell Mol Biol 1994;11(4):439–45.

[118] Morelli S, Ferri C, Polettini E, et al. Plasma endothelin-1 levels, pulmonary hypertension, and lung fibrosis in patients with systemic sclerosis. Am J Med 1995;99(3):255–60.

[119] Fonseca C, Renzoni E, Sestini P, et al. Endothelin axis polymorphisms in patients with scleroderma. Arthritis Rheum 2006;54(9):3034–42.

[120] Verrecchia F, Mauviel A, Farge D. Transforming growth factor-beta signaling through the Smad proteins: role in systemic sclerosis. Autoimmun Rev 2006;5(8):563–9.

[121] Varga J. Scleroderma and Smads: dysfunctional Smad family dynamics culminating in fibrosis. Arthritis Rheum 2002;46(7):1703–13.

[122] Crilly A, Hamilton J, Clark CJ, et al. Analysis of transforming growth factor beta1 gene polymorphisms in patients with systemic sclerosis. Ann Rheum Dis 2002;61(8):678–81.

[123] Sugiura Y, Banno S, Matsumoto Y, et al. Transforming growth factor beta1 gene polymorphism in patients with systemic sclerosis. J Rheumatol 2003;30(7):1520–3.

[124] Bradham DM, Igarashi A, Potter RL, et al. Connective tissue growth factor: a cysteine-rich mitogen secreted by human vascular endothelial cells is related to the SRC-induced immediate early gene product CEF-10. J Cell Biol 1991;114(6):1285–94.

[125] Shimo T, Nakanishi T, Kimura Y, et al. Inhibition of endogenous expression of connective tissue growth factor by its antisense oligonucleotide and antisense RNA suppresses proliferation and migration of vascular endothelial cells. J Biochem (Tokyo) 1998;124(1):130–40.

[126] Leask A, Abraham DJ. All in the CCN family: essential matricellular signaling modulators emerge from the bunker. J Cell Sci 2006;119(Pt 23):4803–10.

[127] Igarashi A, Nashiro K, Kikuchi K, et al. Connective tissue growth factor gene expression in tissue sections from localized scleroderma, keloid, and other fibrotic skin disorders. J Invest Dermatol 1996;106(4):729–33.

[128] Igarashi A, Nashiro K, Kikuchi K, et al. Significant correlation between connective tissue growth factor gene expression and skin sclerosis in tissue sections from patients with systemic sclerosis. J Invest Dermatol 1995;105(2):280–4.

[129] Leask A, Sa S, Holmes A, et al. The control of CCN2 (CTGF) gene expression in normal and scleroderma fibroblasts. Mol Pathol 2001;54(3):180–3.

[130] Fonseca C, Lindahl GE, Ponticos M, et al. A polymorphism in the CTGF promoter region associated with systemic sclerosis. N Engl J Med 2007;357(12):1210–20.

[131] Zhou X, Tan FK, Reveille JD, et al. Association of novel polymorphisms with the expression of SPARC in normal fibroblasts and with susceptibility to scleroderma. Arthritis Rheum 2002;46(11):2990–9.

[132] Zhou X, Tan FK, Guo X, et al. Attenuation of collagen production with small interfering RNA of SPARC in cultured fibroblasts from the skin of patients with scleroderma. Arthritis Rheum 2006;54(8):2626–31.

[133] Zhou X, Tan FK, Guo X, et al. Small interfering RNA inhibition of SPARC attenuates the profibrotic effect of transforming growth factor beta1 in cultured normal human fibroblasts. Arthritis Rheum 2005;52(1):257–61.

[134] Lagan AL, Pantelidis P, Renzoni EA, et al. Single-nucleotide polymorphisms in the SPARC gene are not associated with susceptibility to scleroderma. Rheumatology (Oxford) 2005;44(2):197–201.

[135] Plenge RM, Seielstad M, Padyukov L, et al. TRAF1-C5 as a risk locus for rheumatoid arthritis—a genomewide study. N Engl J Med 2007;357(12):1199–209.

[136] Remmers EF, Plenge RM, Lee AT, et al. STAT4 and the risk of rheumatoid arthritis and systemic lupus erythematosus. N Engl J Med 2007;357(10):977–86.

[137] Samani NJ, Erdmann J, Hall AS, et al. Genomewide association analysis of coronary artery disease. N Engl J Med 2007;357(5):443–53.

[138] Genome-wide association study of 14,000 cases of seven commondiseases and 3,000 shared controls. Nature 2007;447(7145):661–78.

[139] Zhou X, Tan FK, Wang N, et al. Genome-wide association study for regions of systemic sclerosis susceptibility in a Choctaw Indian population with high disease prevalence. Arthritis Rheum 2003;48(9):2585–92.

[140] Whitfield ML, Finlay DR, Murray JI, et al. Systemic and cell type-specific gene expression patterns in scleroderma skin. Proc Natl Acad Sci U S A 2003;100(21):12319–24.

[141] Tan FK, Hildebrand BA, Lester MS, et al. Classification analysis of the transcriptosome of nonlesional cultured dermal fibroblasts from systemic sclerosis patients with early disease. Arthritis Rheum 2005;52(3):865–76.

[142] Gardner H, Shearstone JR, Bandaru R, et al. Gene profiling of scleroderma skin reveals robust signatures of disease that are imperfectly reflected in the transcript profiles of explanted fibroblasts. Arthritis Rheum 2006;54(6):1961–73.

[143] Pannu J, Gardner H, Shearstone JR, et al. Increased levels of transforming growth factor beta receptor type I and up-regulation of matrix gene program: a model of scleroderma. Arthritis Rheum 2006;54(9):3011–21.

[144] Pannu J, Nakerakanti S, Smith E, et al. Transforming growth factor-beta receptor type I-dependent fibrogenic gene program is mediated via activation of Smad1 and ERK1/2 pathways. J Biol Chem 2007;282(14):10405–13.

[145] Tan FK, Zhou X, Mayes MD, et al. Signatures of differentially regulated interferon gene expression and vasculotrophism in the peripheral blood cells of systemic sclerosis patients. Rheumatology (Oxford) 2006;45(6):694–702.

[146] York MR, Nagai T, Mangini AJ, et al. A macrophage marker, Siglec-1, is increased on circulating monocytes in patients with systemic sclerosis and induced by type I interferons and toll-like receptor agonists. Arthritis Rheum 2007;56(3):1010–20.

ELSEVIER
SAUNDERS

Rheum Dis Clin N Am
34 (2008) 41–55

RHEUMATIC
DISEASE CLINICS
OF NORTH AMERICA

The Pathology of Scleroderma Vascular Disease

Jo Nadine Fleming, MD,
Stephen Mark Schwartz, MD, PhD*

Department of Pathology, 815 Mercer Street, Room 421, Brotman Building, Box 358050, University of Washington, Seattle WA 98109-4717, USA

Systemic sclerosis (scleroderma, SSc) is characterized by three distinct pathologic processes: fibrosis, cellular/humoral autoimmunity, and specific vascular changes [1–4]. Although a mild vasculitis may sometimes be present, the vascular pathology of scleroderma is not necessarily inflammatory and is best characterized as a vasculopathy. The three pathologic processes may occur and progress independently, making diagnosis and treatment challenging.

The focus of this article is on the vasculopathy. The idea that the vasculopathy may be the critical, underlying pathology is not new [5]. Evidence for vascular injury was published as early as 1925 [6] and shown to be present in multiple microvascular beds, including skeletal muscle [7–10]. The single most impressive evidence that the vasculopathy is a systemic process in scleroderma came from the pivotal autopsy study in 1969 by D'Angelo and colleagues [11]. This autopsy study of 58 subjects with matched controls showed that SSc patients had intimal proliferation in the pulmonary arteries, the coronary arteries, and the interlobular arteries of the kidney. The neointima was not inflammatory. Moreover, this autopsy study showed that beyond the intimal hyperplasia of larger arteries, SSc patients were likely to have arteriolar intimal hyperplasia in two or more organs.

Finally, there is a wide spread belief that the injured cell-type responsible for this vasculopathy is the endothelium. The major evidence for this is serologic. SSc is characterized by increased serum levels of von Willebrand factor [12], endothelin [13], and increased numbers of circulating viable and

Funding support was provided by the Scleroderma Research Foundation. Dr. Fleming is a fellow of the Scleroderma Research Foundation.

* Corresponding author.

E-mail address: steves@u.washington.edu (S.M. Schwartz).

dead endothelial cells [14–16]. As this article discusses, the pathologic evidence for endothelial injury as an initiating event is less convincing.

Vascular pathology of scleroderma

The functional changes in the vasculature of patients with SSc are well described by others [17]. The most prominent of these changes is Raynaud's phenomenon, a widespread form of vasospasm that is prodromal or concurrent with other changes in SSc. The focus of this article is on understanding the morphologic changes using current knowledge of vascular biology.

Capillary malformation

Widespread capillary involvement in SSc includes malformation, increased permeability, changes in basement membranes, and rarefaction [5,18,19]. Malformation of nail bed capillaries is readily demonstrated by nail bed microscopy and has been shown to correlate both with disease severity and with extent of internal organ involvement [20]. Much of the capillary morphology has been attributed as a response to vascular endothelial growth factor (VEGF) found early in the course of SSc [21,22]. Although VEGF is well known as an angiogenesis factor, it is important to understand that induction of vascular networks by VEGF is not enough to produce permanent vasculature. New vessels induced by VEGF will regress. In a mouse model, overexpression of VEGF produced malformed, permeable vessels that required pericytes and platelet-derived growth factor, signaling it to stabilize. Without pericyte investment, the poorly formed capillaries regressed [23]. VEGF-induced vessels are widely dilated, surrounded by tissue edema, and eventually form vascular ectasia reminiscent of hemangioma or telangectasia. Given the excess of VEGF present in the SSc patient early in the disease [21,22], the telangectasia and abnormal vasculature suggest that unregulated angiogenesis is responsible for at least part of the vasculopathy in SSc. Elevated angiogenic stimulation, however, does not mean more capillaries. The paradox, as discussed below, is that the authors have found loss of capillaries to be as characteristic of SSc in early onset disease as it is in late onset (Fig. 1A) [24].

The combination of Raynaud's, nail fold capillary abnormalities and hand swelling are independent predictors of the development of SSc [10]. The association of both nail fold abnormalities and Raynaud's phenomenon with SSc may be the strongest evidence that SSc is the end result of one or more forms of primary vascular injury.

Intimal hyperplasia

A common feature of the SSc vasculopathy is a hyperplasia: that is, increase in cell number and matrix, and thickening of the arterial intima [25–27]. The intima is a normal layer of the arterial wall that includes the connective tissue between the endothelium and the internal elastic lamina. Focal intimal thickening, comprised of smooth muscle cells and connective tissue matrix, is a normal component of larger arteries, especially near branch sites [28]. The extensive intimal formation seen in SSc, however, is pathologic.

Pathologic intimal thickening, also called "neointima" or, perhaps misleadingly, "intimal hyperplasia," is a common response to a very wide range of arterial injuries, including the response to angioplasty, emplacement of stents, immune rejection, radiation, and placement of an inflammatory stimulus in the adventitia [28–30]. The term "intimal hyperplasia" may be misleading because of controversy as to the source of the intimal cells, with some papers arguing for origin from the adventitia or from the circulation [31–34]. This controversy is especially important in a potential model for the SSc vasculopathy, transplant atherosclerosis (TPA). TPA is a very common event late in the course of recovery from organ transplantation. Despite the name, TPA responds poorly to immunosuppression and has not been clearly related to an immunologic event [35,36]. Because so many kinds of arterial injury result in intimal hyperplasia, it is possible that the change in the intima is a response to ischemic changes occurring during transplantation. If it is the case that ischemia is responsible for some of the injury associated with TPA, ischemia secondary to Raynaud's phenomenon may be an important part of the process that leads to intimal hyperplasia and rarefaction in scleroderma.

Unfortunately, the stimulus for TPA itself is not clear. Based, however, on the belief that neointimal cells are derived from the media or adventitia in the arterial response to injury, a long list of mediators have been identified that can stimulate movement of smooth muscle cells from the media into the intima, synthesis of matrix, and cell replication within the intima. These mediators of intimal formation include several growth factors, cytokines, and angiotensin [37–40]. In most, but not all models, the neointima does not have any substantial number of inflammatory cells. The most studied example of an inflammatory neointima is atherosclerosis, where the fatty lesions of atherosclerosis plaque begin with intimal monocytosis [30,41].

Intimal hyperplasia of large arteries with loss of caliber is believed to be the primary causes of pulmonary arterial hypertension in SSc [14]. Intimal hyperplasia in smaller arteries may occlude lumens and cause gangrene and capillary rarefaction (below) [42–44], but is typically seen only in malignant hypertension. In milder forms of hypertension, the usual arterial changes are remodeling, that is, changes in the wall-lumen ratio without intimal hyperplasia [45,46].

Finally, intimal hyperplasia could precede and be causal for Raynaud's phenomenon. This idea may not be intuitively obvious; however, there have been extensive studies of vasospasm occurring as a response to neointima [47]. This is best described in the intimal response to adventitial inflammation, raising the possibility that a neointimal response to a transient vasculitis might underlie and precede Raynaud's phenomenon [48]. Experimental models and clinical studies of angina and stroke suggest that formation of a vasospastic intima may be prevented by rho-kinase inhibitors [48]. While the natural assumption is that rho kinase plays a central role in smooth muscle contractility, the kinase has also been implicated in the formation of intima, as well as in the interactions of leukocytes with the

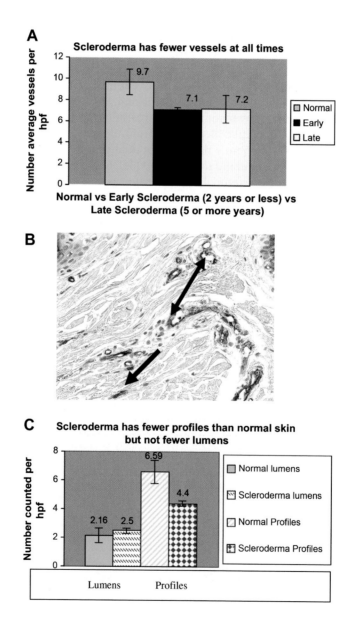

vessel wall [49–52]. Thus, rho kinase inhibition might itself be anti-inflammatory, block vasoactive stimuli, or block intimal formation.

Capillary rarefaction

Although the nail bed changes have sometimes been described as rarefaction, in this article the authors suggest that it is more accurate to describe the nail fold changes as "malformation of capillaries." By definition, rarefaction requires loss of branch levels of the vascular circuit. Loss of branch levels is difficult to find by nail bed microscopy because the capillaries in SSc are so abnormal. Moreover, the need for an actual column of blood to identify vessels by capillary microscopy means that collapsed capillaries, resulting from intimal hyperplasia or vasoconstriction of arterioles, would look like capillary dropout (Fig. 1B).

Skin biopsies from 23 SSc subjects and 24 normal controls were obtained to allow the authors to determine whether capillary loss was present. Morphometry was used to quantify vessels in forearm dermis (see Fig. 1B). The authors characterized the endothelial cells in these same biopsies with immunohistochemistry and RNA in situ hybridization. The results showed decreased capillary counts in dermis from SSc subjects compared with dermis from normal controls (Fig. 1C) [24].

Finally, the residual endothelium of the dermis displays what the authors call an "antiangiogenic phenotype" (Fig. 2) [24]. The three molecules defining this phenotype are implicated in angiogenesis. For example, vascular endothelial (VE) cadherin, a universal endothelial marker responsible for the calcium dependent formation of junctions between endothelial cells, is lost in the residual vasculature of SSc tissue (see Fig. 2A). Formation of intermediate junctions is required for tube formation [53] during the early stages of capillary morphogenesis. Although the authors cannot find any literature on changes in VE cadherin in angiogenesis, its absence would make

Fig. 1. (*A*) The quantification of scleroderma skin included the counting of vessels per high-power field (hpf) in 12 normal and 21 scleroderma skin biopsies stained with CD31. The chart shows the average number of vessels per hpf is significantly decreased in scleroderma when compared with normal controls. Standard error was calculated with the standard deviation divided by the square root of n. (*B*) Representative 20× section of normal skin stained via immunohistochemistry for CD31. "Profiles" or capillaries are defined as groups of cells positive for CD31 with no central lumen (single arrow). "Lumens" are defined as groups of cells positive for CD31 which have central lumens and were counted to estimate numbers of larger vessels (double-headed arrow). (*C*) Reading left to right, the first two bars show average numbers of lumens/hpf in normal and scleroderma biopsies. Average lumens in skin biopsies are not significantly different ($P = .18$). The second two bars show average profiles/hpf in skin biopsies of normal and scleroderma subjects. Average profiles are significantly decreased in scleroderma subjects compared with controls ($P = .009$). The numbers of profiles present in skin biopsies provide an estimate of the numbers of capillaries present, and the results indicate that capillaries are decreased specifically in scleroderma. P values were obtained using students' t-test. Error bars were calculated by dividing the standard deviation by the square root of n.

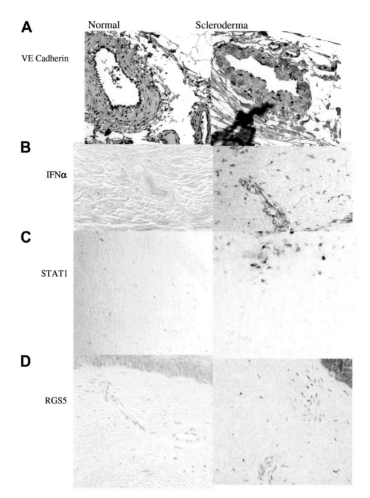

Fig. 2. (*A*) Scleroderma skin (left) shows no sign of vascular endothelial cadherin labeling in many of the endothelial cells. Brown DAB-stained cells are positive for CD123. (*B*) Interferon-α (IFNα) in situ shows a robust signal in scleroderma when compared with normal controls. The normal controls on the left show no pink signal, whereas the antisense probe for IFNα1 on the right has hybridized strongly in the perivascular cells of the horizontal plexus in the scleroderma skin on the right, producing a bright pink color reaction. (*C*) Phosphorylated signal transducer and activator of transcription 1 (STAT1) provide evidence of active interferon signaling in scleroderma skin. Antibody for phosphorylated STAT1 shows brown stain in the nucleus of cells in the superficial horizontal plexus in scleroderma skin, providing evidence of STAT1 phosphorylation, dimerization, and translocation to nucleus in response to stimulus. (*D*) RGS5 mRNA expression is increased in scleroderma. Normal skin on the left shows little or no RGS5 antisense probe in situ hybridization, whereas baseline scleroderma skin on the right shows bright pink color reaction in cells scattered throughout the matrix and in a perivascular distribution.

angiogenesis impossible. The second molecule in this phenotype is inter-feron-α. Interferon-α, has been implicated in SSc because circulating mono-nuclear cells show an expression profile implying that they have been exposed to this cytokine [54]. The data suggest a possible source for the cy-tokine because interferon-α is over-expressed in the SSc dermis (see Fig. 2B, C). Relevant to this discussion, however, interferon-α is a well-known anti-angiogenic molecule [55]. The third component of this phenotype is RGS5. RGS5 is highly expressed in the vessels and connective tissue cells of dermis in SSc (see Fig. 2D). RGS5 is best known as a marker of arteries, and it reg-ulates signaling through certain G-protein–coupled receptors. Elevations of RGS5 should block signaling through a wide range of vasoactive molecules, including two that have been implicated in angiogenesis: angiotensin and en-dothelin. Less well known is that expression of RGS5 correlates with the end of branching morphogenesis during development and tumor angiogenesis [56]. The mechanism of antiangiogenic action of RGS5 is not known.

Reversibility of capillary rarefaction

The authors results suggest that rarefaction is reversible (Fig. 3) [24]. Fol-lowing high-dose immunosuppressive therapy and autologous hematopoi-etic stem cell transplant, five of the seven subjects with SSc had increased capillary counts. This improvement correlated with clinical improvement. It was also observed in the same five subjects that the interferon-α and VE cadherin had returned to normal as other clinical signs in the skin re-gressed. In all seven subjects, RGS5 had returned to normal [24].

Endothelial apoptosis

There is a common assertion that endothelial cell apoptosis is a common, early event in SSc [57]. As noted above, this hypothesis is supported by se-rologic data, evidence for antiendothelial antibodies, evidence for circulat-ing endothelial cells, and the development of rarefaction. Despite this evidence, the authors have not seen pathologic evidence of endothelial cell death or apoptosis in tissue in their own studies or convincing data in the literature. The failure to see apoptosis in vivo may mean that endothelial cell apoptosis in SSc is a very transient process. On the other hand, in the absence of in vivo data it is important to maintain some skepticism, as mo-lecular biologic data suggest that endothelial cells are adapted to resist ap-optosis [58] and, again to the best of the authors' knowledge, there is no evidence from animal models that a primary endothelial injury can result in the syndrome of scleroderma [59,60].

A hypothesis

These data provide the first objective evidence for loss of vessels in SSc, and show that the rarefaction associated with SSc is reversible. Coordinate

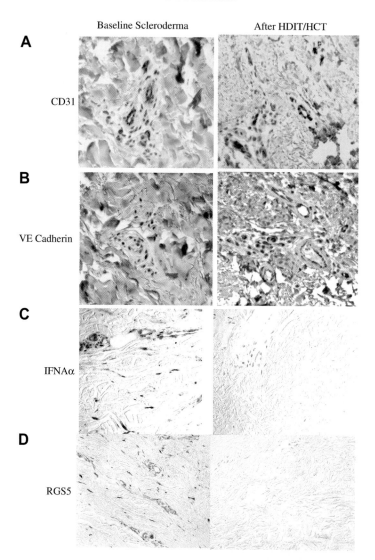

Fig. 3. (*A*) Immunohistochemistry for CD31 before and after high-dose immunosuppressive therapy (HDIT) and autologous hematopoietic stem cell transplant (HCT) is positive in both biopsies, whereas (*B*) when compared with CD31 stained biopsies above, VE cadherin is negative before but positive after HDIT and HCT. (*C*). Baseline biopsies of scleroderma patients before HDIT and autologous HCT all showed cells positive for interferon-α in situ hybridization were associated with the vasculature and scattered in the matrix. After HDIT and autologous HCT, interferon-α mRNA was undetectable in five of seven biopsies. Compared biopsies were run at the same time with the same conditions and probe concentration. (*D*) In situ hybridization for RGS5 shows baseline biopsies positive for increased perivascular stain and some cells scattered in the matrix. Epidermal cells also showed a strong signal. There was little or no detectable RGS5 mRNA after HDIT and autologous HCT in biopsies of all seven subjects.

changes in expression of three molecules already implicated in angiogenesis or antiangiogenesis suggest that control of expression of these three molecules may be part of the underlying mechanism for at least the vascular component of this disease. Because rarefaction has been little studied, these data may have implications for other diseases characterized by loss of capillaries, including hypertension, congestive heart failure, and scar formation [61,62].

Along with others, the authors suggest that the initial event in SSc may be some form of vascular injury [14–16]. Rather than endothelial denudation however, the authors suggest that the initial event could be intimal formation. This unknown event might be the same as the unknown event initiating intimal hyperplasia in transplant atherosclerosis [35,36].

Finally, a comprehensive hypothesis in SSc should include the role of the immune system. There is a new lead to a possible interaction between intimal biology and immunology. Recent studies of dendritic cell formation in the intima and traffic from the intima to regional lymph nodes [63,64], combined with extensive data on novel proteins production in the intima [28], suggest that intimal formation might well be a critical event in exposure of T-cells or B-cells to new epitopes.

Finally, the authors suggest that Raynaud's phenomenon might be a secondary event in this model, dependent on underlying intimal change and vasospasm. As already noted, there is extensive literature on vasospasm resulting from intimal hyperplasia [65]. It is not difficult to imagine that such vasospasm would worsen the injury, creating a vicious cycle driven by downstream ischemia and further vascular injury. In this view, fibrosis would be secondary to the ischemic injury.

Evidence from model systems

Ideally, this hypothesis would lead to an animal model for SSc. The authors will review existing models briefly and discuss their relevance to this hypothesis.

As is the case in human beings, there is little evidence in any animal model for endothelial cell death, and the authors are unaware of an animal model showing a syndrome similar to SSc as a result of endothelial cell death. To the authors' knowledge the only animal model showing endothelial apoptosis with fibrosis is the UCD L200 chicken model of avian SSc. Endothelial cell death occurs only during the initial stage of this genetic disease [66,67], supporting the idea that endothelial cell death initiates the disease. The etiology of avian SSc is not known. Although this model recapitulates some of the aspects of SSc, including intimal hyperplasia, capillary proliferation, and fibrosis, it does not recapitulate capillary rarefaction.

There are a number of profibrotic models for SSc. Unfortunately, vasculature in these models has not been well studied. Chemical exposure to bleomycin or organic solvents also produces robust fibrosis, autoantibodies, and inflammatory changes. Genetic profibrotic models include the tight skin mutations [68,69] and mrl/interferon receptor [70] models, among others [71]. An intriguing exception to the lack of vascular data comes from a recent study of adult mice induced to activate transforming growth factor-beta in their skin as adults [72]. Although the arteries did not show the characteristic intimal hyperplasia of SSc, the investigators claimed to see an increase in arteriolar vascular mass based on morphometric data. Rarefaction was not described, though this may be a difficult criterion in mice, given the absence of vessels comparable to the capillary loops in human skin [73].

Another possible model is chronic graft-versus-host disease (cGVHD). Murine models of cGVHD, although profibrotic, are more inflammatory than SSc and lack the vascular changes that are pathognomic for SSc [74–76]. To date, capillary rarefaction and microvascular abnormalities resembling those seen in SSc have not been seen in cGVHD, and data on intimal hyperplasia is unconvincing. Human cGVHD resembles the fibrotic component of SSc [77,78] and does show intimal hyperplasia [79] and signs of microvascular injury [80].

As already noted, transplant atherosclerosis may be a model for the vasculopathy and may be a much better model for SSc's [81]. In human beings and in animals, a variable number (up to 30%) of organ transplants under go a late loss that is not readily attributed to immune rejection [82]. The affected tissue shows several sclerodermal changes, including fibrosis, intimal hyperplasia, and rarefaction [83,84]. Antiendothelial antibodies are seen early after transplant and capillary rarefaction has long been known to be present in this disease [85–88]. Furthermore, the disease is similar to SSc in that it is difficult to treat by known immunosuppressive strategies. One possible hypothesis is that SSc is a systemic form of transplant vasculopathy.

Evidence from early results with stem cell transplantation

The authors have shown two intriguing findings in a subset of subjects treated with high-dose immunosuppressive therapy and autologous hematopoietic stem cell transplant for SSc: (1) counts of capillary lumens and profiles return to normal in the superficial dermis; and (2) the endothelial immunophenotype normalizes [24]. The question remains: why is the SSc vasculature not regenerating and why does regeneration occur after the stem cell transplant? Perhaps the vessel wall cells are altered by the inflammatory mediators, including interferon or, as suggested above by Mulligan-Kehoe and colleagues [89], by circulating antiangiogenic peptides. The alteration of the vessel wall then creates a condition where angiogenesis is no longer possible. Regeneration after high-dose immunosuppressive therapy and autologous hematopoietic stem cell transplant might reflect removal of a clone producing toxic antibodies, or stem cell transplant may provide replacement cells as suggested by Sata [90] and others [91].

Summary

SSc is a poorly understood connective tissue disease with a characteristic vasculopathy. This vasculopathy has two key features: first, a concentric and often progressively occlusive intimal hyperplasia; and second, a pattern of microvascular injury with an "antiangiogenic phenotype," characteristic gene expression, malformation and rarefaction. In a preliminary study, the authors found that these vascular changes are reversible with autologous transplant of stem cells and high dose immunosuppressive therapy in a subset of subjects.

The authors propose that SSc vasculopathy is the result of an early event involving vascular injury that eventuates in a vicious cycle mediated in part by the immune process. The subsequent vascular malformation and rarefaction may be a function of systemic angiogenic dysregulation, with over expression of VEGF but a lack of proper interactions with smooth muscle cells needed to stabilize and organize blood vessels. Finally, the authors suggest that the pathologic processes in transplant atherosclerosis appear to recapitulate the vascular changes of SSc better than other models.

Acknowledgments

The authors would like to acknowledge the following people who assisted with this manuscript: Simon Corrie, Jeremy Fleming, Richard Nash, David K. Pritchard, Joshua Aaron Sonnen, and Jinnan Wang. We especially wish to thank the patients who enabled us to obtain biopsy material and the Scelroderma Research Foundation for stimulating and supporting this work.

References

[1] Varga J, Korn JH. Pathogenesis: emphasis on human data. In: Clements PJ, Furst DE, editors. Systemic sclerosis. 2nd edition. Los Angeles (CA): Lippincott Williams & Wilkins; 2003. p. 63–98.

[2] Guiducci S, Pignone A, Mattucci-Cerinic M. Raynaud's phenomenon in systemic sclerosis. In: Clements PJ, Furst DE, editors. Systemic sclerosis. 2nd edition. Los Angeles (CA): Lippincott Williams & Wilkins; 2003. p. 221–40.

[3] Handa R, Kumar U, Pandey RM, et al. Raynaud's phenomenon—a prospective study. Journal, Indian Academy of Clinical Medicine 2002;3:35–8.

[4] von Bierbrauer A, Barth P, Willert J, et al. Electron microscopy and capillaroscopically guided nailfold biopsy in connective tissue diseases: detection of ultrastructural changes of the microcirculatory vessels. Br J Rheumatol 1998;37:1272–8.

[5] Campbell PM, LeRoy EC. Pathogenesis of systemic sclerosis: a vascular hypothesis. Semin Arthritis Rheum 1975;4:351–68.

[6] Brown GE, O'Leary PA. Skin capillaries in scleroderma. Arch Intern Med 1925;36:73–88.

[7] Norton WL, Hurd ER, Lewis DC, et al. Evidence of microvascular injury in scleroderma and systemic lupus erythematosus: quantitative study of the microvascular bed. J Lab Clin Med 1968;71:919–33.

[8] Toms SL, Cooke ED. A comparison of the functioning of arteriovenous anastomoses in secondary Raynaud's phenomenon and control subjects in response to local hand warming. Int Angiol 1995;14:74–9.

[9] Rodnan GP, Myerowitz RL, Justh GO. Morphologic changes in the digital arteries of patients with progressive systemic sclerosis (scleroderma) and Raynaud's phenomenon. Medicine (Baltimore) 1980;59:393–408.

[10] Luggen M, Belhorn L, Evans T, et al. The evolution of Raynaud's phenomenon: a longterm prospective study. J Rheumatol 1995;22:2226–32.

[11] D'Angelo WA, Fries JF, Masi AT, et al. Pathologic observations in systemic sclerosis (scleroderma). A study of fifty-eight autopsy cases and fifty-eight matched controls. Am J Med 1969;46:428–40.

[12] Blann AD, Illingworth K, Jayson MI. Mechanisms of endothelial cell damage in systemic sclerosis and Raynaud's phenomenon. J Rheumatol 1993;20:1325–30.

[13] Schachna L, Wigley FM. Targeting mediators of vascular injury in scleroderma. Curr Opin Rheumatol 2002;14:686–93.

[14] Kuwana M, Okazaki Y, Yasuoka H, et al. Defective vasculogenesis in systemic sclerosis. Lancet 2004;364:603–10.

[15] Del Papa N, Colombo G, Fracchiolla N, et al. Circulating endothelial cells as a marker of ongoing vascular disease in systemic sclerosis. Arthritis Rheum 2004;50:1296–304.

[16] Kahaleh MB. Vascular involvement in systemic sclerosis (SSc). Clin Exp Rheumatol 2004; 22:S19–23.

[17] Flavahan NA, Flavahan S, Mitra S, et al. The vasculopathy of Raynaud's phenomenon and scleroderma. Rheum Dis Clin North Am 2003;29:275–91.

[18] Prescott RJ, Freemont AJ, Jones CJ, et al. Sequential dermal microvascular and perivascular changes in the development of scleroderma. J Pathol 1992;166:255–63.

[19] Trotta F, Biagini G, Cenacchi G, et al. Microvascular changes in progressive systemic sclerosis: immunohistochemical and ultrastructural study. Clin Exp Rheumatol 1984;2: 209–15.

[20] Joyal F, Choquette D, Roussin A, et al. Evaluation of the severity of systemic sclerosis by nailfold capillary microscopy in 112 patients. Angiology 1992;43:203–10.

[21] Choi JJ, Min DJ, Cho ML, et al. Elevated vascular endothelial growth factor in systemic sclerosis. J Rheumatol 2003;30:1529–33.

[22] Distler O, Del Rosso A, Giacomelli R, et al. Angiogenic and angiostatic factors in systemic sclerosis: increased levels of vascular endothelial growth factor are a feature of the earliest disease stages and are associated with the absence of fingertip ulcers. Arthritis Res 2002;4: R11.

[23] Dor Y, Djonov V, Keshet E. Induction of vascular networks in adult organs: implications to proangiogenic therapy. Ann N Y Acad Sci 2003;995:208–16.

[24] Fleming JN, Nash RA, McCleod DO, et al. Capillary regeneration in scleroderma; stem cell therapy reverses phenotype? PLoS ONE 2008;3(1):e1452 .

[25] An SF, Fleming KA. Removal of inhibitor(s) of the polymerase chain reaction from formalin fixed, paraffin wax embedded tissues. J Clin Pathol 1991;44:924–7.

[26] Youssef P, Englert H, Bertouch J. Large vessel occlusive disease associated with CREST syndrome and scleroderma. Ann Rheum Dis 1993;52:464–6.

[27] Veale DJ, Collidge TA, Belch JJ. Increased prevalence of symptomatic macrovascular disease in systemic sclerosis. Ann Rheum Dis 1995;54:853–5.

[28] Schwartz SM. The intima: A new soil. Circ Res 1999;85:877–9.

[29] Korshunov VA, Schwartz SM, Berk BC. Vascular remodeling: hemodynamic and biochemical mechanisms underlying Glagov's phenomenon. Arterioscler Thromb Vasc Biol 2007;27: 1722–8.

[30] Schwartz SM, Galis ZS, Rosenfeld ME, et al. Plaque rupture in humans and mice. Arterioscler Thromb Vasc Biol 2007;27:705–13.

[31] Xu Q. Progenitor cells in vascular repair. Curr Opin Lipidol 2007;18:534–9.

[32] Bentzon JF, Weile C, Sondergaard CS, et al. Smooth muscle cells in atherosclerosis originate from the local vessel wall and not circulating progenitor cells in ApoE knockout mice. Arterioscler Thromb Vasc Biol 2006;26(12):2969–702.

[33] Torsney E, Hu Y, Xu Q. Adventitial progenitor cells contribute to arteriosclerosis. Trends Cardiovasc Med 2005;15:64–8.

[34] Liu C, Nath KA, Katusic ZS, et al. Smooth muscle progenitor cells in vascular disease. Trends Cardiovasc Med 2004;14:288–93.

[35] Mitchell RN, Libby P. Vascular remodeling in transplant vasculopathy. Circ Res 2007;100: 967–78.

[36] Rahmani M, Cruz RP, Granville DJ, et al. Allograft vasculopathy versus atherosclerosis. Circ Res 2006;99:801–15.

[37] Raines EW. PDGF and cardiovascular disease. Cytokine Growth Factor Rev 2004;15: 237–54.

[38] Schwartz SM, Reidy MA, de Blois D. Factors important in arterial narrowing. J Hypertens Suppl 1996;14:S71–81.

[39] Charo IF, Taubman MB. Chemokines in the pathogenesis of vascular disease. Circ Res 2004; 95:858–66.

[40] Koyama H, Olson NE, Reidy MA. Cell signaling in injured rat arteries. Thromb Haemost 1999;82:806–9.

[41] Llodra J, Angeli V, Liu J, et al. Emigration of monocyte-derived cells from atherosclerotic lesions characterizes regressive, but not progressive, plaques. Proc Natl Acad Sci U S A 2004;101:11779–84.

[42] Cheng KS, Tiwari A, Boutin A, et al. Carotid and femoral arterial wall mechanics in scleroderma. Rheumatology (Oxford) 2003;42:1299–305.

[43] Guiducci S, Giacomelli R, Cerinic MM. Vascular complications of scleroderma. Autoimmun Rev 2007;6:520–3.

[44] Herrick AL. Vascular function in systemic sclerosis. Curr Opin Rheumatol 2000;12:527–33.

[45] Mulvany MJ. Structural abnormalities of the resistance vasculature in hypertension. J Vasc Res 2003;40(6):558–60.

[46] Kozai T, Shimokawa H, Fukumoto Y, et al. Tyrosine kinase inhibitor markedly suppresses the development of coronary lesions induced by long-term treatment with platelet-derived growth factor in pigs in vivo. J Cardiovasc Pharmacol 1997;29(4):536–45.

[47] Masumoto A, Mohri M, Shimokawa H, et al. Suppression of coronary artery spasm by the Rho-kinase inhibitor fasudil in patients with vasospastic angina. Circulation 2002;105: 1545–7.

[48] Kandabashi T, Shimokawa H, Mukai Y, et al. Involvement of rho-kinase in agonists-induced contractions of arteriosclerotic human arteries. Arterioscler Thromb Vasc Biol 2002;22:243–8.

[49] Shimokawa H, Morishige K, Miyata K, et al. Long-term inhibition of Rho-kinase induces a regression of arteriosclerotic coronary lesions in a porcine model in vivo. Cardiovasc Res 2001;51(1):169–77.

[50] Fukumoto Y, Mohri M, Inokuchi K, et al. Anti-ischemic effects of fasudil, a specific Rho-kinase inhibitor, in patients with stable effort angina. J Cardiovasc Pharmacol 2007;49(3):117–21.

[51] Kandabashi T, Shimokawa H, Miyata K, et al. Inhibition of myosin phosphatase by upregulated rho-kinase plays a key role for coronary artery spasm in a porcine model with interleukin-1beta. Circulation 2000;101(11):1319–23.

[52] Ito A, Shimokawa H, Fukumoto Y, et al. The role of fibroblast growth factor-2 in the vascular effects of interleukin-1 beta in porcine coronary arteries in vivo. Cardiovasc Res 1996;32(3):570–9.

[53] Wallez Y, Vilgrain I, Huber P. Angiogenesis: the VE-cadherin switch. Trends Cardiovasc Med 2006;16:55–9.

[54] Duan H, Fleming J, Pritchard DK, et al. Combined analysis of monocyte and lymphocyte mRNA expression with serum protein profiles in patients with scleroderma. Arthritis Rheum, in press.

[55] Angiolillo AL, Sgadari C, Taub DD, et al. Human interferon-inducible protein 10 is a potent inhibitor of angiogenesis in vivo. J Exp Med 1995;182:155–62.

[56] Cho H, Kozasa T, Bondjers C, et al. Pericyte-specific expression of RGS5: implications for PDGF and EDG receptor signaling during vascular maturation. FASEB J 2003;17:440–2.

[57] Jun JB, Kuechle M, Harlan JM, et al. Fibroblast and endothelial apoptosis in systemic sclerosis. Curr Opin Rheumatol 2003;15:756–60.

[58] Skurk C, Maatz H, Kim HS, et al. The Akt-regulated forkhead transcription factor FOXO3a controls endothelial cell viability C through modulation of the caspase-8 inhibitor FLIP. J Biol Chem 2004;279(2):1513–25.

[59] Schouten M, Wiersinga WJ, Levi M, et al. Inflammation, endothelium, and coagulation in sepsis. J Leukoc Biol 2007; [epub ahead of print].

[60] Winn RK, Harlan JM. The role of endothelial cell apoptosis in inflammatory and immune diseases. J Thromb Haemost 2005;3(8):1815–24.

[61] Houben AJ, Beljaars JH, Hofstra L, et al. Microvascular abnormalities in chronic heart failure: a cross-sectional analysis. Microcirculation 2003;10:471–8.

[62] Antonios TF, Singer DR, Markandu ND, et al. Rarefaction of skin capillaries in borderline essential hypertension suggests an early structural abnormality. Hypertension 1999;34: 655–8.

[63] Randolph GJ, Angeli V, Swartz MA. Dendritic-cell trafficking to lymph nodes through lymphatic vessels. Nat Rev Immunol 2005;5:617–28.

[64] Liu X, Zhu S, Wang T, et al. Paclitaxel modulates TGFß Signaling in scleroderma skin grafts in immunodeficient mice. PLoS Med 2005;2:e354.

[65] Shimokawa H, Rashid M. Development of Rho-kinase inhibitors for cardiovascular medicine. Trends Pharmacol Sci 2007;28(6):296–302.

[66] Sgonc R. The vascular perspective of systemic sclerosis: of chickens, mice and men. Int Arch Allergy Immunol 1999;120:169–76.

[67] Sgonc R, Gruschwitz MS, Dietrich H, et al. Endothelial cell apoptosis is a primary pathogenetic event underlying skin lesions in avian and human scleroderma. J Clin Invest 1996;98: 785–92.

[68] Christner PJ, Peters J, Hawkins D, et al. The tight skin 2 mouse. An animal model of scleroderma displaying cutaneous fibrosis and mononuclear cell infiltration. Arthritis Rheum 1995;38:1791–8.

[69] Dodig TD, Mack KT, Cassarino DF, et al. Development of the tight-skin phenotype in immune-deficient mice. Arthritis Rheum 2001;44:723–7.

[70] Le Hir M, Martin M, Haas C. A syndrome resembling human systemic sclerosis (scleroderma) in MRL/lpr mice lacking interferon-gamma (IFN-gamma) receptor (MRL/lprgammaR-/-). Clin Exp Immunol 1999;115:281–7.

[71] Zhang Y, Gilliam AC. Animal models for scleroderma: an update. Curr Rheumatol Rep 2002;4:150–62.

[72] Sonnylal S, Denton CP, Zheng B, et al. Postnatal induction of transforming growth factor beta signaling in fibroblasts of mice recapitulates clinical, histologic, and biochemical features of scleroderma. Arthritis Rheum 2006;56:334–44.

[73] Braverman IM. The cutaneous microcirculation. J Investig Dermatol Symp Proc 2000;5:3–9.

[74] Zhang Y, McCormick LL, Desai SR, et al. Murine sclerodermatous graft-versus-host disease, a model for human scleroderma: cutaneous cytokines, chemokines, and immune cell activation. J Immunol 2002;168:3088–98.

[75] Ruzek MC, Jha S, Ledbetter S, et al. A modified model of graft-versus-host-induced systemic sclerosis (scleroderma) exhibits all major aspects of the human disease. Arthritis Rheum 2004;50:1319–31.

[76] Jaffee BD, Claman HN. Chronic graft-versus-host disease (GVHD) as a model for scleroderma. I. Description of model systems. Cell Immunol 1983;77:1–12.

[77] Andrews ML, Robertson I, Weedon D. Cutaneous manifestations of chronic graft-versus-host disease. Australas J Dermatol 1997;38:53–62.

[78] Farmer ER. Human cutaneous graft-versus-host disease. J Invest Dermatol 1985;85: 124s–8s.

[79] Aractingi S, Chosidow O. Cutaneous graft-versus-host disease. Arch Dermatol 1998;134: 602–12.

[80] Biedermann BC, Sahner S, Gregor M, et al. Endothelial injury mediated by cytotoxic T lymphocytes and loss of microvessels in chronic graft versus host disease. Lancet 2002;359: 2078–83.

[81] Ertault-Daneshpouy M, Leboeuf C, Lemann M, et al. Pericapillary hemorrhage as criterion of severe human digestive graft-versus-host disease. Blood 2004;103:4681–4.

[82] Hillebrands JL, Klatter FA, Rozing J. Origin of vascular smooth muscle cells and the role of circulating stem cells in transplant arteriosclerosis. Arterioscler Thromb Vasc Biol 2003;23: 380–7.

[83] Weis M, von Scheidt W. Cardiac allograft vasculopathy a review. Circulation 1997;96: 2069–77.

[84] Karnovsky MJ, Russell ME, Hancock W, et al. Chronic rejection in experimental cardiac transplantation in a rat model. Clin Transplant 1994;8:308–12.

[85] Hruban RH, Beschorner WE, Baumgartner WA, et al. Accelerated arteriosclerosis in heart transplant recipients is associated with a T-lymphocyte-mediated endothelialitis. Am J Pathol 1990;137:871–82.

[86] Denton MD, Davis SF, Baum MA, et al. The role of the graft endothelium in transplant rejection: evidence that endothelial activation may serve as a clinical marker for the development of chronic rejection. Pediatr Transplant 2000;4:252–60.

[87] Koglin J, Russell ME. Alloimmune-mediated apoptosis: comparison in mouse models of acute and chronic cardiac rejection. Transplantation 1999;67:904–9.

[88] Crisp SJ, Dunn MJ, Rose ML, et al. Antiendothelial antibodies after heart transplantation: the accelerating factor in transplant-associated coronary artery disease? J Heart Lung Transplant 1994;13:81–91.

[89] Mulligan-Kehoe MJ, Drinane MC, Mollmark J, et al. Antiangiogenic plasma activity in patients with systemic sclerosis. Arthritis Rheum 2007;56:3448–58.

[90] Sata M. Role of circulating vascular progenitors in angiogenesis, vascular healing, andpulmonary hypertension: lessons from animal models. Arterioscler Thromb Vasc Biol 2006;26: 1008–14.

[91] Goldschmidt-Clermont PJ. Loss of bone marrow-derived vascular progenitor cells leads to inflammation and atherosclerosis. Am Heart J 2003;146:S5–12.

ELSEVIER
SAUNDERS

Rheum Dis Clin N Am
34 (2008) 57–71

RHEUMATIC
DISEASE CLINICS
OF NORTH AMERICA

Vascular Disease in Scleroderma: Mechanisms of Vascular Injury

Bashar Kahaleh, MD

*Division of Rheumatology and Immunology, University of Toledo Medical Center,
3120 Glendale Avenue, Toledo, OH 43617, USA*

Vascular endothelial injury in systemic sclerosis (SSc) includes a spectrum of changes that involve predominantly the microcirculation and arterioles. These changes range from endothelial activation with increased expression of adhesion molecules to capillary necrosis, intimal proliferation of arterioles, and occlusion of blood vessels. The pathologic changes in the blood vessels adversely impact the physiology of many organ systems, with a reduction in the size of microvascular beds leading to decreased organ blood flow and ultimately to a state of chronic ischemia. Current hypotheses in SSc vascular disease suggest a possible chemical or infectious trigger. An enhanced vasoconstrictive tendency in the disease may contribute to the pathogenesis by mechanisms related to ischemia-reperfusion–associated free radical injury. Activation of cellular and humoral immunity may lead to vascular injury through the production of autoantibodies and the release of products of activated T cells that can directly damage the endothelium. A variety of circulating markers reflecting the degree of vascular injury have been described, including plasma von Willebrand factor, certain cytokines, and soluble adhesion molecules. The working hypothesis in the pathogeneses of SSc vascular disease is shown in (Fig. 1).

Vascular disease in scleroderma

Vascular involvement in SSc includes a spectrum of changes that involve predominantly the microcirculation and arterioles [1,2]. The microvascular changes include a reduction in the number of capillaries and the presence of avascular areas. The most marked abnormalities appear in the arteriolar segments of capillary beds. Morphologic capillary changes can be visualized in the nail fold when examined with the dissecting stereomicroscope. Specific

E-mail address: bashar.kahaleh@utoledo.edu

0889-857X/08/$ - see front matter © 2008 Elsevier Inc. All rights reserved.
doi:10.1016/j.rdc.2007.12.004   *rheumatic.theclinics.com*

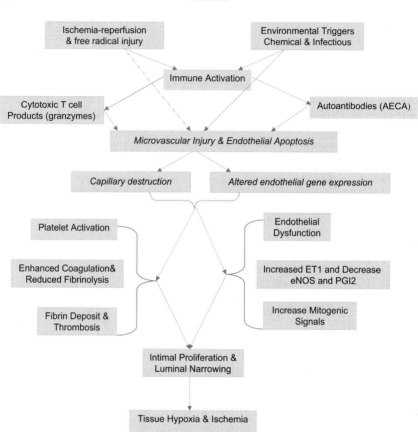

Fig. 1. Endothelial apoptosis and dysfunction are central to the development of vascular disease in SSc. The initial trigger for endothelial injury is not known; however, reperfusion injury, autoantibodies (particularly anti-endothelial antibodies that directly injure the cells or have a role in antibody-dependent cytotoxicity), infectious agents, and environmental factors can all initiate endothelial injury in a genetically predisposed host. Endothelial cells and their fragments appear in the circulation. Furthermore, reduced endothelial nitric oxide synthase (eNOS) and prostacyclin (PGI$_2$) synthase expression and increased endothelin-1 (ET-1) production by the dysfunctional endothelial cells set the stage for the subsequent events in the vascular wall, including platelet activation, fibrin deposits, intimal proliferation, vascular wall thickness, and tissue ischemia.

capillary patterns in SSc were initially described in 1925 [3] and were characterized and popularized later with the use of nail fold capillaroscopy, which helps in the diagnosis of SSc, particularly in the preclinical stages [4].

On the ultrastructural level, the earliest changes in the edematous stage of the disease consist of large gaps between the endothelial cells, vacuolization of endothelial cell cytoplasm with an increase in the number of basal lamina–like layers, and occasional entrapment of lymphocytes and cellular vesicles [5]. Further signs of nuclear injury with signs of cellular apoptosis occur in more advanced stages. Swelling of the intima and intimal proliferation with mononuclear cell infiltration are seen in the early stages and consist of infiltrating macrophages and activated T and B cells with a predominance of CD4+ T cells. Milder degrees of vascular changes can be seen in clinically uninvolved skin mainly in the papillary dermal layer in association with increased numbers of adhering platelets to the dermal microvasculature [6]. It is not known whether these changes precede the development of tissue fibrosis or are independent of it. Similar changes in the capillaries are reported in all involved organs, including the muscles, lungs, heart, kidneys, and choroid membranes, demonstrating the widespread nature of capillary changes in SSc, even in sites not affected with fibrosis [7]. Significant intimal proliferation and accumulation of proteoglycan in the arterioles and small-sized arteries are common [1,2]. It is likely that the underlying abnormality of the vessel wall is the result of an increase in the synthesis of glycosamino-glycans and collagen by intimal and adventitial fibroblasts in a manner similar to skin fibrosis that results from uncontrolled activity of the dermal fibroblast; however, the molecular mechanism responsible for this critical neointimal lesion is not known.

Arterial occlusion in SSc is common, particularly in the ulnar arteries in patients with the limited form of SSc and in association with anti-centromere antibodies (Fig. 2). In the arteries, intimal proliferation of a uniform and symmetric nature forms a neointima indistinguishable from that formed in other autoimmune diseases, in chronic homograft rejection, and in accelerated atherosclerosis such as restenosis after coronary bypass.

Endothelial injury and apoptosis

Endothelial cell injury is identified as an early and central event in the pathogenesis of SSc vasculopathy. An apoptotic alteration in endothelial cells was first described on ultrastructural examination of SSc biopsy specimens in the early stages of the disease in association with the inflammatory stage, suggesting a causal association [2]. It was later noted in the University of California at Davis lines 200/206 chickens that spontaneously develop disease resembling SSc [8]. Endothelial cell apoptosis is not unique to SSc. It is frequently observed in diseases with prominent vascular involvement, such as atherosclerotic vascular lesions, graft rejection, thrombotic thrombocytopenic purpura, and the hemolytic uremic syndrome [9,10].

Although the fate of apoptotic endothelial cells is not clear, immature dendritic cells and macrophages may engulf apoptotic cells and subsequently present cellular antigens to CD8+ T cells [11], perpetuating tissue injury. Moreover, apoptotic endothelial cells can activate the alternate complement and coagulant cascades, leading to vascular microthrombosis and further tissue compromise [12,13]. The mechanism of endothelial cell apoptosis in SSc is not known. Experimental studies have identified multiple pathways that may

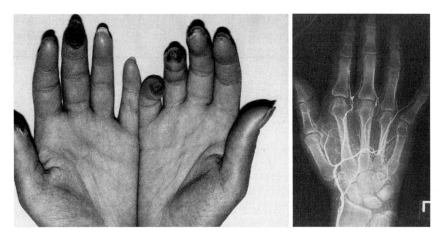

Fig. 2. (*Left*) Multiple ischemic digital ulcers in a 33-year-old patient with a 3-month history of sclerodactyly and a 10-year history of Raynaud's phenomenon. Positive anti-centromere and anti-endothelial cell antibodies were noted. (*Right*) Arteriogram of the left hand. Occlusion of the distal ulnar artery approximately 2.0 cm proximal to the articular surface of the distal ulna with collateral vessels at the point of occlusion was noted. The superficial palmer arch is occluded. Diffuse occlusive disease in the digital arteries is prominent.

lead to endothelial cell apoptosis, including infectious agents, cytotoxic T cells, antibody-dependent cellular cytotoxicity, anti-endothelial antibodies, and ischemia-reperfusion injury.

Viral triggers

Viruses have long been held to be of pathogenetic importance in the evolution of autoimmune connective tissue disorders. In SSc, a viral trigger is proposed because of increased levels of antibodies to human cytomegalovirus (hCMV), and because of the known association of this virus with intimal proliferation and vasculopathy in graft rejection and coronary artery bypass restenosis [14]. It seems likely that CMV does not cause a persisting virion-producing infection in SSc patients because the characteristic cytomegalic changes are not seen. A partially aborted latent hCMV reactivation is a more likely possibility in which immediate early (IE1and 2) CMV genes drive host gene expression. The circumstances that eventuate in reactivation are unclear. hCMV can induce transforming growth factor beta (TGF-β) (and thereby several collagen genes) and adhesion molecule expression in vitro. Moreover, a CMV immune response may be responsible for triggering events leading to vascular damage by the induction of endothelial cell apoptosis. The evidence suggests that some anti-topoisomerase I antibodies recognize an epitope (VTLGGAGIWLPP) contained within the hCMV-derived UL94 protein, suggesting a molecular mimicry mechanism [15]. The UL94 epitope shows homology with NAG-2 (tetraspan novel antigen-2), a cell surface molecule highly expressed on endothelial cells. Affinity purified anti-UL94 peptide antibodies induce endothelial cell apoptosis; therefore, the immune response to hCMV may be linked to the pathogenesis of SSc through a particular set of anti-hCMV antibodies that specifically interacts with a normally expressed endothelial cell surface receptor sharing similarity with the UL94 viral protein [16].

Cytotoxic T-cell involvement in endothelial cell apoptosis is suggested by histologic and experimental findings in the disease. It is known that the apoptosis of endothelial cells results from their interaction with cytotoxic T cells by fas or granzyme/perforin-related mechanisms [17]. The CD4+ T cells induce endothelial cell apoptosis by a fas-related mechanism as seen in cytolytic T-cell killing of vascular endothelium in the rejection reaction. The granzyme/perforin system mediates endothelial cell apoptosis by the major cytotoxic cells, the CD8+ T cells, natural killer cells, and lympho-kine-activated killer cells. Granzymes gain access to the cells following cellular membrane damage by perforin. The mechanism whereby granzymes induce endothelial cell apoptosis, although not well documented, bypasses the caspase cascade and is fas independent. Viral infection of the endothelium may trigger cytotoxic T cells when endothelial cells express viral antigen. What is intriguing is the fact that certain viral infections of the vascular endothelium may prime cytolytic T cells to kill noninfected innocent bystander endothelial cells [18], a development that may explain the widespread endothelial injury in the disease. Involvement of cytotoxic T cells in SSc is suggested by the presence of a 60-kDa protein in SSc sera that was originally described as an endothelial cytotoxic factor. This factor was characterized as the granular enzyme granzyme A. Granzyme A was detected in SSc sera and in the perivascular spaces in SSc skin, suggesting involvement of the granzyme/perforin system in the disease [19]. Furthermore, granzyme gene expression in SSc skin and in circulating lymphocytes was also shown, suggesting local antigen activation of cytotoxic T cells. Granzymes are activation products of a variety of cytotoxic cell types, including CD4+ and CD8+ cytotoxic T cells, natural killer cells, and γδ-TCR bearing lymphocytes. The latter cell types have been shown to accumulate in the perivascular spaces in the early stages of the disease and are also reported to bind and kill endothelial cells in vitro [20].

Antibody-dependent cellular cytotoxicity of vascular endothelium is reported in as many as 40% of SSc patients [21,22]. The effector cells express Fc receptors and are non-T and non-adherent lymphocytes, whereas the antibody is an IgG with endothelial cell specificity (AECA) that mediates endothelial cell cytotoxicity via the Fas pathway. Endothelial cell cytotoxicity is seen in the presence of AECA-positive SSc sera and activated natural killer cells and could be inhibited by an anti-Fas ligand antibody. Moreover, immunofluorescence analysis of cryosections from SSc skin show Fas (CD95) expression by endothelial cells, supporting the in vitro findings [23].

The antigen specificity of the antibody is not known. The cytotoxicity is reported to be prominent in patients with severe and extensive visceral disease.

Nonetheless, this mode of cytotoxicity is not specific to SSc, because similar observations are noted in other vascular and connective tissue diseases.

Anti-endothelial antibodies (AECA) are present in 40% to 50% of SSc sera and are mostly of the IgG1 isotype. The antibody titers correlate negatively with pulmonary diffusion capacity and positively with pulmonary hypertension and with digital ischemic ulcers [24,25], suggesting a pathologic role in the development of vascular disease. Evidence suggests that exposure of endothelial cells to AECA in vitro results in up-regulation of the adhesion molecules ICAM-1, VCAM-1, and E-selectin, leading to enhanced leukocyte adhesion and promotion of inflammatory trafficking in the vessel wall [26]. This effect is mediated by AECA induction of interleukin-1 (IL-1) synthesis by endothelial cells. AECA can also mediate endothelial cell cytotoxicity by direct complement activation. Some AECA are reported to induce endothelial cell apoptosis independent of the fas–fas ligand pathway [27]. This characteristic is clearly shown in the chicken model of SSc (UCD-200), in which serum transfer into normal chicken embryos results in binding of antibodies to the microvasculature in the chorioallantoic membrane in association with endothelial apoptosis [28]. The exact identity of the endothelial cell antigen is not known; however, a topoisomerase 1 specificity for some AECA has been suggested [29]. SSc sera containing anti-centromere antibodies or anti-topoisomerase I antibodies can induce endothelial cell apoptosis in association with increased gene expression of transcripts for the proapoptotic protease caspase 3 as well as the SSc autoantigen fibrillin 1 [30].

It is not clear whether AECA are truly endothelial cell specific and whether they react with the same antigens. Indeed, Western blot analysis of endothelial cell protein extracts showed an average of 10 reacting bands in each AECA-positive serum, and in most examples, extracts from fibroblasts reacted with AECA, sometimes even more so than with endothelial cells [31].

Ischemia-reperfusion injury may initiate or perpetuate the vascular disease in SSc by mechanisms related to Raynaud's phenomena. Ischemia-reperfusion injury is an inflammatory process that results from an interaction between humoral and cellular components including the complement, cytokine, and contact-activated cascades. Platelets and neutrophils adhere to the endothelium following reperfusion injury. In general, soon after the start of reperfusion, endothelial dysfunction of the ischemic vascular bed develops. The initial endothelial dysfunction appears to be related to adhesion molecule expression and the recruitment of neutrophils and platelets [32]. Tumor necrosis factor alpha (TNF-α) and IL-1 are released during ischemia-reperfusion and contribute to up-regulation of adhesion molecule expression. Other cytokines released in the process of reperfusion include IL-8 that helps in the recruitment of neutrophils and monocytes, IL-1 convertase that may induce endothelial cell apoptosis, and endothelin-1 (ET-1) that enhances vasospasm and vascular injury [33].

Endothelial cell injury is believed to be mediated by superoxide radicals formed by endothelial cells and neutrophils, perhaps via the hypoxanthine-xanthine oxidase pathway. Superoxide inhibits the release of nitric oxide (NO), prostacyclin, tissue plasminogen activator, protein S, and heparin sulfate from endothelial cells, leading to impairment of vascular tone control and thrombo-resistance within the microvasculature [34]. Endothelial cell dysfunction can be prevented or treated by direct NO donors. Inhaled NO can reduce the adhesive properties, vasoconstriction, and permeability of injured blood vessels in NO-depleted tissue, suggesting the presence of blood-borne molecules that have NO carrying capacity [35]. Moreover, NO inhibits or attenuates endothelial cell apoptosis by inhibition of NF-kappa B binding activities and increased expression of Bcl-2. Complement activation may also have a decisive role in endothelial cell injury after ischemia-reperfusion injury, because the soluble complement receptor CR1 significantly reduces tissue injury by blocking complement deposition [36]. Moreover, intracellular oxygen-derived free radicals activate NF-kappa B–mediated complement C3b deposition on microvascular endothelial cell membrane [37]. Localized ischemia-reperfusion vascular insult may lead to remote vascular dysfunction as noted in the pulmonary vascular beds after mesenteric ischemia-reperfusion [38]. TGF-β appears to be an important and remarkably effective protective agent in this setting. TGF-β acts by preserving endothelial function, particularly in the maintenance of endothelium-derived relaxing factor formation. This observation may explain the reported enhanced expression of TGF-β in the vessels of primary and secondary Raynaud's phenomena [39].

Vascular dysfunction

The earliest signs of vascular dysfunction in SSc include enhanced vascular permeability and dysregulated control of vascular tone. The propensity for vasospasm in SSc is well known and best illustrated by Raynaud's phenomenon, which results from digital arterial closure after cold exposure. The arterial closure is believed to be the end result of an imbalance in endothelial signals (increased endothelin release and an impaired endothelial-dependent vasodilatory mechanism, NO). Although vascular injury undoubtedly contributes to all aspects of dysregulated vascular tone control, increased endothelin synthesis and release and impaired NO are directly related to endothelial cell dysfunction. Platelet activation and enhanced coagulation with reduced fibrinolytic activity lead to fibrin deposits and contribute to the intimal proliferation and luminal narrowing.

Endothelin

The potent vasoconstrictor peptide ET-1 first isolated from vascular endothelial cells and the related isoforms 2 and 3 mediate endothelium-dependent vasoconstriction and are potent mitogens for smooth muscle cells and fibroblasts [40]. ET-1 is a 21 linear amino acid peptide in a unique structure related to a group of snake venoms [41]. ET-1 is produced from a pre-propeptide that is converted to endothelin by an endothelin-converting enzyme. Many substances including thrombin, epinephrine, TNF-α, TGF-β, angiotensin II, and hypoxia stimulate the release of ET-1 from endothelial cells.

Increased plasma levels of endothelin have been associated with several vascular disorders, including Raynaud's phenomenon and SSc, particularly diffuse SSc, pulmonary hypertension, lung fibrosis, and SSc renal crisis [42,43]. Increased ET-1 expression in association with increased numbers of ET-1 receptors, particularly the B receptors, is seen in SSc skin and lung tissue [44]. Endothelin is also a fibrotic cytokine because it enhances fibroblast proliferation and synthesis of types I and III collagen and decreases expression of matrix metalloproteinase-1 [45].

The critical role that ET-1 has in the pathogenesis of SSc vascular disease is illustrated by the efficacy of the dual endothelin receptor antagonist bosentan in the prevention of digital ulcers and in improvement of symptoms of pulmonary hypertension [46,47].

Endothelial-dependent relaxation (nitric oxide)

NO is a unique signaling molecule that has an important role in the regulation of cardiovascular, nervous, renal, immune, and other system interactions. NO synthase catalyzes the five-electron oxidation of L-arginine to equimolar quantities of NO and L-citrulline [48]. The release of NO from the vascular endothelium represents a powerful vasodilator signal to the underlying smooth muscle. This release occurs continuously and increases when membrane receptors on the endothelial cells are activated by soluble stimuli (including acetylcholine, bradykinin, ADP, substance P, and serotonin), or when the calcium channels are opened by increased shear stress leading to activation of the calcium-dependent endothelial NO synthase [49]. The target of NO in the vascular wall is the soluble guanylate cyclase in smooth muscle cells. Activation of guanylate cyclase leads to accumulation of cyclic GMP that triggers smooth muscle relaxation and results in vasodilatation [50].

Deficient endothelial-dependent relaxation in SSc is suggested by impaired maximal responses to endothelial-dependent vasodilators with normal responses to endothelial-independent dilators [51]. This impairment is directly related to a reduction in endothelial nitric oxide synthase (eNOS) gene expression and NO release in SSc skin and microvascular endothelial cells derived from involved and uninvolved skin biopsies in the steady state and after shear stress [52].

The consequences of impaired endothelial NO release are related not only to defects in vascular tone control but may also mediate other pathologic events, because NO inhibits platelet aggregation and is a potent chemical barrier that protects endothelial cells from oxidation injury. NO also limits cytokine-induced endothelial activation and monocyte adhesion and inhibits the endothelial release of the chemoattractants IL-6 and IL-8 [53]. These diverse biologic actions suggest that NO is a potent and important regulator of inflammatory trafficking within the vessel wall, a process frequently seen in SSc. Furthermore, NO inhibits smooth muscle cell proliferation through elevation of cyclic GMP and inhibition of the mitogenic peptides TGF-β and PDGF. Impaired NO production may contribute to the pathogenesis of arteriolar intimal proliferation in SSc; therefore, it may have a significant role in the pathophysiology of the disease and particularly in the genesis of intimal proliferation and structural vascular lesions.

Platelets

Platelet activation in SSc is well established. Elevated plasma levels of the platelet-specific proteins β-thromboglobulin and platelet factor-4 have been noted and proposed as markers of progression from primary Raynaud's phenomenon on to SSc [54]. Ultrastructural examination of SSc platelets showed evidence of in vivo activation and granular release. Enhanced platelet activation was demonstrated in vitro by increased spontaneous whole blood platelet aggregation and the aggregation induced by ADP and collagen, and by increased platelet adhesion to collagen. Platelet activation may be viewed as secondary to endothelial dysfunction. Several of the endothelial cell–derived mediators inhibit platelet aggregation and activation, including prostacyclin (PGI_2), NO, heparin, and thrombomodulin. Impaired endothelial function may directly result in platelet activation. Platelet activation in SSc may contribute to the occlusive arterial disease by the release of growth factors and to tissue fibrosis because platelet products stimulate glycosaminoglycan synthesis, particularly by SSc fibroblasts [55].

Coagulation and fibrinolysis

Endothelial cells are essential for several important antithrombotic properties that are responsible for maintaining blood fluidity. These properties are directly related to the synthesis and release of specific molecules by the vascular endothelium. These molecules include NO, PGI_2, thrombomodulin, and plasminogen activator. A balance between the production and release of opposing molecules appears to be critical for maintaining normal coagulation and fibrinolytic potentials. Microvascular thrombosis and enhanced fibrin deposition are frequently encountered in SSc, suggesting defective endothelial control of coagulation and fibrinolysis. A comprehensive study of SSc patients showed significant activation of the coagulation system with reduced parameters of fibrinolytic activities [56]. The conclusions in this study were in agreement with the histologic findings in SSc, in which excessive fibrin deposits are commonly seen in association with thrombosis in the microvessels. No controlled trial using anticoagulation or fibrinolytic-enhancing therapy in SSc has been accomplished to date. The reported improvement in the symptoms of Raynaud's phenomenon and the parameters of fibrinolysis after therapy with stanozolol or with recombinant tissue plasminogen activator lends support to the proposed impairment of fibrinolysis in SSc.

Circulating markers of vascular disease

An increase in the circulating level of von Willebrand factor was the first proposed marker for endothelial cell injury in SSc. A decrease in the level of angiotensin-converting enzyme (ACE) was later identified as another marker that correlates inversely with von Willebrand factor levels. Other markers were later suggested (Table 1).

von Willebrand factor

Endothelial cells and megakaryocytes synthesize von Willebrand factor. In the endothelium, von Willebrand factor is secreted constitutively or stored in endothelial specific sites (the Weibel-Palade bodies). In the platelets, it resides in the α-granules with other platelet constituents. Factor VIII circulates in the plasma complex with von Willebrand factor; it can bind to basement membrane, collagen, and heparin. Increased plasma concentrations of von Willebrand factor have been observed in SSc by several investigators [57,58]. Plasma levels have been positively correlated with the extent of visceral involvement and disease prognosis [59]. Some studies have demonstrated differences in the levels between limited and diffuse forms of SSc, whereas others have not. Striking elevations of von Willebrand factor are reported in patients with isolated pulmonary hypertension without pulmonary fibrosis [60].

Table 1
Circulating markers of scleroderma vascular disease

Marker	Endothelial cell specific	Endothelial cell activation	Endothelial cell injury	Clinical correlation[a]
von Willebrand factor	−	+	+	+
ACE	−	−	+	−
Platelet products	−	+	+	+
Thrombomodulin	+	−	+	−
s-E-selectin	+	+	−	−
s-ICAM-1	−	+	−	−
Endothelin	−	+	+	+
Circulating endothelial cells	+	−	+	+

[a] Marker has been associated with certain clinical manifestations of the disease.

Thrombomodulin is an endothelial cell membrane-associated glycoprotein that inhibits several procoagulant actions of thrombin and has a role in the regulation of intravascular coagulation. Injured endothelial cells release fragments of thrombomodulin at a rate directly related to the degree of cellular injury; therefore, the plasma level of thrombomodulin is an excellent marker of endothelial cell injury. Elevated levels of serum soluble thrombomodulin in circulating multiple molecular weight fragments, which appear to be proteolytically degraded forms of cellular thrombomodulin, are reported in SSc [61]. Moreover, the thrombomodulin level is highest in the active phase of the disease and correlates with anti–Scl-70 and dermal endothelial cell expression of the protein [62].

ACE, a dipeptidyl carboxypeptidase located on the luminal surface of the endothelium, is a key component of the renin-angiotensin system. Decreased plasma ACE activity has been reported in SSc patients [63]. ACE levels are inversely related to levels of von Willebrand factor. Reductions in ACE levels are also noted in patients with primary Raynaud's phenomenon [64].

Soluble adhesion molecules

Increases in circulating E-selectin levels, also known as ELAM-1, are reported in patients with SSc and other connective tissue diseases. In SSc, increased levels are seen not only in early acute stages of the disease but also in chronic atrophic disease [65]. Increased circulating levels of intercellular adhesion molecule-1 (s-ICAM-1) are also noted in SSc. Patients with diffuse rapidly progressive disease have the highest levels; however, no association has been observed between the extent of skin or internal organ involvement and circulating levels [66]. This molecule has an important role in the activation and migration of lymphocytes across the endothelium and basement membranes and in adherence to target tissues [67].

Circulating endothelial cells

Recent innovations in cell isolation and immunohistochemical evaluation have allowed the isolation of circulating fully differentiated endothelial cells and bone marrow–derived endothelial progenitor cells. An increased circulating endothelial cell number that correlated with the overall disease activity score and with pulmonary hypertension was described [68].

Summary

The etiology and pathogenesis of SSc remain unknown. Nonetheless, signs of vascular injury and devascularization of involved organs in association with evidence of profound endothelial dysfunction are well documented. Countless central issues in the pathogenic process of SSc remain poorly understood. Issues related to the initial trigger in the disease, the nature of immune activation, mechanisms of intimal proliferation, and the relationship of vascular injury to tissue fibrosis are some of the unresolved essential questions. The fact that the vascular tree, particularly the microcirculation, is the target tissue in this disease is now well established. It is likely that the immune process is aimed at the destruction of microvessels, leading to the clinically recognized state of chronic organ ischemia and tissue underperfusion in SSc. Identification of the initial vascular trigger of immune stimulation is fundamental to understanding the disease. Chemical modifications of the endothelium, reperfusion injury by mechanisms of Raynaud's phenomenon, or viral infection of endothelial cells are some of the proposed triggers. The microvascular damage in the disease, which includes endothelial cell apoptosis, may not be related to the direct effect of virus replication but may be linked to immune-mediated endothelial injury triggered by viral infection. Knowledge of the immune mechanisms in disease pathogenesis may offer an opportunity to develop a multiple step strategy for therapeutic intervention.

References

[1] Norton WL, Nardo JM. Vascular disease in progressive systemic sclerosis (scleroderma). Ann Intern Med 1970;73:317–24.
[2] Fleischmajer R, Perlish JS. Capillary alterations in scleroderma. J Am Acad Dermatol 1980; 2:161–70.
[3] Brown GE, O'Leary PA. The skin capillaries in Raynaud's disease. Arch Intern Med 1925; 36:161–70.
[4] Maricq HR, Leroy EC, D'Angelo WA. Diagnostic potential of in vivo capillary microscopy in scleroderma and related disorders. Arthritis Rheum 1980;23:183–9.
[5] Fleischmajer R, Perlish JS, Shaw KV, et al. Skin capillary changes in early systemic scleroderma: electron microscopy and "in vitro" autoradiography with tritiated thymidine. Arch Dermatol 1976;112:1553–7.
[6] Freemont AJ, Hoyland J, Fielding P, et al. Studies of the microvascular endothelium in uninvolved skin of patients with systemic sclerosis: direct evidence for a generalized microangiopathy. Br J Dermatol 1992;126:561–8.
[7] Grassi W, Core P, Carlino G, et al. Labial capillary microscopy in systemic sclerosis. Ann Rheum Dis 1993;52:564–9.
[8] Sgnonc R, Gruschwitz MS, Dietrich H, et al. Endothelial cell apoptosis is a primary pathogenetic event underlying skin lesions in avian and human scleroderma. J Clin Invest 1996;98: 785–92.
[9] Chen F, Eriksson P, Kimura T, et al. Apoptosis and angiogenesis are induced in the unstable coronary atherosclerotic plaque. Coron Artery Dis 2005;16(3):191–7.
[10] Mitra D, Steiner M, Staiano-Coico L, et al. Plasma from patients with idiopathic and human immunodeficiency virus-associated thrombotic thrombocytopenic purpura induces apoptosis in microvascular endothelial cells. Blood 1996;87(8):3245–54.
[11] Francisco LM, Sauter B, Roy P, et al. Immature dendritic cells phagocytose apoptotic T lymphocytes. J Exp Med 1998;88:1359–68.
[12] Greeno EW, Bach RR, Moldow CF. Apoptosis is associated with increased cell surface tissue factor procoagulant activity. Lab Invest 1996;75(2):281–9.
[13] Tsuji S, Kaji K, Nagasawa S. Activation of the alternative pathway of human complement by apoptotic human umbilical vein endothelial cells. J Biochem 1994;116(4):794–800.

[14] Pandey JP, LeRoy EC. Human cytomegalovirus and the vasculopathies of autoimmune diseases (especially scleroderma), allograft rejection, and coronary restenosis. Arthritis Rheum 1998;41(1):10–5.

[15] Zaia JA. Epidemiology and pathogenesis of cytomegalovirus disease. Semin Hematol 1990; 2:5–10.

[16] Lunardi C, Bason C, Corrocher R, et al. Induction of endothelial cell damage by hCMV molecular mimicry. Trends Immunol 2005;26(1):19–24.

[17] Madge LA, Li JH, Choi J, et al. Inhibition of phosphatidylinositol 3-kinase sensitizes vascular endothelial cells to cytokine-initiated cathepsin-dependent apoptosis. J Biol Chem 2003; 278(23):21295–306.

[18] Waldman WJ, Knight DA, Adams PW. Cytolytic activity against allogeneic human endothelia: resistance of cytomegalovirus-infected cells and virally activated lysis of uninfected cells. Transplantation 1998;66(1):66–7.

[19] Kahaleh MB, Fan PS. Mechanism of serum mediated endothelial injury in scleroderma: identification of granular enzyme in scleroderma skin and sera. Clin Immunol Immunopathol 1997;83:32–40.

[20] Kahaleh MB, Fan PS, Otsuka T. Gamma delta receptor bearing T cells in scleroderma: enhanced interaction with vascular endothelial cells in vitro. Clin Immunol 1999;91(2): 188–95.

[21] Sgonc R, Gruschwitz MS, Boeck G, et al. Endothelial cell apoptosis in systemic sclerosis is induced by antibody-dependent cell-mediated cytotoxicity via CD95. Arthritis Rheum 2000; 43(11):2550–62.

[22] Wusirika R, Ferri C, Marin M, et al. The assessment of anti-endothelial cell antibodies in scleroderma-associated pulmonary fibrosis. Am J Clin Pathol 2003;120(4):596–606.

[23] Belizna C, Duijvestijn A, Hamidou M, et al. Antiendothelial cell antibodies in vasculitis and connective tissue disease. Ann Rheum Dis 2006;65(12):1545–50.

[24] Pignone A, Scaletti C, Matucci-Cerinic M, et al. Anti-endothelial cell antibodies in systemic sclerosis: significant association with vascular involvement and alveolo-capillary impairment. Clin Exp Rheumatol 1998;16(5):527–32.

[25] Negi VS, Tripathy NK, Misra R, et al. Antiendothelial cell antibodies in scleroderma correlate with severe digital ischemia and pulmonary arterial hypertension. J Rheumatol 1998;25:462–6.

[26] Carvalho D, Savage CO, Black CM, et al. IgG antiendothelial cell autoantibodies from scleroderma patients induce leukocyte adhesion to human vascular endothelial cells in vitro: induction of adhesion molecule expression and involvement of endothelium-derived cytokines. J Clin Invest 1996;97(1):111–9.

[27] Bordron A, Dueymes M, Levy Y, et al. The binding of some human antiendothelial cell antibodies induces endothelial cell apoptosis. J Clin Invest 1998;101(10):2029–35.

[28] Worda M, Sgonc R, Dietrich H, et al. In vivo analysis of the apoptosis-inducing effect of anti-endothelial cell antibodies in systemic sclerosis by the chorioallantoic membrane assay. Arthritis Rheum 2003;48:2605–14.

[29] Garcia de la Pena-Lefebvre P, Chanseaud Y, Tamby MC, et al. IgG reactivity with a 100-kDa tissue and endothelial cell antigen identified as topoisomerase 1 distinguishes between limited and diffuse systemic sclerosis patients. Clin Immunol 2004;111(3):241–51.

[30] Ahmed SS, Tan FK, Arnett FC, et al. Induction of apoptosis and fibrillin 1 expression in human dermal endothelial cells by scleroderma sera containing anti-endothelial cell antibodies. Arthritis Rheum 2006;54(7):2250–62.

[31] Magro CM, Ross P, Marsh CB, et al. The role of anti-endothelial cell antibody-mediated microvascular injury in the evolution of pulmonary fibrosis in the setting of collagen vascular disease. Am J Clin Pathol 2007;127(2):237–47.

[32] Christen S, Finckh B, Lykkesfeldt J, et al. Oxidative stress precedes peak systemic inflammatory response in pediatric patients undergoing cardiopulmonary bypass operation. Free Radic Biol Med 2005;38(10):1323–32.

[33] Bohm F, Settergren M, Gonon AT, et al. The endothelin-1 receptor antagonist bosentan protects against ischaemia/reperfusion-induced endothelial dysfunction in humans. Clin Sci (Lond) 2005;108(4):357–63.

[34] Szocs K. Endothelial dysfunction and reactive oxygen species production in ischemia/reperfusion and nitrate tolerance. Gen Physiol Biophys 2004;23(3):265–95.

[35] Fox-Robichaud A, Payne D, Hasan SU, et al. Inhaled NO as a viable antiadhesive therapy for ischemia/reperfusion injury of distal microvascular beds. J Clin Invest 1998;101(11): 2497–505.

[36] Lehmann TG, Koeppel TA, Kirschfink M, et al. Complement inhibition by soluble complement receptor type 1 improves microcirculation after rat liver transplantation. Transplantation 1998;66:717–22.

[37] Collard CD, Agah A, Stahl GL. Complement activation following reoxygenation of hypoxic human endothelial cells: role of intracellular reactive oxygen species, NF-kappa B and new protein synthesis. Immunopharmacology 1998;39(1):39–50.

[38] Fullerton DA, Eisenach JH, Friese RS, et al. Impairment of endothelial-dependent pulmonary vasorelaxation after mesenteric ischemia/reperfusion. Surgery 1996;120(5):879–84.

[39] Gabrielli A, Di Loreto C, Taborro R, et al. Immunohistochemical localization of intracellular and extracellular associated TGF beta in the skin of patients with systemic sclerosis (scleroderma) and primary Raynaud's phenomenon. Clin Immunol Immunopathol 1993; 68(3):340–9.

[40] Yanagisawa M, Kurihara H, Kimura S, et al. A novel potent vasoconstrictor peptide produced by vascular endothelial cells. Nature 1988;332:411–5.

[41] Inoue A, Yanagisawa M, Kimura S. The human endothelin family: three structurally and pharmacologically distinct isopeptides predicted by three separate genes. Proc Natl Acad Sci U S A 1989;86:2863–7.

[42] Kahaleh MB. Endothelin, an endothelial-dependent vasoconstrictor in scleroderma: enhanced production and profibrotic action. Arthritis Rheum 1991;34:978–83.

[43] Yamane K, Miyanchi T, Suzuki N, et al. Significance of plasma endothelin-1 levels in patients with systemic sclerosis. J Rheumatol 1992;19:1566–71.

[44] Vancheeswaran R, Azam A, Black C, et al. Localization of endothelin-1 and its binding sites in scleroderma skin. J Rheumatol 1994;21(7):1268–76.

[45] Clozel M, Salloukh H. Role of endothelin in fibrosis and anti-fibrotic potential of bosentan. Ann Med 2005;37(1):2–12.

[46] Korn JH, Mayes M, Matucci-Cerinic M, et al. Digital ulcers in systemic sclerosis: prevention by treatment with bosentan, an oral endothelin receptor antagonist. Arthritis Rheum 2004; 50:3985–93.

[47] Rubin LJ, Badesch DB, Barst RJ, et al. Bosentan therapy for pulmonary arterial hypertension. N Engl J Med 2002;346(12):896–903.

[48] Bush PA, Gonzalez NE, Griscavage JM, et al. Nitric oxide synthase from cerebellum catalyzes the formation of equimolar quantities of nitric oxide and citrulline from l-arginine. Biochem Biophys Res Commun 1992;185:960–6.

[49] Kuo L, Davis MJ, Chilian WM. Endothelial modulation of arteriolar tone. News Physiol Sci 1992;7:5–9.

[50] Wanstall JC, Homer KL, Doggrell SA. Evidence for, and importance of, cGMP-independent mechanisms with NO and NO donors on blood vessels and platelets. Curr Vasc Pharmacol 2005;3(1):41–53.

[51] Anderson ME, Moore TL, Hollis S, et al. Endothelial-dependent vasodilation is impaired in patients with systemic sclerosis, as assessed by low dose iontophoresis. Clin Exp Rheumatol 2003;21(3):403.

[52] Tmito M, Fan P, Santoro T, et al. Impaired response to mechanical fluid shear stress (MFSS) by scleroderma (SSc) microvascular endothelial cells (MVEC) from involved and uninvolved skin. Arthritis Rheum 1997;40:S297.

[53] Berk BC, Abe JI, Min W, et al. Endothelial atheroprotective and anti-inflammatory mechanisms. Ann N Y Acad Sci 2001;947:93–109.

[54] Kahaleh MB, Osborn I, LeRoy EC. Elevated levels of circulating platelet aggregates and beta-thromboglobulin in scleroderma. Ann Intern Med 1982;96:610–3.

[55] Falanga V, Alstadt SP. Effect of a platelet release fraction on glycosaminoglycan synthesis by cultured dermal fibroblasts from patients with progressive systemic sclerosis. Br J Dermatol 1988;118:339–45.

[56] Mattuci-Cerinic M, Valentinie G, Sorano GG, et al. Blood coagulation, fibrinolysis, and markers of endothelial dysfunction in systemic sclerosis. Semin Arthritis Rheum 2003; 32(5):285–95.

[57] Kahaleh MB, Osborn I, LeRoy EC. Increased factor VIII/von Willebrand factor antigen and von Willebrand factor activity in scleroderma and in Raynaud's phenomenon. Ann Intern Med 1981;94:482–4.

[58] Herrick AL, Illingworth K, Blann A, et al. Von Willebrand factor, thrombomodulin, thromboxane, beta-thromboglobulin and markers of fibrinolysis in primary Raynaud's phenomenon and systemic sclerosis. Ann Rheum Dis 1996;55(2):122–7.

[59] Greaves M, Malia RG, Milford Ward A, et al. Elevated von Willebrand factor antigen in systemic sclerosis: relationship to visceral disease. Br J Rheumatol 1988;27(4):281–5.

[60] Matucci-Cerinic M, Pignone A, Iannone F, et al. Clinical correlations of plasma angiotensin converting enzyme (activity in systemic sclerosis): a longitudinal study of plasma ACE endothelial injury and lung involvement. Respir Med 1990;84(4):283–7.

[61] Stratton R, Pompon L, Coghlan J, et al. Soluble thrombomodulin concentration is raised in scleroderma associated pulmonary hypertension. Ann Rheum Dis 2000;59(2):132–4.

[62] Mizutani H, Hayashi T, Nouchi N, et al. Increased endothelial and epidermal thrombomodulin expression and plasma thrombomodulin level in progressive systemic sclerosis. Acta Med Okayama 1996;50(6):293–7.

[63] Matucci-Cerinic M, Borsotti M, Barbieri R, et al. Angiotensin converting enzyme (ACE) in scleroderma. Clin Rheumatol 1987;6(2):300–1.

[64] Matucci-Cerinic M, Jaffa A, Kahaleh B. Angiotensin converting enzyme: an in vivo and in vitro marker of endothelial injury. J Lab Clin Med 1992;120(3):428–33.

[65] Carson CW, Beall LD, Hunder GG, et al. Serum ELAM-1 is increased in vasculitis, scleroderma, and systemic lupus erythematosus. J Rheumatol 1993;20(5):809–14.

[66] Sfikakis PP, Tesar J, Baraf H, et al. Circulating intercellular adhesion molecule-1 in patients with systemic sclerosis. Clin Immunol Immunopathol 1993;68(1):88–92.

[67] Oppenheimer-marks N, Davis LS, Lipsky PE. Differential utilization of ICAM-1 and VCAM-1 during the adhesion and transendothelial migration of human T lymphocytes. J Immunol 1991;147:398–321.

[68] Del Papa N, Colombo G, Fracchiolla N, et al. Circulating endothelial cells as a marker of ongoing vascular disease in systemic sclerosis. Arthritis Rheum 2004;50(4):1296–304.

ELSEVIER
SAUNDERS

Rheum Dis Clin N Am
34 (2008) 73–79

RHEUMATIC
DISEASE CLINICS
OF NORTH AMERICA

Vascular Disease in Scleroderma: Angiogenesis and Vascular Repair

Mary Jo Mulligan-Kehoe, PhD[a,b],
Michael Simons, MD[a,c,d],*

[a]Angiogenesis Research Center, Dartmouth-Hitchcock Medical Center, Dartmouth Medical
School, Borwell 530 E, 1 Medical Center Drive, Lebanon, NH 03756, USA
[b]Department of Medicine, Vascular Section, Dartmouth-Hitchcock Medical Center,
Dartmouth Medical School, 1 Medical Center Drive, Lebanon, NH 03756, USA
[c]Department of Medicine, Cardiology Section, Dartmouth-Hitchcock Medical Center,
Dartmouth Medical School, 1 Medical Center Drive, Lebanon, NH 03756, USA
[d]Department of Pharmacology and Toxicology, Dartmouth-Hitchcock Medical Center,
Dartmouth Medical School, 1 Medical Center Drive, Lebanon, NH 03756, USA

The healing of the ongoing tissue injury that is a hallmark of scleroderma requires generation of new vasculature, mostly at the capillary level. Typically, wound healing is accompanied by extensive angiogenesis driven by vascular endothelial growth factor (VEGF) produced by injured tissues and invading inflammatory cells [1]. The situation in scleroderma is not different; indeed, analysis of skin biopsies from affected and even unaffected areas in patients who have systemic sclerosis (SSc) is consistent with a pro-inflammatory state and increased VEGF production [2–4]. In addition to pro-angiogenic factors, anti-angiogenic factors also have a role in vascular regeneration. Currently, most naturally occurring angiogenic factors are thought to be products of breakdown of the extracellular matrix and other circulating proteins. Endostatin is a cleavage product of collagen XVIII, whereas angiostatin is a product of plasminogen cleavage. Other extracellular matrix–derived inhibitors include tumstatin and canstatin among others (Table 1). Recent evidence suggests that the presence of anti-angiogenic factors in patients with scleroderma may be an important element in the abnormal vascular regeneration seen in this disease [5].

This work was supported in part by NIH grants HL069948 (MJMK), HL53793, and 62289 (MS), and a grant from the Scleroderma Research Foundation (MS).

* Corresponding author. Angiogenesis Research Center, Dartmouth-Hitchcock Medical Center, Dartmouth Medical School, Borwell 530 E, 1 Medical Center Drive, Lebanon, NH 03756.
E-mail address: michael.simons@dartmouth.edu (M. Simons).

Table 1
Anti-angiogenic factors cleaved from endogenous proteins

Angiogenesis inhibitor	Native protein	Reference
aaAntithrombin	Antithrombin	[42]
Alphastatin	Fibrinogen, α chain	[43]
Angiostatin	Plasminogen	[27]
Arrestin	A1 (IV) collagen	[44]
Canstatin	A2 (IV) collagen	[45]
cbeta(2)gp1	Beta(2)-glycoprotein-1	[46]
Endostatin	A1 (XV) collagen	[47]
	A1 (XVIII) collagen	
Endorepellin	Perlecan	
Prolactin (16 kDa fragment)	Prolactin	[48]
rPAI-1$_{23}$	Plasminogen activator inhibitor-1	[49]
rhLK68	Apolipoprotein (a)	[50]
Thrombospondin-1 fragments	Thrombospondin-1	[51]
Tissue inhibitor of metalloproteinases TIMP-2	TIMP-2	[52]
Tumstatin	Collagen IV	[45]

In addition to the regeneration of damaged vasculature, vasculature maintenance is another key event in scleroderma pathophysiology. The process of active maintenance of the normal vasculature is poorly understood; however, observed pulmonary hemorrhage and thrombosis in patients exposed to anti-VEGF drugs [6,7] suggests that at least the normal capillary bed requires continuous VEGF stimulation. Factors regulating arterial and venous integrity and maintenance are completely unknown at this time. The loss of pulmonary arterial vasculature observed in scleroderma is certainly consistent with a defective maintenance of the normal vasculature.

Bone marrow–derived cells in systemic sclerosis vascular repair

Certain subsets of bone marrow–derived mononuclear cells are thought to home to sites of vascular injury and ischemia where they cooperate with existing endothelial cells in vascular healing [8]. Some investigators have considered that SSc patients may have abnormal levels of these bone marrow–derived cell populations that impact the replacement of damaged endothelial cells in ischemic or injured tissue. For example, SSc patients with more advanced disease have fewer circulating CD133+ and CD34+ cells [9] when compared with patients with less advanced disease [10]. Recent studies have examined bone marrow–derived mesenchymal stem cells from SSc patients to determine whether endothelial differentiation of these cells is altered following vascular damage, which may explain the impaired vascular repair processes [11]. Flow cytometry analyses of phenotype markers have shown that the percentages of VEGFR2-positive mesenchymal stem cells and endothelial-like mesenchymal stem cells in SSc patients are significantly less than in controls. VEGF- and SDF-1–stimulated migration and tubulogenesis of mesenchymal stem cells and endothelial-like mesenchymal stem cells from SSc patients are also significantly less than in controls. These studies suggest that abnormalities in bone marrow mononuclear cell responsiveness and function may account for some of the impairment of angiogenesis and tissue repair in SSc.

The pro- to anti-angiogenic switch

One of the earliest vascular abnormalities observed in scleroderma is Raynaud's phenomenon. In the early stages of the disease, microscopic analysis of the nail fold beds demonstrates the presence of tortuous, giant capillary loop clusters that are surrounded by normal capillary loops of varied shapes with some detectable microhemorrhages, reminiscent of immature newly formed vasculature during an angiogenic response. The short lived pro-angiogenic response is followed by an extensive reduction in capillary density, leaving large avascular areas [12]. The dramatic switch from pro- to anti-angiogenic characteristics suggests that the angiogenic process becomes impaired.

The avascular areas may be the direct result of extensive local tissue hypoxia [13]. Indeed, intradermal skin oxygenation measurements show that hypoxic tissue is more prevalent in SSc patients than in normal subjects, and there is an increase in levels of HIF-1α, a hypoxia-inducible transcriptional factor [13].

The defective angiogenesis is not limited to nail beds. Analysis of skin tissues demonstrates increased VEGF, VEGFR1, and VEGFR2 expression levels in skin samples from patients who have SSc [2,4]. The cumulative data support an initial VEGF-related pro-angiogenic event in SSc patients but suggest that the angiogenic process is aborted.

Anti-angiogenesis and vascular homeostasis

The presence of widespread angiogenic abnormalities, even in ostensibly uninvolved tissues in SSc patients, suggests the presence of circulating anti-angiogenic factors. Vascular homeostasis requires both pro- and anti-angiogenic factors. The pro-angiogenic factors are secreted molecules that promote endothelial cell proliferation, migration, and tubulogenesis [14,15]. Many anti-angiogenic molecules are cleavage products of a number of extracellular proteins [16,17]. The activity of the pro- and anti-angiogenic factors is tightly regulated in quiescent tissues. If their activity becomes altered under pathologic conditions, abnormal growth of the vasculature or defective repair processes may occur [18].

Gene expression levels of pro- and anti-angiogenic factors that are differentially regulated in SSc patients have been analyzed by DNA microarrays. One study which screened a 14,000 gene array for proteases in normal and SSc microvascular endothelial cells detected distinct differences in the tissue kallikren gene family in the SSc group [19]. Pro-angiogenic kallikrens 9, 11, and 12 were down-regulated in SSc patients, whereas anti-angiogenic kallikren 3 was up-regulated. The microarray data were validated in normal microvascular endothelial cells that were first treated with antibodies against kallikrens 9, 11, and 12 and then analyzed in migration, proliferation, and tubulogenesis functional assays. All three antibodies blocked the angiogenic activity of the treated cells. Tissue kallikren is a serine protease that cleaves kininogen and thereby regulates the kininogen-kinin pathway that has an important role in the clotting cascade [20,21]. It also contributes to angio-genesis [21,22] and potentially to recovery from tissue ischemia [23]. Other researchers have shown that tissue kallikren is increased in the serum of SSc patients, suggesting a microvascular involvement [24].

Another DNA microarray study examined the expression of 14,000 genes in microvascular endothelial cells isolated from skin biopsies obtained from SSc patients with diffuse disease and control subjects [25]. Gene expression levels were analyzed and then categorized into functional groups based on gene ontology. Genes that are important for endothelial cell migration and extracellular matrix coupling were found to be down-regulated in SSc endothelial cells when compared with controls [25].

Overlapping pathways: hemostasis and angiogenesis

The plasminogen activator pathway and angiogenesis have key roles in wound healing. A prominent feature of SSc is abnormal wound healing in the skin and internal organs that causes scarring and sclerosis [18]. Plasmin-ogen is a precursor of pro-angiogenic plasmin [26] and anti-angiogenic angiostatin [27]; therefore, it has a complicated role in the regulation of vascular homeostasis. Plasminogen can be cleaved at the carboxy terminus by plasminogen activator to produce plasmin, a proteolytic and fibrinolytic protease. Its proteolytic activity activates many key pro-angiogenic factors, including VEGF [28], transforming growth factor-beta [29], and matrix met-alloproteinases (MMPs) [30]. Plasminogen can also be cleaved within its amino terminus kringle domains by several proteases [31–34]. The cleaved kringle domain fragments are angiostatins of various sizes that possess var-ied anti-angiogenic activity. Alterations in plasminogen processing can have a profound effect on angiogenic homeostasis.

Plasmin activity is reduced in scleroderma while the amount of circulat-ing angiostatin is increased in plasma [35]. This pro-/anti-angiogenic imbal-ance is manifested by reduced migration and proliferation of normal human microvascular dermal endothelial cells when exposed to the plasma of pa-tients with SSc. Mixing studies suggest that the effect is likely due to a circu-lating inhibitor and the reduced amount of pro-angiogenic activities. Indeed, exposure of normal microvascular dermal endothelial cells to angiostatin in amounts detected in SSc plasma results in a significant impairment of these cells' migration and ability to form vascular structures in collagen [35]. Other studies have also detected increased angiostatin levels in tight skin mouse models that mimic SSc vascular defects found in humans [36]. Still others have found that the plasma of SSc patients contains increased levels of endostatin, another endogenous angiogenesis inhibitor derived from the breakdown of a matrix protein [37].

The plasminogen activator pathway is further implicated in SSc studies that have examined the importance of urokinase plasminogen activator receptor (uPAR) in endothelial cells isolated from the skin biopsies of SSc patients. uPAR has an important roll in cell motility through its binding interactions with urokinase plasminogen activator (uPA) [38] and vitronectin [39]. The proteolytic activity of MMP-12 cleaves uPAR to result in loss of uPAR-stimulated cell motility function. Microvascular endothelial cells from SSc patients have elevated levels of MMP-12 and cleaved uPAR [40]. Furthermore, cleaved uPAR in SSc microvascular endothelial cells results in loss of an integrin-mediated uPAR connection with the actin cytoskeleton that accounts for loss of motility of these cells in SSc [41].

The emerging data suggest several abnormalities in regulation of angiogenic responses in scleroderma. To date, the evidence is suggestive of the presence of circulating inhibitors likely due to extracellular matrix breakdown and abnormal plasminogen processing. It is likely that further studies will demonstrate not only abnormal vascular repair but also abnormal maintenance of the existing vascular integrity. If correct, these new insights should lead to development of new scleroderma therapies.

References

[1] Eming SA, Krieg T. Molecular mechanisms of VEGF-A action during tissue repair. J Investig Dermatol Symp Proc 2006;11(1):79–86.

[2] Davies CA, Jeziorska M, Freemont AJ, et al. The differential expression of VEGF, VEGFR-2, and GLUT-1 proteins in disease subtypes of systemic sclerosis. Hum Pathol 2006;37(2): 190–7.

[3] Higley H, Persichitte K, Chu S, et al. Immunocytochemical localization and serologic detection of transforming growth factor beta 1: association with type I procollagen and inflammatory cell markers in diffuse and limited systemic sclerosis, morphea, and Raynaud's phenomenon. Arthritis Rheum 1994;37(2):278–88.

[4] Mackiewicz Z, Sukura A, Povilenaite D, et al. Increased but imbalanced expression of VEGF and its receptors has no positive effect on angiogenesis in systemic sclerosis skin. Clin Exp Rheumatol 2002;20(5):641–6.

[5] Mulligan-Kehoe MJ, Simons M. Current concepts in normal and defective angiogenesis: implications for systemic sclerosis. Curr Rheumatol Rep 2007;9(2):173–9.

[6] Burger RA. Experience with bevacizumab in the management of epithelial ovarian cancer. J Clin Oncol 2007;25(20):2902–8.

[7] Kindler HL, Friberg G, Singh DA, et al. Phase II trial of bevacizumab plus gemcitabine in patients with advanced pancreatic cancer. J Clin Oncol 2005;23(31):8033–40.

[8] Gill M, Dias S, Hattori K, et al. Vascular trauma induces rapid but transient mobilization of VEGFR2(+)AC133(+) endothelial precursor cells. Circ Res 2001;88(2):167–74.

[9] Kuwana M, Okazaki Y, Yasuoka H, et al. Defective vasculogenesis in systemic sclerosis. Lancet 2004;364(9434):603–10.

[10] Del Papa N, Quirici N, Soligo D, et al. Bone marrow endothelial progenitors are defective in systemic sclerosis. Arthritis Rheum 2006;54(8):2605–15.

[11] Cipriani P, Guiducci S, Miniati I, et al. Impairment of endothelial cell differentiation from bone marrow-derived mesenchymal stem cells: new insight into the pathogenesis of systemic sclerosis. Arthritis Rheum 2007;56(6):1994–2004.

[12] Cutolo M, Pizzorni C, Sulli A. Nailfold video-capillaroscopy in systemic sclerosis. Z Rheumatol 2004;63(6):457–62.

[13] Distler O, Distler JH, Scheid A, et al. Uncontrolled expression of vascular endothelial growth factor and its receptors leads to insufficient skin angiogenesis in patients with systemic sclerosis. Circ Res 2004;95(1):109–16.

[14] Simons M. Angiogenesis: where do we stand now? Circulation 2005;111(12):1556–66.

[15] Simons M, Ware JA. Therapeutic angiogenesis in cardiovascular disease. Nat Rev Drug Discov 2003;2(11):863–71.

[16] Lu H, Dhanabel M, Volk R, et al. Kringle 5 causes cell cycle arrest and apoptosis of endothelial cells. Biochem Biophys Res Commun 1999;258(3):668–73.

[17] Staton CA, Lewis CE. Angiogenesis inhibitors found within the haemostasis pathway. J Cell Mol Med 2005;9(2):286–302.

[18] Wigley FM, Flavahan NA. Raynaud's phenomenon. Rheum Dis Clin North Am 1996;22(4):765–81.

[19] Giusti B, Serrati S, Margheri F, et al. The antiangiogenic tissue kallikrein pattern of endothelial cells in systemic sclerosis. Arthritis Rheum 2005;52(11):3618–28.

[20] Bhoola KD, Figueroa CD, Worthy K. Bioregulation of kinins: kallikreins, kininogens, and kininases. Pharmacol Rev 1992;44(1):1–80.

[21] Schmaier AH, McCrae KR. The plasma kallikrein/kinin systems: its evolution from contact activation. J Thromb Haemost 2007;5:2323–9.

[22] Plendl J, Snyman C, Naidoo S, et al. Expression of tissue kallikrein and kinin receptors in angiogenic microvascular endothelial cells. Biol Chem 2000;381(11):1103–15.

[23] Emanueli C, Madeddu P. Targeting kinin receptors for the treatment of tissue ischaemia. Trends Pharmacol Sci 2001;22(9):478–84.

[24] Del Rosso A, Distler O, Milia AF, et al. Increased circulating levels of tissue kallikrein in systemic sclerosis correlate with microvascular involvement. Ann Rheum Dis 2005;64(3):382–7.

[25] Giusti B, Fibbi G, Margheri F, et al. A model of anti-angiogenesis: differential transcriptosome profiling of microvascular endothelial cells from diffuse systemic sclerosis patients. Arthritis Res Ther 2006;8(4):R115.

[26] Pepper MS. Role of the matrix metalloproteinase and plasminogen activator–plasmin systems in angiogenesis. Arterioscler Thromb Vasc Biol 2001;21(7):1104–17.

[27] Cao Y, Ji RW, Davidson D, et al. Kringle domains of human angiostatin: characterization of the anti-proliferative activity on endothelial cells. J Biol Chem 1996;271(46):29461–7.

[28] Keck RG, Berleau L, Harris R, et al. Disulfide structure of the heparin binding domain in vascular endothelial growth factor: characterization of posttranslational modifications in VEGF. Arch Biochem Biophys 1997;344(1):103–13.

[29] Ihn H. The role of TGF-beta signaling in the pathogenesis of fibrosis in scleroderma. Arch Immunol Ther Exp (Warsz) 2002;50(5):325–31.

[30] Jinnin M, Ihn H, Mimura Y, et al. Effects of hepatocyte growth factor on the expression of type I collagen and matrix metalloproteinase-1 in normal and scleroderma dermal fibroblasts. J Invest Dermatol 2005;124(2):324–30.

[31] Lijnen HR, Ugwu F, Bini A, et al. Generation of an angiostatin-like fragment from plasminogen by stromelysin-1 (MMP-3). Biochemistry 1998;37(14):4699–702.

[32] O'Reilly MS, Wiederschain D, Stetler-Stevenson WG, et al. Regulation of angiostatin production by matrix metalloproteinase-2 in a model of concomitant resistance. J Biol Chem 1999;274(41):29568–71.

[33] Patterson BC, Sang QA. Angiostatin-converting enzyme activities of human matrilysin (MMP-7) and gelatinase B/type IV collagenase (MMP-9). J Biol Chem 1997;272(46):28823–5.

[34] Stathakis P, Fitzgerald M, Matthias LJ, et al. Generation of angiostatin by reduction and proteolysis of plasmin: catalysis by a plasmin reductase secreted by cultured cells. J Biol Chem 1997;272(33):20641–5.

[35] Mulligan-Kehoe MJ, Drinane MC, Mollmark J, et al. Antiangiogenic plasma activity in patients with systemic sclerosis. Arthritis Rheum 2007;56(10):3448–58.

[36] Weihrauch D, Xu H, Shi Y, et al. Effects of D-4F on vasodilation, oxidative stress, angiostatin, myocardial inflammation, and angiogenic potential in tight-skin mice. Am J Physiol 2007;293(3):H1432–41.

[37] Dziankowska-Bartkowiak B, Waszczykowska E, Dziankowska-Zaboroszczyk E, et al. Decreased ratio of circulatory vascular endothelial growth factor to endostatin in patients with systemic sclerosis: association with pulmonary involvement. Clin Exp Rheumatol 2006; 24(5):508–13.

[38] Vassalli JD, Baccino D, Belin D. A cellular binding site for the Mr 55,000 form of the human plasminogen activator, urokinase. J Cell Biol 1985;100(1):86–92.

[39] Wei Y, Waltz DA, Rao N, et al. Identification of the urokinase receptor as an adhesion receptor for vitronectin. J Biol Chem 1994;269(51):32380–8.

[40] D'Alessio S, Fibbi G, Cinelli M, et al. Matrix metalloproteinase 12-dependent cleavage of urokinase receptor in systemic sclerosis microvascular endothelial cells results in impaired angiogenesis. Arthritis Rheum 2004;50(10):3275–85.

[41] Margheri F, Manetti M, Serrati S, et al. Domain 1 of the urokinase-type plasminogen activator receptor is required for its morphologic and functional, beta2 integrin-mediated connection with actin cytoskeleton in human microvascular endothelial cells: failure of association in systemic sclerosis endothelial cells. Arthritis Rheum 2006;54(12):3926–38.

[42] O'Reilly MS, Pirie-Shepherd S, Lane WS, et al. Antiangiogenic activity of the cleaved conformation of the serpin antithrombin. Science 1999;285(5435):1926–8.

[43] Staton CA, Brown NJ, Rodgers GR, et al. Alphastatin, a 24-amino acid fragment of human fibrinogen, is a potent new inhibitor of activated endothelial cells in vitro and in vivo. Blood 2004;103(2):601–6.

[44] Colorado PC, Torre A, Kamphaus G, et al. Anti-angiogenic cues from vascular basement membrane collagen. Cancer Res 2000;60(9):2520–6.

[45] Kamphaus GD, Colorado PC, Panka DJ, et al. Canstatin, a novel matrix-derived inhibitor of angiogenesis and tumor growth. J Biol Chem 2000;275(2):1209–15.

[46] Beecken WD, Engl T, Ringel EM, et al. An endogenous inhibitor of angiogenesis derived from a transitional cell carcinoma: clipped beta2-glycoprotein-I. Ann Surg Oncol 2006; 13(9):1241–51.

[47] O'Reilly MS, Boehm T, Shing Y, et al. Endostatin: an endogenous inhibitor of angiogenesis and tumor growth. Cell 1997;88(2):277–85.

[48] Ferrara N, Clapp C, Weiner R. The 16K fragment of prolactin specifically inhibits basal or fibroblast growth factor stimulated growth of capillary endothelial cells. Endocrinology 1991;129(2):896–900.

[49] Mulligan-Kehoe MJ, Wagner R, Wieland C, et al. A truncated plasminogen activator inhibitor-1 protein induces and inhibits angiostatin (kringles 1-3), a plasminogen cleavage product. J Biol Chem 2001;276(11):8588–96.

[50] Kim JS, Chang JH, Yu HK, et al. Inhibition of angiogenesis and angiogenesis-dependent tumor growth by the cryptic kringle fragments of human apolipoprotein(a). J Biol Chem 2003;278(31):29000–8.

[51] Tolsma SS, Volpert OV, Good DJ, et al. Peptides derived from two separate domains of the matrix protein thrombospondin-1 have anti-angiogenic activity. J Cell Biol 1993;122(2): 497–511.

[52] Stetler-Stevenson WG, Seo DW. TIMP-2: an endogenous inhibitor of angiogenesis. Trends Mol Med 2005;11(3):97–103.

ELSEVIER
SAUNDERS

Rheum Dis Clin N Am
34 (2008) 81–87

RHEUMATIC
DISEASE CLINICS
OF NORTH AMERICA

Regulation of Vascular Reactivity in Scleroderma: New Insights into Raynaud's Phenomenon

Nicholas A. Flavahan, PhD

Department of Anesthesiology and Critical Care Medicine, Johns Hopkins University, Ross Research Building R370, 720 Rutland Avenue, Baltimore, MD 21205, USA

Cold-induced vasoconstriction in the cutaneous circulation is normally a protective response that acts to reduce heat loss [1]. Cold exposure initiates cutaneous vasoconstriction by a reflex increase in sympathetic nerve activity and by a direct action on the blood vessel to enhance sympathetic constriction [1]. The major sympathetic neurotransmitter, norepinephrine, initiates cutaneous vasoconstriction by activating two distinct families of receptors on vascular smooth muscle (VSM) cells, α_1 and α_2-adrenoceptors (ARs) [2–5]; however, cold exposure amplifies constriction mediated by only one of these subtypes, the α_2-AR, while simultaneously reducing the activity of the other, the α_1-AR [6–8]. Although α_1-ARs are ubiquitous, the functional activity of α_2-ARs is most prominent on VSM of cutaneous blood vessels including human digital arteries [2,4,9,10], reflecting their important involvement in thermoregulation. The effect of cold on cutaneous arteries is dramatically increased in Raynaud's phenomenon, leading to vasospastic attacks. Local inhibition of α_2-ARs inhibits cold-induced cutaneous vasoconstriction in healthy humans and prevents the vasospastic attacks of Raynaud's phenomenon [11–13].

Although α_2-ARs represent a family of three different subtypes (α_{2A}, α_{2B}, α_{2C}), only one subtype, the α_{2C}-AR, appears to be "thermosensitive" [3,8,14]. Initial studies on α_{2C}-ARs suggested that they may be "silent" or "vestigial" receptors [15]. Indeed, unlike α_{2A}-ARs and α_{2B}-ARs, which are directed to the plasma membrane, α_{2C}-ARs are predominantly localized to endoplasmic reticulum/Golgi compartments [14,16–18]. Although intracellular α_{2C}-ARs

This article was supported by grants from the NIH (HL080119 and OH008531) and the Peninsula Community Foundation.

E-mail address: nflavah1@jhmi.edu

doi:10.1016/j.rdc.2007.12.005

are functionally competent, they do not cycle to the cell surface and are not accessible to physiologic agonists [17,18]. One exception is certain neurons and neuronal cell lines (eg, PC12), in which α_{2C}-ARs are targeted to the plasma membrane and are functional [18]. α_{2C}-ARs are expressed in cutaneous VSM and are essential for the thermoregulatory function of cutaneous arteries [8]. Constriction to α_2-AR stimulation at warm temperatures is mediated by α_{2A}-ARs, with no apparent contribution from α_{2C}-ARs [8], whereas during cold exposure, the augmented α_2-AR response is mediated entirely by α_{2C}-ARs [8]. Cold causes a remarkable functional and spatial rescue of α_{2C}-ARs from the *trans*Golgi to the cell surface, where they can respond to stimulation [3,14,19,20]. Although α_{2C}-ARs are important effectors in the cutaneous vascular response to cooling, they do not appear to respond directly to cold; therefore, they should be considered "thermoeffectors" rather than "thermosensors."

Cold signaling in cutaneous arteries

Immediately upon cooling, there is increased generation of reactive oxygen species (ROS) from VSM mitochondria in cutaneous arteries from the mouse tail [20]. Indeed, this increase represents the earliest detectable cold-induced response in cutaneous arteries, suggesting that the mitochondria may be the thermosensor responsible for initiating cold-induced vasoconstriction in cutaneous blood vessels. These mitochondrial ROS do not appear to be pathogenic but instead activate novel REDOX signaling through the RhoA/Rho kinase (ROCK) pathway [19]. A similar REDOX signaling pathway has been linked to oxygen-induced constriction of the ductus arteriosus [21]. RhoA is a member of the Ras family of small GTP-binding proteins [22,23] and has a central role in regulating actin-myosin–dependent processes in VSM, including contractility and motility [22,24]. Actin-myosin interaction is determined by the phosphorylation status of regulatory myosin light chains (MLCs), which reflects the relative activities of MLC kinase and MLC phosphatase [24]. Activation of RhoA and its effector, Rho kinase, (ROCK) inhibits MLC phosphatase, causing increased phosphorylation of MLC and contraction of VSM in the absence of an increase in intracellular calcium concentration [24,25]. This mechanism, termed *calcium sensitization*, can contribute to VSM and blood vessel contraction; however, in the mouse tail artery, cold-induced activation of ROS/Rho/ROCK was not directed to generalized constriction but to selective amplification of the α_{2C}-AR response [19]. Indeed, inhibition of ROCK by pharmacologic (fasudil, Y27632, or H-1152) or molecular approaches (RNA interference to reduce protein expression) prevented the cold-induced mobilization of α_{2C}-ARs to the cell surface [19]; therefore, under these experimental conditions, the ROS/Rho/ROCK pathway contributed to cold-induced constriction by an indirect manner to facilitate delivery of constrictor α_{2C}-ARs to the cell surface [19,20]. Under normal conditions, cold exposure actually caused vasodilation in the absence of α_2-AR stimulation, and there was no evidence that cold-induced activation of ROS/Rho/ROCK initiated direct constriction of these cutaneous arteries [8,19]. Cold-induced dilation most likely negated the direct influence of ROS/RhoA/ROCK on the contractile process, ensuring that their role in facilitating α_{2C}-AR translocation predominated during cold exposure. Interestingly, in permeabilized cutaneous tail arteries, cold increased the "calcium sensitivity" of constriction in the absence of agonist stimulation [19], confirming that under some circumstances ROS/Rho/ROCK can contribute directly to cold-induced constriction [24].

The role of the Rho/ROCK pathway in mediating cold-induced vasoconstriction in the cutaneous circulation has been confirmed in several studies [26–28]. In vivo analysis of the cutaneous circulation of mice and humans demonstrated an important role of ROCK activity in mediating the cold-induced increase in adrenergic and α_{2C}-AR vasoconstrictor activity [26–28]. Interestingly, during prolonged exposure to local cooling in human volunteers (> 30 minutes), a large component of the cold-induced constriction was independent of adrenergic receptors but was still dependent on ROCK [27,28]; therefore, in humans, cold-induced activation of the Rho/ROCK pathway may initiate constriction mediated by both indirect (α_{2C}-ARs) and direct (calcium sensitization) pathways [27,28]. Cold-induced cutaneous dilation, which may restrain this non-adrenergic response in the mouse model, was observed only during the initial response to cold and was not evident during prolonged cooling in these human volunteers [27,28]. A component of the late non-adrenergic cutaneous vasoconstriction to local cooling in humans may be mediated by a cold-induced decrease in nitric oxide (NO) dilator signaling [29]. Impaired NO activity could result in part from the cold-induced generation of ROS, which can inactivate NO, or from cold-induced activation of Rho/ROCK, which can inhibit NO signaling at multiple sites [30,31].

Cold-induced cutaneous constriction is restrained by simultaneous cold-induced cutaneous vasodilation, which can be observed in vitro and in vivo [6,7,28]. In addition to stimulating constriction through the Rho/ROCK pathway, increased generation of mitochondrial ROS in VSM can initiate vasodilation. Mitochondrial ROS can increase the frequency of calcium sparks, which are highly localized intracellular calcium $[Ca^{2+}]_i$ transients generated in response to the opening of Ca^{2+} release channels on the sarcoplasmic reticulum in VSM [32]. Although Ca^{2+} sparks elevate $[Ca^{2+}]_i$ to micromolar concentrations in the local vicinity of the release site, they do not contribute directly to global $[Ca^{2+}]_i$ because of their transient and localized nature [32]. Calcium sparks activate large conductance calcium-activated potassium channels (K_{Ca}) inducing membrane hyperpolarization and relaxation [32]. It is tempting to speculate that this mechanism may contribute to cold-induced vasodilation in cutaneous and other blood vessels, and that the same thermosensor (ie, VSM mitochondria) initiates both cold-induced vasoconstriction and cold-induced vasodilation. Indeed, the ability of mitochondrial ROS to couple to these divergent pathways may determine whether the response to cold is vasodilation, as observed in deep blood vessels, or a combination of vasodilation and vasoconstriction, as observed in cutaneous blood vessels.

Stress signaling and Raynaud's phenomenon

Raynaud's phenomenon can be of idiopathic origin or can occur in response to mechanical (hand-arm vibration syndrome or vibration white finger), immunologic (autoimmune disease), or chemical stress (antineoplastic chemotherapeutic agents including bleomycin) in cutaneous blood vessels [13]. It is intriguing that these pathologic stressors act to amplify what is a normal physiologic stress response to cold exposure.

Indeed, α_{2C}-ARs may function as stress receptors within cutaneous arteries [10,33]. Stimuli that mimic arterial injury or inflammation cause a dramatic and selective increase in α_{2C}-AR expression in cutaneous VSM, which is associated with partial mobilization of α_{2C}-ARs to the cell surface [10,33]. Although these receptors appear to be carefully regulated in VSM, resulting in their intracellular retention under normal conditions, in response to physiologic or pathophysiologic stress they can be up-regulated or relocated to the cell surface. α_{2C}-ARs may have signaling qualities that are desirable under conditions of vascular stress but less beneficial under normal circumstances. For example, unlike α_{2A} or other cell-surface receptors, α_{2C}-ARs are resistant to agonist-induced desensitization [34–36]; therefore, α_{2C}-ARs may have a functional advantage for responses that require prolonged activation (eg, vascular remodeling, prejunctional regulation) but may not be beneficial for normal vascular function. Although such unusual regulation may not be required for agonists that are present only during stress, norepinephrine is always present in the blood vessel wall. This remarkable regulation may provide a unique ability for norepinephrine to engage in certain vascular responses; however, inappropriate regulation of α_{2C}-ARs may precipitate pathologic changes in the blood vessel wall, including enhanced cold-induced vasoconstriction and Raynaud's phenomenon. Interestingly, although the female sex hormone estrogen increases expression of α_{2C}-ARs in cutaneous VSM, it increases α_{2}-AR vasoconstriction only during cold exposure [37]. Increased expression of α_{2C}-ARs may act to increase a mobile pool of intracellular α_{2C}-ARs and thereby selectively increase cold-induced vasoconstriction.

The other signaling components involved in cold-induced vasoconstriction (ROS, Rho/ROCK) are also known to have increased activity during pathologic stress and the development of vascular disease [30,31]. It is tempting to consider that Raynaud's phenomenon may arise from altered activity of components of the signal transduction pathway involved in the thermosensor or thermoeffector function (including ROS, Rho, ROCK, α_{2C}-ARs) of cutaneous arteries.

A mechanism-based therapeutic approach to Raynaud's phenomenon

Although multiple mechanisms may contribute to the amplified cold-induced vasoconstriction of Raynaud's phenomenon, it is unlikely that the cutaneous arteries have developed a distinct thermosensor when compared with control arteries. Therapies targeting the signal transduction pathway responsible for cold-induced constriction of cutaneous arteries (ROS/Rho/ROCK) should provide an effective mechanism-based therapeutic intervention for this condition. Given the complexities of ROS and REDOX signaling, the most promising candidate may be ROCK, especially considering that several pharmaceutical companies are developing inhibitors for these enzymes [30,31]. Because of the role of ROCK in regulating numerous pathologic processes including vasoconstriction, vascular remodeling, and fibrosis, ROCK inhibitors may be especially beneficial in treating scleroderma. Many of the cholesterol-independent or "pleiotropic" vascular protective effects of 3-hydroxy-3-methylglutaryl (HMG)-CoA reductase inhibitors (statins) are thought to result from their ability to inhibit Rho/ROCK signaling in the blood vessel wall [30,31]. The promising preliminary results obtained with statins in Raynaud's phenomenon and scleroderma [38–41] may herald an even more impressive outcome for ROCK inhibitors.

References

[1] Vanhoutte PM. Physical factors of regulation. In: Bohr DF, Somlyo AP, Sparks HV, editors. Handbook of physiology. Washington (DC): American Physiological Society; 1980. p. 443–74.

[2] Flavahan NA, Cooke JP, Shepherd JT, et al. Human postjunctional alpha-1 and alpha-2 adrenoceptors: differential distribution in arteries of the limbs. J Pharmacol Exp Ther 1987;241:361–5.

[3] Hein L, Altman JD, Kobilka BK. Two functionally distinct alpha2-adrenergic receptors regulate sympathetic neurotransmission. Nature 1999;402:181–4.

[4] Flavahan NA, Rimele TJ, Cooke JP, et al. Characterization of postjunctional alpha-1 and alpha-2 adrenoceptors activated by exogenous or nerve-released norepinephrine in the canine saphenous vein. J Pharmacol Exp Ther 1984;230:699–705.

[5] Flavahan NA, McGrath JC. Are human vascular alpha-adrenoceptors atypical ? [letter] J Cardiovasc Pharmacol 1984;6:208–10.

[6] Flavahan NA, Lindblad LE, Verbeuren TJ, et al. Cooling and alpha 1- and alpha 2-adrenergic responses in cutaneous veins: role of receptor reserve. Am J Physiol 1985;249:H950–5.

[7] Flavahan NA, Vanhoutte PM. Effect of cooling on alpha-1 and alpha-2 adrenergic responses in canine saphenous and femoral veins. J Pharmacol Exp Ther 1986;238:139–47.

[8] Chotani MA, Flavahan S, Mitra S, et al. Silent alpha(2C)-adrenergic receptors enable cold-induced vasoconstriction in cutaneous arteries. Am J Physiol Heart Circ Physiol 2000;278: H1075–83.

[9] Flavahan NA, Vanhoutte PM. Alpha-1 and alpha-2 adrenoceptor: response coupling in canine saphenous and femoral veins. J Pharmacol Exp Ther 1986;238:131–8.

[10] Chotani MA, Mitra S, Su BY, et al. Regulation of alpha(2)-adrenoceptors in human vascular smooth muscle cells. Am J Physiol Heart Circ Physiol 2004;286:H59–67.

[11] Lindblad LE, Ekenvall L. Alpha 2-adrenoceptor inhibition in patients with vibration white fingers. Kurume Med J 1990;37(Suppl):S95–9.

[12] Freedman RR, Baer RP, Mayes MD. Blockade of vasospastic attacks by alpha 2-adrenergic but not alpha 1-adrenergic antagonists in idiopathic Raynaud's disease. Circulation 1995;92: 1448–51.

[13] Block JA, Sequeira W. Raynaud's phenomenon. Lancet 2001;357:2042–8.

[14] Jeyaraj SC, Chotani MA, Mitra S, et al. Cooling evokes redistribution of α2C-adrenoceptors from Golgi to plasma membrane in transfected HEK293 cells. Mol Pharmacol 2001;60: 1195–200.

[15] MacDonald E, Kobilka BK, Scheinin M. Gene targeting: homing in on alpha 2-adrenoceptor-subtype function. Trends Pharmacol Sci 1997;18:211–9.

[16] Philipp M, Brede M, Hein L. Physiological significance of alpha(2)-adrenergic receptor sub-type diversity: one receptor is not enough. Am J Physiol Regul Integr Comp Physiol 2002; 283:R287–95.

[17] Daunt DA, Hurt C, Hein L, et al. Subtype-specific intracellular trafficking of alpha2-adrenergic receptors. Mol Pharmacol 1997;51:711–20.

[18] Hurt CM, Feng FY, Kobilka B. Cell-type specific targeting of the alpha 2c-adrenoceptor: evidence for the organization of receptor microdomains during neuronal differentiation of PC12 cells. J Biol Chem 2000;275:35424–31.

[19] Bailey SR, Eid AH, Mitra S, et al. Rho kinase mediates cold-induced constriction of cutaneous arteries: role of alpha2C-adrenoceptor translocation. Circ Res 2004;94:1367–74.

[20] Bailey SR, Mitra S, Flavahan S, et al. Reactive oxygen species from smooth muscle mito-chondria initiate cold-induced constriction of cutaneous arteries. Am J Physiol Heart Circ Physiol 2005;289(1):H243–50.

[21] Kajimoto H, Hashimoto K, Bonnet SN, et al. Oxygen activates the Rho/Rho-kinase path-way and induces RhoB and ROCK-1 expression in human and rabbit ductus arteriosus by increasing mitochondria-derived reactive oxygen species: a newly recognized mechanism for sustaining ductal constriction. Circulation 2007;115:1777–88.

[22] Hall A. Rho GTPases and the actin cytoskeleton. Science 1998;279:509–14.

[23] Fukata Y, Amano M, Kaibuchi K. Rho-Rho-kinase pathway in smooth muscle contraction and cytoskeletal reorganization of non-muscle cells. Trends Pharmacol Sci 2001;22:32–9.

[24] Somlyo AP, Somlyo AV. Ca2+ sensitivity of smooth muscle and nonmuscle myosin II: modulated by G proteins, kinases, and myosin phosphatase. Physiol Rev 2003;83:1325–58.

[25] Riento K, Ridley AJ. Rocks: multifunctional kinases in cell behaviour. Nat Rev Mol Cell Biol 2003;4:446–56.

[26] Honda M, Suzuki M, Nakayama K, et al. Role of alpha2C-adrenoceptors in the reduction of skin blood flow induced by local cooling in mice. Br J Pharmacol 2007;152:91–100.

[27] Thompson-Torgerson CS, Holowatz LA, Flavahan NA, et al. Rho kinase-mediated local cold-induced cutaneous vasoconstriction is augmented in aged human skin. Am J Physiol Heart Circ Physiol 2007;293:H30–6.

[28] Thompson-Torgerson CS, Holowatz LA, Flavahan NA, et al. Cold-induced cutaneous vasoconstriction is mediated by Rho kinase in vivo in human skin. Am J Physiol Heart Circ Physiol 2007;292:H1700–5.

[29] Hodges GJ, Zhao K, Kosiba WA, et al. The involvement of nitric oxide in the cutaneous vasoconstrictor response to local cooling in humans. J Physiol 2006;574:849–57.

[30] Liao JK, Seto M, Noma K. Rho kinase (ROCK) inhibitors. J Cardiovasc Pharmacol 2007; 50:17–24.

[31] Rikitake Y, Liao JK. Rho GTPases, statins, and nitric oxide. Circ Res 2005;97:1232–5.

[32] Xi Q, Cheranov SY, Jaggar JH. Mitochondria-derived reactive oxygen species dilate cerebral arteries by activating Ca2+ sparks. Circ Res 2005;97:354–62.

[33] Chotani MA, Mitra S, Eid AH, et al. Distinct cyclic AMP signaling pathways differentially regulate α2C-adrenoceptor expression: role in serum induction in human arteriolar smooth muscle cells. Am J Physiol Heart Circ Physiol 2005;288:H69–76 [Epub 2004 Sep 2].

[34] Eason MG, Liggett SB. Subtype-selective desensitization of alpha 2-adrenergic receptors: different mechanisms control short and long term agonist-promoted desensitization of alpha 2C10, alpha 2C4, and alpha 2C2. J Biol Chem 1992;267:25473–9.

[35] Jewell-Motz EA, Liggett SB. G protein-coupled receptor kinase specificity for phosphorylation and desensitization of alpha2-adrenergic receptor subtypes. J Biol Chem 1996;271: 18082–7.

[36] Jewell-Motz EA, Donnelly ET, Eason MG, et al. Role of the amino terminus of the third intracellular loop in agonist-promoted downregulation of the alpha2A-adrenergic receptor. Biochemistry 1997;36:8858–63.

[37] Eid AH, Maiti K, Mitra S, et al. Estrogen increases smooth muscle expression of alpha2C-adrenoceptors and cold-induced constriction of cutaneous arteries. Am J Physiol Heart Circ Physiol 2007;293:H1955–61.

[38] Kuwana M. Potential benefit of statins for vascular disease in systemic sclerosis. Curr Opin Rheumatol 2006;18:594–600.

[39] Derk CT, Jimenez SA. Statins and the vasculopathy of systemic sclerosis: potential therapeutic agents? Autoimmun Rev 2006;5:25–32.

[40] Furukawa S, Yasuda S, Amengual O, et al. Protective effect of pravastatin on vascular endothelium in patients with systemic sclerosis: a pilot study. Ann Rheum Dis 2006;65: 1118–20.

[41] Kuwana M, Kaburaki J, Okazaki Y, et al. Increase in circulating endothelial precursors by atorvastatin in patients with systemic sclerosis. Arthritis Rheum 2006;54:1946–51.

ELSEVIER
SAUNDERS

Rheum Dis Clin N Am
34 (2008) 89–114

RHEUMATIC
DISEASE CLINICS
OF NORTH AMERICA

Diagnosis and Management of Scleroderma Peripheral Vascular Disease

Ariane Herrick, MD, FRCP

*Rheumatic Diseases Centre, University of Manchester,
Salford Royal NHS Foundation Trust, Salford M6 8HD, UK*

Peripheral vascular involvement occurs in almost all patients who have systemic sclerosis (SSc), because it is rare for them not to experience Raynaud's phenomenon (episodic color changes of the digits, usually in response to cold exposure or stress). The feet as well as the hands are commonly affected.

In primary (idiopathic) Raynaud's phenomenon (PRP), digital vasospasm is entirely reversible and does not progress to tissue injury [1]. However, in patients who have SSc, digital ischemia can result in digital ulcers, digital pitting (which is an American Rheumatism Association criterion for SSc [2]), and sometimes gangrene necessitating amputation. Digital ischemia in SSc can be so severe for many reasons, including abnormalities of neuroendothelial control mechanisms (leading to an imbalance of vasoconstriction over vasodilation), structural abnormalities of the vasculature involving both microvessels and the digital arteries, and intravascular factors, including a procoagulant tendency and oxidative stress [3]. Many of these factors are potentially amenable to therapeutic intervention. A key challenge for clinicians is gauging the severity and extent of peripheral vascular involvement in each patient who has SSc and formulating an appropriate investigation and management plan that may vary throughout the disease course.

This article considers the assessment and management of SSc-related peripheral vascular disease and highlights the importance of identifying coexisting proximal artery disease.

Dr. Herrick has consulted for and spoken at meetings sponsored by Actelion Pharmaceuticals Ltd.

E-mail address: ariane.herrick@manchester.ac.uk

doi:10.1016/j.rdc.2007.11.006

Microvascular versus macrovascular disease

Vascular abnormalities have long been recognized as being central to the pathogenesis of SSc, and SSc has been suggested to be primarily a vascular disease [4,5]. Both structural and functional changes occur, which interrelate [6]. Structural changes affect digital microcirculation (well demonstrated with nailfold capillaroscopy) (Fig. 1) and the digital arteries, in which the most characteristic histologic lesion is marked intimal hyperplasia/fibrosis (Fig. 2) [7].

Although involvement of peripheral arteries proximal to the digital arteries was previously believed to be unusual, in the past 15 years considerable interest has been shown in the suggestion that patients who have SSc have an increased prevalence of large vessel disease [8–10]. Studies investigating the prevalence of lower limb large vessel disease have shown conflicting results. Veale and colleagues [8] reported that 10 of 46 patients (21.7%) who had SSc who participated in a questionnaire-based study experienced claudication, compared with 4.5% of the population of a neighboring region in Scotland. The same investigators then reported ankle–brachial pressure indices (ABPI) of less than 0.9 in 9 of 53 patients who had SSc (17%) but in none of 43 controls, with 21 (40%) patients who had SSc having an ABPI of less than 1.0 compared with 4 (10%) controls [9]. However, a later study of 119 patients who had SSc reported that only 12% had an ABPI of less than 1.0, but this study did not include a control group [11]. A recent study found no differences in ABPIs between 53 patients who had SSc and 43 controls, despite higher intima-media thickness (an index of atherosclerotic carotid artery disease) in the SSc group [12].

If macrovascular disease is increased in SSc, it may be from the SSc disease process or because of an increased prevalence of atheromatous disease as reported in other rheumatic diseases. Despite whether the prevalence of large vessel peripheral arterial disease is increased in SSc, atheromatous disease is

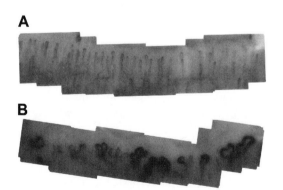

Fig. 1. Nailfold capillaroscopy showing (*A*) normal capillaries in a healthy control subject and (*B*) grossly abnormal capillaries in a patient who has SSc, showing enlarged loops, areas of avascularity, and loss of the normal capillary architecture.

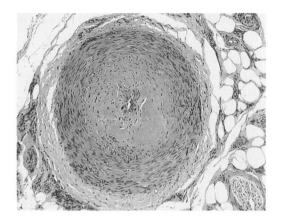

Fig. 2. Digital artery from a patient who has SSc (amputation specimen) showing marked intimal hyperplasia and almost complete occlusion of the lumen. (*Courtesy of* A.J. Freemont, FRCP, FRCPath, Manchester, UK.)

common, especially in older patients, and the coexistence of proximal and small vessel disease in SSc is potentially limb-threatening. It is important not to miss, for example, a subclavian or superficial femoral artery stenosis that may be amenable to angioplasty or surgery.

Upper and lower limb arteriographic studies in patients who have SSc, mostly with critical digital ischemia, have shown a combination of proximal and digital arterial disease, although in small numbers of patients. Hasegawa and colleagues [13] described arteriographic findings in eight patients who had SSc and severe digital ischemia; seven had digital artery occlusions, but four also had arterial occlusions proximal to the digits, and in three the ulnar artery was involved. These authors reviewed the earlier literature on arteriographic findings in SSc [13]. Three previous groups of investigators reported ulnar artery occlusion on angiography in patients who had SSc: in 11 of 31 patients [14], 10 of 24 hands (12 patients) [15], and 9 of 29 patients [16]. In contrast, radial artery involvement was only rarely reported. Ulnar artery disease was also reported in a retrospective study by Stafford and colleagues [17], who found that 10 of 19 patients who had SSc had ulnar arterial wall abnormalities on Doppler ultrasound, and by Taylor and colleagues [18], who reported ulnar artery involvement in all 15 patients (9 had bilateral involvement) who underwent arteriography based on severe digital ischemia/ulceration and a positive Allen's test (all 15 patients also had digital artery disease). Why the ulnar artery should be involved more than the radial artery is unknown.

The message to clinicians is that the possibility of proximal vessel disease should always be considered in patients who have SSc and severe digital ischemia, because it may be amenable to limb-saving angioplasty or surgical revascularization. Also, patients should be assessed for risk factors for atherosclerotic disease.

Diagnosis

Two aspects of the approach to diagnosis are considered: (1) diagnosis of an underlying scleroderma-spectrum disorder in patients who present with Raynaud's phenomenon/digital ischemia and (2) diagnosis/assessment of severe digital ischemia/ulceration in patients who have an established diagnosis of SSc. Although the main contributor to disease pathogenesis is a non-inflammatory microangiopathy in most patients who have SSc-related peripheral vascular disease, other possibilities should always be considered, such as (1) concomitant proximal vessel disease, (2) vasculitis, which is unusual in SSc but has been described [19,20], and (3) thrombotic disease, for example as part of a concomitant antiphospholipid syndrome, which is rare but has been described in association with SSc [21].

Other factors to consider are whether an ischemic ulcer is infected and whether an area of calcinosis is present beneath an ulcer (Fig. 3), which may contribute to delayed healing.

In peripheral vascular disease, as in most other medical conditions, diagnosis is made based on the history, examination, and investigations.

History

The diagnosis of Raynaud's phenomenon is usually based on the patient's history, color changes of the hands (classically triphasic, but may be biphasic

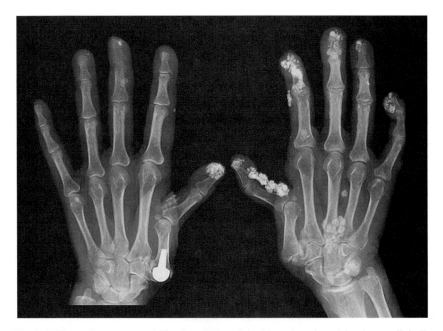

Fig. 3. Diffuse subcutaneous calcification. Although in this patient the calcinosis was clinically obvious, less severe cases of calcinosis may be visible only on radiography.

or uniphasic) in response to cold exposure or stress. However, clearly this approach involves some subjectivity [22]. In epidemiologic research, a set of color charts, combined with a simple questionnaire, may increase sensitivity and specificity [23].

Is an underlying scleroderma-spectrum disorder present?

Specific pointers toward an underlying connective tissue disease (versus PRP) include later age of onset and a history of digital ulcers. The feet and hands may be affected in PRP and Raynaud's phenomenon associated with a scleroderma-spectrum disorder. Patients who have limited cutaneous SSc often have a long history of Raynaud's phenomenon, which becomes more severe before SSc is diagnosed. A full history must be taken, including a full systems enquiry to identify symptoms such as difficulty swallowing, which could be suggestive of an underlying connective tissue disease.

Is the digit critically ischemic or at risk of becoming so, and if so why?

Permanent discoloration of the digit and increased pain are the main symptoms of critical ischemia.

Examination

Is an underlying scleroderma-spectrum disorder present?

In patients presenting with Raynaud's phenomenon, findings on examination of the hands and feet pointing toward an underlying scleroderma-spectrum disorder include sclerodactyly, digital pitting, digital ulceration, and (rarely) gangrene. Sometimes large dilated nailfold capillary loops (well demonstrated on capillaroscopy as described below) are visible.

Is the digit critically ischemic or at risk of becoming so, and if so why?

In patients who have established SSc or other scleroderma-spectrum disorder, features to look for include permanent discoloration (usually cyanosis or pallor) (Fig. 4), digital ulceration (Fig. 5), extreme tenderness

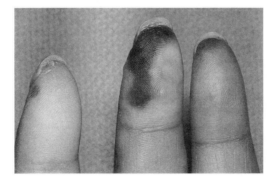

Fig. 4. Critical digital ischemia in a patient who has SSc. (*Courtesy of* Salford Royal NHS Foundation Trust, Salford, UK, with permission. Copyright © Salford Royal NHS Foundation Trust.)

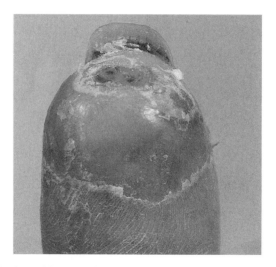

Fig. 5. Digital tip ulcer, with surrounding infection, in a patient who has SSc. The fingertip was extremely tender. (*Courtesy of* Salford Royal NHS Foundation Trust, Salford, UK, with permission. Copyright © Salford Royal NHS Foundation Trust.)

at the site of ulceration (which might represent a focus of necrotic tissue requiring surgical debridement or underlying bone infection), and gangrene. If any evidence of critical ischemia is seen, the distal pulses must be checked, which should be easily palpable in patients who have SSc experiencing an exacerbation of symptoms because of microangiopathy. Absence of one or more peripheral pulses suggests a large (proximal) vessel problem, which demands further investigation. Signs of vasculitis, such as a vasculitic rash, should be sought, although they are very rarely associated with SSc.

Investigations

This section discusses the approach to investigating peripheral vascular disease, whereas the subsequent section describes the different imaging modalities used in clinical practice and research. Investigations complement the history and examination.

Is an underlying scleroderma-spectrum disorder present?

In patients who have PRP, the antinuclear antibody should be either negative or only weakly positive (titre < 1/100), the erythrocyte sedimentation rate should be normal, and the nailfold capillaries should be normal [1]. Therefore, antinuclear antibody, erythrocyte sedimentation rate, and nailfold microscopy (discussed below) are part of the routine assessment of patients referred with Raynaud's phenomenon. Other autoantibodies, for example anticentromere antibody, are highly specific (but not sensitive) for an underlying connective tissue disease and may be assayed when the index of suspicion of an underlying scleroderma-spectrum disorder is high. Abnormal nailfold microscopy has been reported to be the best predictor of underlying connective tissue disease [24,25].

Thermography is also useful in assessing patients who have Raynaud's phenomenon. Patients who have underlying connective tissue disease tend to have characteristic patterns of temperature response to different hot or cold stimuli. However, its use is currently restricted to specialist centers. Laser Doppler imaging (which measures microvascular flow) and finger systolic pressures may also help separate patients who have PRP from those who have underlying structural vascular disease, but are currently research tools and not used in routine clinical practice.

Investigation of the patient who has a severely/critically ischemic digit

In the clinic, the most useful test is the assessment of the peripheral pulses with Doppler ultrasound. This test is an extension of the clinical examination; if the pulses are difficult to feel, then Doppler ultrasound will establish whether significant large vessel disease is likely, requiring further investigation, such as with angiography. In the lower limbs, the ABPI is usually reported; less than 0.9 is abnormal and the value is inversely proportional to the severity of peripheral vascular disease [26].

A vasculitic screen and testing for a lupus anticoagulant and anticardiolipin antibodies should be considered. A plain radiograph of the affected digit may show underlying calcinosis (see Fig. 3) or suggest osteomyelitis (Fig. 6).

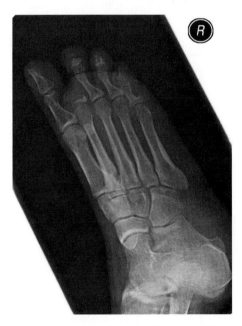

Fig. 6. Radiograph showing osteomyelitis of the tip of the right third toe in a patient who has SSc. The second toe has been amputated.

However, plain radiograph cannot exclude bone infection, and an MRI scan should be requested if the index of suspicion is high (Fig. 7).

Anticentromere antibody is associated with severity of digital ischemia in patients who have SSc [27,28].

Assessment of peripheral vascular disease severity

The definition and measurement of peripheral vascular disease activity and severity in patients who have SSc are currently the subjects of much debate and research [29]. The peripheral vasculature is one of nine organ systems of the disease severity score proposed by Medger and colleagues [30], assessed by the presence or absence of Raynaud's phenomenon requiring vasodilators, digital pitting, digital-tip ulcers, and gangrene. The Raynaud's Condition Score is increasingly being used in clinical trials, which is a self-assessment score (0–10) incorporating frequency, duration, and severity of attacks [29].

In patients who have SSc, laboratory outcome measures for monitoring digital vascular disease progression and treatment response are currently restricted to the research setting. Capillary microscopy, thermography, laser Doppler, and finger systolic blood pressure measurements have all been advocated [31], but all require further validation. Finger systolic pressure

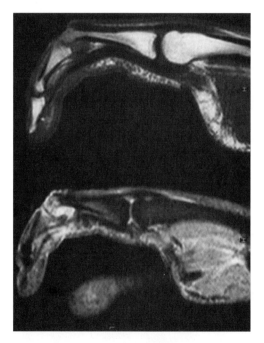

Fig. 7. MRI images in a patient who has SSc and flexion contracture, showing osteomyelitis beneath an ulcer overlying the proximal interphalangeal joint. The top image is a T1 weighted image showing cortical loss of the head of the proximal phalanx and low signal within the bone marrow and surrounding soft tissue. The lower image is a STIR sequence showing areas of high signal at the same areas. These findings are consistent with bone infection.

measurements at different finger temperatures give an index of digital artery involvement [32,33]. Because these techniques are being continually refined and new applications developed, the separation between clinical and research methodologies is somewhat arbitrary and likely to change over the next 5 to 10 years.

Imaging of peripheral vascular disease

Different imaging modalities are complementary because they examine different aspects of vascular structure and function. Those selected for further discussion are relevant to the rheumatologist because they inform management or are important research tools. These modalities include (1) nailfold capillaroscopy, which assesses microvascular structure; (2) thermography, which gives an indirect assessment of small and large vessel function; (3) conventional (radiographic), MRI, and CT angiography, all of which assess large vessel structure; and (4) laser Doppler imaging, which assesses microvascular function.

Nailfold capillaroscopy

Widefield microscopy
Method. Nailfold capillaroscopy is entirely noninvasive. At the nailfold, capillaries run parallel to the epidermis and can be examined under a light microscope at a magnification of ×12 to ×14 [34]. A drop of oil is applied to improve visualization. The distal row of capillaries normally appears as hairpin loops (Fig. 1a), formed by the column of red blood cells moving through the capillary (the actual walls of the capillary are not visible). Although ideally all nail beds should be examined, if this is not possible (eg, because of time constraints), then experts have suggested 'it has been suggested...' that it is probably best to examine at least the ring fingers [35]. If widefield microscopy is not available, the nailfold capillaries can usually be visualized using an opthalmoscope [36] or handheld dermatoscope [37], again after a drop of oil is applied.

Applications. Nailfold microscopy is a well-established technique for predicting underlying connective tissue disease in patients presenting with Raynaud's phenomenon [38,39], in whom abnormal capillaroscopy has been estimated to confer a relative risk for developing SSc on the order of 13 [40]. Although subtle changes on capillaroscopy have been reported in patients who have PRP [41,42], a scleroderma pattern should not occur. The capillary abnormalities occurring in scleroderma-spectrum disorders were by Maricq and colleagues over 30 years ago [43] and include enlarged capillary loops, areas of avascularity disruption of the normal capillary bed and areas of haemorrhage [34]. Since then, other investigators have undertaken cross-sectional studies of nailfold capillaroscopy at different magnifications. Many of these studies have been qualitative, but some have been semiquantitative or included measurement of capillary dimensions [44–51].

Videomicroscopy

Method. Videomicroscopy is an extension of the widefield technique in which the microscope, connected to a video camera, incorporates a light-emitting diode/fiberoptic light source. The magnification ($\times 200$–$\times 600$) is very much higher than with the widefield technique, allowing measurement of dimensions of individual capillaries, such as arterial, venous, and apical loop width, and of capillary density [42]. These dimensions can be averaged over an entire nailfold or over (for example) five consecutive capillaries [52].

Using commercially available systems, only a small section of the nailbed is visualized at a time because of the high magnification. More recently developed systems are entirely digitized and newly developed software allows a mosaic of images to be constructed, combining the advantages of high magnification with a panoramic image of the whole nail bed and allowing nail beds to be tracked over time [53].

Application. Some specialist centers use videomicroscopy rather than widefield microscopy to assess patients who have Raynaud's phenomenon or SSc. Cutola and colleagues [39] proposed classifying scleroderma-spectrum capillary abnormalities into early, active, and late; an association may exist between capillaroscopy pattern and disease subtype and autoantibody status [54]. A key challenge is to be able to monitor digital microvascular disease progression and treatment response and thereby exploit this unique window into the digital microcirculation [55].

Thermography

Method

Infrared thermography is a noninvasive technique that measures surface temperature, and is therefore an indirect measure of blood flow, in both small and large vessels. It requires expensive equipment that should ideally be used in a temperature- and humidity-controlled laboratory. Therefore, its use is restricted to specialist centers, although it has been suggested that portable radiometry may provide a less-expensive option [56].

Applications

Dynamic imaging, examining rewarming response to a cold challenge, may differentiate between healthy controls and patients who have PRP or SSc [57–60], although results are conflicting. Cherkas and colleagues [61] reported that a cold challenge test did not help to differentiate between 175 patients who had Raynaud's phenomenon and 404 controls in a population setting, and Schufried and colleagues [62] similarly reported that the precold challenge (ie, baseline) temperatures were more useful than dynamic measurements in distinguishing between individuals who had Raynaud's phenomenon and those who did not. In patients who have Raynaud's phenomenon, a heat challenge may be more specific of underlying connective tissue disease than parameters derived from the cold challenge [63]. In a retrospective study, a temperature gradient between any fingertip and the dorsum of the hand of greater than 1°C (fingers cooler) at a room temperature of 30°C was found to have a positive predictive value of 70% and a negative predictive value of 82% in identifying patients in whom Raynaud's phenomenon was associated with SSc [64]. Prospective studies are now required. As with many tests of vascular physiology, concerns exist about the reproducibility of these dynamic protocols, with large intrasubject standard deviations [63]. Therefore, investigators who include thermography as an outcome measure in studies of vasoactive treatments should include details about reproducibility of their protocol.

Angiography

Methods

Angiographic techniques have evolved considerably in recent years, and large vessels may now be assessed using conventional (radiographic), MRI, or CT angiography.

Radiographic angiography provides excellent visualization of the vessel lumen, showing stenosis, occlusions, aneurysms, and other irregularities (Fig. 8). However, it is invasive and involves a high contrast and radiation load. Modern methods, such as digital subtraction angiography, improve image quality with smaller doses of contrast. MRI angiography does not involve arterial puncture, and visualizes not only the lumen but also the vessel wall and surrounding structures. Spiral CT angiography also allows three-dimensional imaging of vessels and surrounding structures. Scanning times are shorter than for MRI, but it involves ionizing radiation and intravenous contrast.

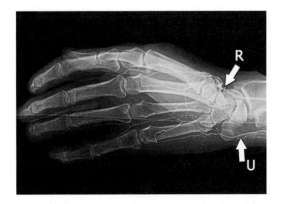

Fig. 8. Arteriogram of the right hand in a patient who has SSc showing occluded distal ulnar artery (U) with collateral circulation and occluded radial artery (R) with collateral circulation. Acro-osteolysis of several of the fingertips has occurred.

Applications

The main indication for angiography in patients who have SSc is to identify whether a proximal lesion is amenable to angioplasty or surgery in evaluating severe digital ischemia [13]. MRI angiography will usually show this, obviating the need for intra-arterial angiography. Contrast-enhanced MRI angiography of the hand is being advocated to visualize the vasculature before surgery [65], but this technique has been little applied in patients who have SSc, and surgeons are still likely to request intra-arterial angiography to demarcate the anatomy of these more distal arteries if they are considering arterial reconstruction of the wrist or hand. Therefore, conventional radiographic angiography remains the gold standard, and a patient with lower limb arterial disease has the advantage, because if a lesion is detected, it may be treated by angioplasty during the same procedure.

Laser Doppler

Method

Laser Doppler measures microvascular perfusion. Single-probe laser Doppler flowmetry suffers from its large site-to-site variation, which limits the usefulness of the technique in comparing blood flow between sites and monitoring change over time. Laser Doppler imaging (LDI), or scanning laser Doppler, measures blood flow over an area rather than at a single point [66]. Another advantage is that it does not require direct contact between the probe and the skin (which might affect blood flow). Thermographic and LDI results correlate poorly, and therefore the two methods cannot substitute for each other [67].

Applications

The use of laser Doppler in patients who have SSc is currently confined to research [68,69]. Many investigators have used laser Doppler flowmetry to assess treatment response, as in a recent study of phosphodiesterase inhibition [70]. As with thermography, longitudinal studies must include estimates of reproducibility. Recent developments in LDI, including faster scanning speeds and the use of different wavelengths to probe different levels of microcirculation, increase its potential usefulness in studying pathophysiology and monitoring disease progression and treatment response. For example, studies with dual-wavelength LDI recently suggested that the microvascular functional abnormality of SSc is confined to the digits (as opposed to affecting the hand more proximally) [71].

Conclusions

The assessment of peripheral vascular disease in patients who have suspected or established SSc depends on a careful history and examination complemented by a small panel of investigations, including vascular imaging. In patients presenting with critical ischemia, a high index of suspicion of concomitant large vessel disease must be present, because failure to diagnose this may miss a lesion amenable to intervention.

Management

The first principle of management is to establish the diagnosis. Raynaud's phenomenon in the patient who has SSc is almost invariably part of the disease process (vasospasm against the background of a noninflammatory microangiopathy), but in the context of severe/critical peripheral ischemia, other possibilities should be considered, especially proximal vessel disease but also vasculitis or a coagulopathy. Although this section provides a broad overview of management, it will emphasize recent advances since the management of peripheral vascular disease was last reviewed in *Rheumatic Disease Clinics of North America* [72], with some discussion of future treatment approaches. Management will be considered under the headings of general (nondrug) measures, drug treatment, surgery, and management of the severe digital ischemic episode, with or without ulceration.

General (nondrug) measures

Patient education in keeping warm and avoiding cold exposure is very important, as described in information leaflets produced by patient support groups. Patients should be strongly advised to stop smoking because, in patients who have SSc, cigarette smoking is a risk factor for severity of digital ischaemia [73], and should, if possible, avoid drugs with vasoconstrictive effects. For patients who develop digital ulcers, optimal wound care is clearly an important part of management. However, topical therapies/dressings for SSc-related digital ulcers have been little researched.

Drug treatment

The number of clinical trials of drug treatment in SSc-related Raynaud's phenomenon is disappointing, and the clinical trials that exist usually involve only small numbers of patients. For instance, a meta-analysis of calcium channel blockers [74], the group of drugs most commonly used in SSc-associated Raynaud's phenomenon, included data on only 109 patients from eight trials. Clinical trials of Raynaud's phenomenon are complicated by a large placebo effect, the need to study patients over the winter months, and a lack of objective outcome measures. Therefore, a key challenge is to develop robust outcome measures that are sensitive to change; this would facilitate clinical trials by allowing them to be adequately powered with smaller numbers of patients than is currently possible.

The drugs used in SSc-associated peripheral vascular disease have one or more of the following properties: (1) enhance vasodilation, (2) inhibit vasoconstriction, (3) reduce endothelial injury, and (4) inhibit platelet aggregation/procoagulant tendency [3].

Although a good rationale exists for using drugs in combination, currently no evidence base supports this approach, and clinical trials examining different combinations will probably not be undertaken in the foreseeable future. However, the pragmatic approach is to combine therapies when a single drug is ineffective, especially if the different drugs prescribed have complementary actions.

Calcium channel blockers

Calcium channel blockers act on vascular smooth muscle to cause arterial vasodilation. They also have antiplatelet effects [75] and may reduce oxidative stress [76]. They are generally considered first-line treatment in SSc-related Raynaud's phenomenon. In their meta-analysis, Thompson and colleagues [74] suggested that the mean reduction in Raynaud's attacks over 2 weeks was 8.3, with a greater than 35% improvement over placebo in attack severity. Although side effects such as flushing and edema are common, these may be minimized by using a sustained-release preparation and commencing with a low dosage. The concern also exists that by reducing lower esophageal sphincter pressure, calcium channel blockers may exacerbate upper gastrointestinal problems [77]. Sustained-release nifedipine and amlodipine are commonly prescribed, and other dihydropyridines are also used [78].

Angiotensin-converting enzyme inhibitors and angiotensin II receptor antagonists

A strong rationale exists for using angiotensin-converting enzyme (ACE) inhibitors and angiotensin II receptor antagonists in SSc-related peripheral vascular disease. Angiotensin II is not only vasoconstrictive but also profibrotic, and, in addition to preventing vasoconstriction, ACE inhibitors have effects on endothelial function [79] and vascular remodeling [80].

However, few studies have been conducted on ACE inhibition in Raynaud's phenomenon. A recent multicenter, double-blind, placebo-controlled trial of 210 patients who had either limited cutaneous SSc (186 patients) or antibody-positive Raynaud's (24 patients) reported that 2 to 3 years of treatment with the ACE inhibitor quinapril conferred no benefit on peripheral vascular manifestations [81]. Losartan, 50 mg/d, an angiotensin II type 1 receptor antagonist, was found in an open-label, randomized, parallel-group trial of 12 weeks of treatment to reduce frequency and severity of Raynaud's attacks, whereas nifedipine, 20 mg daily, was not associated with significant benefit [82]. The effect of losartan was greater in patients who had PRP (12 patients treated with losartan) than in those who had SSc (14 treated with losartan) [82]. A larger double-blind study is required to establish the role of angiotensin II receptor antagonists in SSc-related peripheral vascular disease, but in the meantime, these or ACE inhibitors seem a reasonable choice if calcium channel blockers are either ineffective or not tolerated.

α-Adrenergic blockers

α-Adrenergic blockers also have been little studied in Raynaud's phenomenon. A Cochrane review in 1998 included two trials and concluded that prazosin had modest efficacy compared with placebo in Raynaud's secondary to SSc [83]. Considerable interest has recently been shown in the α_{2C}-adrenoceptor, which is cold sensitive [84]. Although very much in the future, selective blockade of α_{2C}-adrenoceptors may be an exciting new avenue of therapy [85].

Prostanoids

Prostanoids may confer benefit in SSc-related peripheral vascular disease through several mechanisms. They are powerful vasodilators, they inhibit platelet aggregation, they may have effects on vascular remodeling [86], and intravenous iloprost has been shown to suppress the profibrotic cytokine, connective tissue growth factor [87], and circulating levels of adhesion molecules [88].

In the United Kingdom, intravenous prostanoids are the mainstay of management for acute digital ischemia. A meta-analysis examining prostaglandin analogs in SSc concluded that intravenous iloprost, a stable analog of prostacyclin (PGI2, epoprostenol), was effective in reducing both frequency and severity of ischemic attacks and in the healing of digital ulceration [89]. A retrospective study of 15 children who had connective tissue disease (six who had SSc) reported that iloprost was a safe and effective treatment for digital ischemia/ulceration [90].

Several different regimes for iloprost administration have been studied [91–94], but the one that is probably most used involves daily infusions of 0.5 to 2.0 ng/kg per minute for 5 days, each infusion lasting 6 hours [92]. Intravenous prostanoids require hospitalization, and an oral preparation would clearly be preferable. However, trials of oral prostanoids in SSc-related Raynaud's have been disappointing [95,96]. Longer-term clinical trials of oral prostanoids are required to establish whether these provide symptomatic relief or vascular protection in SSc-related peripheral vascular disease. Currently, oral prostanoids are not generally available for prescription.

Supplementation of the L-arginine/nitric oxide pathway, including with phosphodiesterase inhibitors

Nitric oxide (NO) is a potent vasodilator. Several groups of investigators have examined its administration in patients who had primary and secondary Raynaud's, either directly through NO donation or its precursor L-arginine [97,98]. Topical glyceryl trinitrate, an NO donor, administered through patch, was effective in both primary and SSc-related Raynaud's phenomenon but had side effects because of its systemic absorption [99]. Therefore, the feasibility of using topical NO donors to produce local but not systemic vasodilation has been examined in short-term physiologic studies [100–102]. The purely local effect of topical glyceryl trinitrate was shown by the fact that blood flow was increased in the treated but not the adjacent finger

[102]. Considerable interest currently exists in developing and trialing systems of topical NO donation in patients who have Raynaud's phenomenon, and therapeutic studies of topical treatment will probably be published in the next 5 years.

Phosphodiesterase type 5 inhibitors enhance the effect of NO through inhibiting degradation of cyclic guanosine monophosphate. Several recent studies and case reports describe benefit in Raynaud's phenomenon [70,103–105], although Friedman and colleagues [106] reported that a single dose of tadalafil did not inhibit cold-induced vasoconstriction in a study of 20 patients who had Raynaud's (18 of whom had PRP). In a double-blind, placebo-controlled crossover study that included 16 patients who had secondary Raynaud's (14 who had SSc), Fries and colleagues [104] reported benefit from 4 weeks of treatment with sildenafil, 50 mg twice daily. In these 16 patients, frequency of attacks, cumulative attack duration, and Raynaud's Condition Score were reduced, and capillary perfusion increased on sildenafil compared with placebo, although the study was not truly blinded, because all patients correctly guessed their order of treatment [104]. An earlier double-blind clinical trial of cilostazol, a phosphodiesterase type 3 inhibitor used to treat intermittent claudication [26], reported an increase in brachial artery diameter in PRP and Raynaud's secondary to connective tissue disease (7 of 20 patients who had connective tissue disease had SSc) but no improvement in symptoms after 6 weeks of treatment [107]. Further clinical trials of longer duration are required to establish the role of phosphodiesterase inhibition in SSc-related digital ischemia.

Endothelin-1 receptor antagonists

Endothelin (ET)-1 has been strongly implicated in the pathogenesis of SSc. It is a potent vasoconstrictor, is profibrotic, and has effects on vascular remodeling [108,109]. Its expression is increased in sclerodermatous skin [110].

The effects of ET-1 are mediated through ET_A and ET_B receptors, and recently considerable interest has been shown in ET-1 receptor antagonism as a treatment for digital ischemia in SSc. Two recent large multicenter, double-blind controlled clinical trials [111,112] (the second, which included 188 patients, so far reported only in abstract form [112]) examined the effects of bosentan, a nonpeptide antagonist of both the ET_A and ET_B receptors, on SSc-related digital ulcers. Both studies showed that bosentan reduced the number of new digital ulcers but had no effect on the healing of existing ulcers. In the study by Korn and colleagues [111] of 122 patients who had SSc, the number of new ulcers during the 16-week study period was 1.4 in the bosentan group versus 2.7 in the placebo-treated group, with the effect being more marked in those who had digital ulcers on study entry, who were more likely to develop new ulcers (1.8 in the bosentan subgroup, and 3.6 in the placebo subgroup). The number of patients with four or more new ulcers was markedly reduced in those treated with bosentan, and hand function improved

[111]. Therefore, ET-1 antagonism should be considered, especially in patients who have multiple recurrent ulcers refractory to other therapies.

Other vasodilator therapies

Serotonin is a vasoconstrictor, therefore serotonin antagonists may have benefit in treating SSc. However, a meta-analysis suggested that ketanserin, a serotonin receptor antagonist, did not confer clinical benefit in patients who have SSc-related Raynaud's phenomenon [113]. Moreover, katanserin is no longer available in the United States or United Kingdom because of its side effect profile.

Another approach to opposing the actions of serotonin is to inhibit its uptake. An open label, crossover pilot study of 53 patients suggested that fluoxetine, a selective serotonin reuptake inhibitor, was beneficial in both primary and secondary Raynaud's phenomenon [114]. Attack frequency and severity were significantly reduced during the 6-week treatment period with fluoxetine but not with nifedipine [114]. Serotonin reuptake inhibitors therefore warrant further study.

Other drug therapies

Because of the complex pathogenesis of SSc, various possible therapeutic targets exist in SSc-related peripheral vascular disease, including antioxidant therapy and antithrombotic/antiplatelet agents. In the author's opinion, these have not been adequately researched and currently evidence is insufficient to recommend either approach.

Antioxidants

Despite considerable evidence that oxidative stress is implicated in the pathogenesis of SSc [115], few controlled clinical trials have examined the effects of antioxidants in Raynaud's phenomenon. Twelve weeks of treatment with 500 mg of probucol was associated with a reduction in the frequency and severity of Raynaud's attacks and a rise in oxidation lag time in a parallel group study of 40 patients who had Raynaud's phenomenon (20 of whom had SSc) [116]. However, neither 10 weeks of treatment with a combination of micronutrient antioxidants and allopurinol (which blocks superoxide by way of xanthine oxidase) [117] nor 3 weeks of vitamin E alone [118] conferred benefit in patients who had SSc, although most patients in these studies had well-established disease and it is likely that for antioxidant therapy to be effective it must be given early, before irreversible vascular injury has occurred.

Drugs with antithrombotic effects

Platelet activation is well described in patients who have SSc. Although it therefore seems reasonable to give low-dose aspirin to patients who have severe digital ischemia or digital ulceration based on the fact that this may improve digital microvascular perfusion, antiplatelet agents have been little studied in SSc [119]. Several drugs used in treating SSc-related digital ischemia, including prostanoids and calcium channel blockers, have antiplatelet effects. Open studies have suggested that low molecular weight heparin [120] and tissue plasminogen activator followed by warfarin [121] may confer benefit in severe Raynaud's, but it is difficult to recommend these therapies without further data from studies involving larger numbers of patients.

Botulinum toxin

Recently, it has been suggested that botulinum toxin may confer benefit in severe vasospasm [122]. However, further studies are required before this treatment can be recommended

Surgery

Only few patients are treated surgically. The most common form of surgery is debridement of infected or necrotic tissue. In this clinical context it is best to seek a surgical opinion early, because once bone infection is established, amputation is more likely to be necessary.

Cervical sympathectomy is now only rarely recommended for SSc-related Raynaud's phenomenon. However, experience has recently increased in digital artery (palmar) sympathectomy [123–127]. Some benefit is likely to come from the adventitial strip/mechanical decompression rather than from the sympathectomy itself [123]. Decompression arteriolysis of the radial and ulnar arteries proximal to the wrist and vascular reconstruction may also be performed concurrently, if indicated [18,125]. Taylor and colleagues [18] reported that all of their eight patients who underwent ulnar artery revascularization concurrently with digital sympathectomy experienced ulcer healing. Digital artery sympathectomy is a highly specialized procedure that should be performed only in specialist centers, because a significant proportion of patients who have connective tissue disease develop postoperative complications [126].

If patients have proximal arterial disease, angioplasty or proximal vascular reconstruction may be indicated and should be discussed with vascular surgical colleagues. Finally, if an area of calcinosis is underlying a nonhealing ulcer, surgery should be considered to debulk the calcinosis [127], although the risks and benefits of digital surgery set against the background of a compromised blood supply must be carefully explained to the patient.

Therapy of an acute exacerbation of digital ischemia/ulceration

When patients who have SSc develop a severe exacerbation of digital ischemia—a permanently cyanosed, painful digit, or digital ulceration (see Figs. 4 and 5; Fig. 9)—this is a medical emergency usually requiring hospitalization. These patients have a high risk of losing the digit. Ideally, an open-door policy should be established to allow early assessment and treatment.

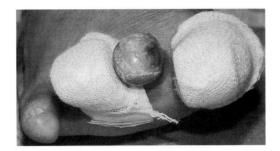

Fig. 9. Infected, necrotic ulceration of the right second toe in a patient who has SSc. The toe is cyanosed. The fourth toe has been amputated. (*Courtesy of* Salford Royal NHS Foundation Trust, Salford, UK, with permission. Copyright © Salford Royal NHS Foundation Trust.)

The key points in management are intravenous prostanoids, antibiotics if an infection is suspected, consideration of surgical debridement of any collection of pus or necrotic/ischemic tissue (to be suspected if the fingertip is exquisitely tender), and adequate analgesia. SSc-related digital ischemia is often excruciatingly painful and opiates may be required temporarily. A temporary sympathetic block could be considered if patients remain in severe pain [128], although local anesthetic blocks for acute digital ischemia have not been formally studied in clinical trials.

Although severe digital ischemia/ulceration in patients who have connective tissue disease usually has a microvascular basis, patients who have SSc are at increased risk for macrovascular disease and therefore large vessel occlusion, and other possible causes for digital ischemia (vasculitis/thrombosis), should always be considered.

Conclusions

In most patients, the treatment goal is to control symptoms using a combination of nondrug measures and vasodilators, but this can be difficult in severe disease because currently available treatments are not ideal. Calcium channel blockers are the first line in drug treatment. A key issue is whether vascular protective drugs, such as ACE inhibitors, prostanoids, or ET-1 receptor antagonists, should be prescribed to prevent vascular disease progression. The answer to this question must await controlled clinical trials. Critical ischemia/ulceration is a medical emergency usually requiring hospitalization.

Summary

Diagnosis and management of peripheral vascular disease in patients who have SSc present different challenges according to the clinical context. In patients presenting with Raynaud's phenomenon, whether an underlying scleroderma-spectrum disorder exists must be established. If not, the patient can be reassured, but if so, the patient is likely to require long-term follow-up. In patients who have SSc and severe/critical ischemia, treatable contributory causes, especially proximal vessel disease, must be excluded.

In the past 5 years, considerable progress has been made, with new treatments being researched in physiologic studies and clinical trials. The networking of clinicians with an interest in SSc has been a major step forward, allowing multicenter studies involving large numbers of patients. The development and validation of new outcome measures for monitoring peripheral vascular disease progression and treatment response will further facilitate future trials. Increased understanding of the underlying SSc disease process and how to measure the associated peripheral vascular disease is leading—and will continue to lead—to new approaches to therapy.

Acknowledgment

I am grateful to Dr. Charles Hutchinson for the radiology images.

References

[1] LeRoy EC, Medsger TA. Raynaud's phenomenon: a proposal for classification. Clin Exp Rheumatol 1992;10:485–8.
[2] Masi AT, Rodnan GP, Medsger TA, et al. Preliminary criteria for the classification of systemic sclerosis (scleroderma). Arthritis Rheum 1980;23:581–90.
[3] Herrick AL. Pathogenesis of Raynaud's phenomenon. Rheumatology 2005;44:587–96.
[4] Campbell PM, LeRoy EC. Pathogenesis of systemic sclerosis: a vascular hypothesis. Semin Arthritis Rheum 1975;4:351–68.
[5] LeRoy EC. Systemic sclerosis. A vascular perspective. Rheum Dis Clin North Am 1996;22: 675–94.
[6] Herrick AL. Vascular function in systemic sclerosis. Curr Opin Rheumatol 2000;12:527–33.
[7] Rodnan GP, Myerowitz RL, Justh GO. Morphological changes in the digital arteries of patients with progressive systemic sclerosis (scleroderma) and Raynaud phenomenon. Medicine 1980;59:393–408.
[8] Veale DJ, Collidge TA, Belch JJF. Increased prevalence of symptomatic macrovascular disease in systemic sclerosis. Ann Rheum Dis 1995;54:853–5.
[9] Ho M, Veale D, Eastmond C, et al. Macrovascular disease and systemic sclerosis. Ann Rheum Dis 2000;59:39–43.
[10] Youseff P, Brama T, Englert H, et al. Limited scleroderma is associated with increased prevalence of macrovascular disease. J Rheumatol 1995;22:469–72.
[11] Wan MC, Moore T, Hollis S, et al. Ankle brachial pressure index in systemic sclerosis: influence of disease subtype and anticentromere antibody. Rheumatology 2001;40: 1102–5.
[12] Bartoli F, Angotti C, Fatini C, et al. Angiotensin-converting enzyme I/D polymorphism and macrovascular disease in systemic sclerosis. Rheumatology 2007;46:772–5.
[13] Hasegawa M, Nagai Y, Tamura A, et al. Arteriographic evaluation of vascular changes of the extremities in patients with systemic sclerosis. Br J Dermatol 2006;155:1159–64.
[14] Dabich I, Bookstein JJ, Zweifler A, et al. Digital arteries in patients with scleroderma: arteriographic and plethysmographic study. Arch Intern Med 1972;130:708–14.

[15] Janevski B. Arteries of the hand in patients with scleroderma. Diagn Imaging Clin Med 1986;55:262–5.

[16] Stucker M, Quinna S, Memmel U, et al. Macroangiopathy of the upper extremities in progressive systemic sclerosis. Eur J Med Res 2000;5:295–302.

[17] Stafford L, Englert H, Gover J, et al. Distribution of macrovascular disease in scleroderma. Ann Rheum Dis 1998;57:476–9.

[18] Taylor MH, McFadden JA, Bolster MB, et al. Ulnar artery involvement in systemic sclerosis (scleroderma). J Rheumatol 2002;29:102–6.

[19] Oddis CV, Eisenbeis CH, Reidbord HE, et al. Vasculitis in systemic sclerosis: association with Sjögren's syndrome and the CREST syndrome. J Rheumatol 1987;14:942–8.

[20] Sari-Kouzel H, Herrick AL, Freemont AJ, et al. Giant cell arteritis in a patient with limited cutaneous systemic sclerosis. Rheumatology 1999;38:479–80.

[21] Shapiro LS. Large vessel arterial thrombosis in systemic sclerosis associated with antiphospholipid antibodies. J Rheumatol 1990;17:685–8.

[22] Brennan P, Silman A, Black C, et al. Validity and reliability of three methods used in the diagnosis of Raynaud's phenomenon. Br J Rheumatol 1993;32:357–61.

[23] Maricq HR, Weinrich MC. Diagnosis of Raynaud's phenomenon assisted by color charts. J Rheumatol 1988;15:454–9.

[24] Harper FE, Maricq HR, Turner RE, et al. A prospective study of Raynaud phenomenon and early connective tissue disease. Am J Med 1982;72:883–8.

[25] Spencer-Green G. Outcomes in primary Raynaud phenomenon. A meta-analysis of the frequency, rates, and predictors of transition to secondary diseases. Arch Intern Med 1998;158:595–600.

[26] White C. Intermittent claudication. N Engl J Med 2007;356:1241–50.

[27] Wigley FM, Wise RA, Miller R, et al. Anticentromere antibody as a predictor of digital ischemic loss in patients with systemic sclerosis. Arthritis Rheum 1992;35:688–93.

[28] Herrick AL, Haeney M, Hollis S, et al. Anticardiolipin, anticentromere and anti-Scl-70 antibodies in patients with systemic sclerosis and severe digital ischaemia. Ann Rheum Dis 1994;53:540–2.

[29] Merkel PA, Herlyn K, Martin RW, et al. Measuring disease activity and functional status in patients with scleroderma and Raynaud's phenomenon. Arthritis Rheum 2002;46: 2410–20.

[30] Medsger TA, Silman AJ, Steen VD, et al. A disease severity scale for systemic sclerosis: development and testing. J Rheumatol 1999;26:2159–67.

[31] Herrick AL, Clark S. Quantifying digital vascular disease in patients with primary Raynaud's phenomenon and systemic sclerosis. Ann Rheum Dis 1998;57:70–8.

[32] Neilson SL. Raynaud phenomenon and finger systolic pressure during cooling. Scand J Clin Lab Invest 1978;38:765–70.

[33] Maricq HR, Weinrich MC, Valter I, et al. Digital vascular responses to cooling in subjects with cold sensitivity, primary Raynaud's phenomenon, or scleroderma-spectrum disorders. J Rheumatol 1996;23:2068–78.

[34] Maricq HR. Widefield capillary microscopy. Technique and rating scale for abnormalities seen in scleroderma and related disorders. Arthritis Rheum 1981;24:1159–65.

[35] Houtman PM, Kallenberg CGM, Fidler V, et al. Diagnostic significance of nailfold capillary patterns in patients with Raynaud's phenomenon. J Rheumatol 1986;13:556–63.

[36] Anders HJ, Sigl T, Schattenkirchner M. Differentiation between primary and secondary Raynaud's phenomenon: a prospective study comparing nailfold capillaroscopy using an opthalmoscope or stereomicroscope. Ann Rheum Dis 2001;60:407–9.

[37] Bergman R, Sharony L, Shapira D, et al. The handheld dermatoscope as a nail-fold capillaroscopic instrument. Arch Dermatol 2003;139:1027–30.

[38] Maricq HR, Weinberger AB, LeRoy EC. Early detection of scleroderma-spectrum disorders by in vivo capillary microscopy. J Rheumatol 1982;9:289–91.

[39] Cutolo M, Grassi W, Matucci Cerinic M. Raynaud's phenomenon and the role of capillaro-scopy. Arthritis Rheum 2003;11:3023–30.

[40] Carpentier PH, Maricq HR. Microvasculature in systemic sclerosis. Rheum Dis Clin North Am 1990;16:75–91.

[41] Statham BN, Rowell NR. Quantification of the nail fold capillary abnormalities in systemic sclerosis and Raynaud's syndrome. Acta Derm Venereol (Stockh) 1986;66:139–43.

[42] Bukhari M, Herrick AL, Moore T, et al. Increased nailfold capillary dimensions in primary Raynaud's phenomenon and systemic sclerosis. Br J Rheumatol 1996;35:1127–31.

[43] Maricq HR, LeRoy EC. Patterns of finger capillary abnormalities in connective tissue disease by 'wide-field' microscopy. Arthritis Rheum 1973;16:619–28.

[44] Lee P, Leung FY, Alderdice C, et al. Nailfold capillary microscopy in the connective tissue diseases: a semiquantitative assessment. J Rheumatol 1983;10:930–8.

[45] Lee P, Sarkozi J, Bookman AA, et al. Digital blood flow and nailfold capillary microscopy in Raynaud's phenomenon. J Rheumatol 1986;13:564–9.

[46] Lefford F, Edwards JCW. Nailfold capillary microscopy in connective tissue disease: a quantitative morphological analysis. Ann Rheum Dis 1986;45:741–9.

[47] Ter Borg EJ, Piersma-Wichers G, Smit AJ, et al. Serial nailfold capillary microscopy in primary Raynaud's phenomenon and scleroderma. Semin Arthritis Rheum 1994;24: 40–7.

[48] Michoud E, Poensin D, Carpentier PH. Digitized nailfold capillaroscopy. Vasa 1994;23: 35–42.

[49] Kabasakal Y, Elvins DM, Ring EFJ, et al. Quantitative nailfold capillaroscopy findings in a population with connective tissue disease and in normal healthy controls. Ann Rheum Dis 1996;55:507–12.

[50] Wildt M, Hesselstrand R, Scheja A, et al. Capillary density in patients with systemic sclerosis, as determined by microscopy counts and compared with computer-based analy-sis. Clin Exp Rheumatol 1999;17:219–22.

[51] Nagy Z, Czirjak L. Nailfold digital capillaroscopy in 447 patients with connective tissue disease and Raynaud's disease. J Eur Acad Dermatol Venereol 2004;18:62–8.

[52] Bukhari M, Hollis S, Moore T, et al. Quantitation of microcirculatory abnormalities in patients with primary Raynaud's phenomenon and systemic sclerosis by video capillaro-scopy. Rheumatology 2000;39:506–12.

[53] Anderson ME, Allen PD, Moore T, et al. Computerized nailfold video capillaroscopy— a new tool for the assessment of Raynaud's phenomenon. J Rheumatol 2005;32:841–8.

[54] Cutolo M, Pizzorni C, Tuccio M, et al. Nailfold videocapillaroscopic patterns and serum autoantibodies in systemic sclerosis. Rheumatology 2004;43:719–26.

[55] Moore TL, Vail A, Herrick AL. Assessment of digital vascular structure and function in response to bosentan in patients with systemic sclerosis-related Raynaud's phenomenon. Rheumatology 2007;46:363–4.

[56] Cherkas LF, Howell K, Carter L, et al. The use of portable radiometry to access Raynaud's phenomenon: a practical alternative to thermal imaging. Rheumatology 2001;40:1384–7.

[57] Kyle V, Parr G, Salisbury R, et al. Prostaglandin E1 vasospastic disease and thermography. Ann Rheum Dis 1985;44:73–8.

[58] Darton K, Black CM. Pyroelectric vidicon thermography and cold challenge quantify the severity of Raynaud's phenomenon. Br J Rheumatol 1991;30:190–5.

[59] O'Reilly D, Taylor L, El-Hadidy K, et al. Measurement of cold challenge responses in primary Raynaud's phenomenon and Raynaud's phenomenon associated with systemic sclerosis. Ann Rheum Dis 1992;51:1193–6.

[60] Foerster J, Kuerth A, Neiderstrasser E, et al. A cold-response index for the assessment of Raynaud's phenomenon. J Dermatol Sci 2007;45:113–20.

[61] Cherkas LF, Carter L, Spector T, et al. Use of thermographic criteria to identify Raynaud's phenomenon in a population setting. J Rheumatol 2003;30:720–2.

[62] Schufried O, Vacariu G, Lang T, et al. Thermographic parameters in the diagnosis of secondary Raynaud's phenomenon. Arch Phys Med Rehabil 2000;81:495–9.

[63] Clark S, Hollis S, Campbell F, et al. The 'distal-dorsal difference' as a possible predictor of secondary Raynaud's phenomenon. J Rheumatol 1999;26:1125–8.

[64] Anderson ME, Moore TL, Lunt M, et al. The 'distal-dorsal difference': a thermographic parameter by which to differentiate between primary and secondary Raynaud's phenomenon. Rheumatology 2007;46:533–8.

[65] Connell DA, Koulouris G, Thorn DA, et al. Contrast-enhanced MR angiography of the hand. Radiographics 2002;22:583–99.

[66] Murray A, Herrick AL, King TA. Laser Doppler imaging: a developing technique for application in the rheumatic diseases. Rheumatology 2004;43:1210–8.

[67] Clark S, Dunn G, Moore T, et al. Comparison of thermography and laser Doppler imaging in the assessment of Raynaud's phenomenon. Microvasc Res 2003;66:73–6.

[68] Seifalian AM, Stansby G, Jackson A, et al. Comparison of laser Doppler perfusion imaging, laser Doppler flowmetry, and thermographic imaging for assessment of blood flow in human skin. Eur J Vasc Surg 1994;8:65–9.

[69] Clark S, Campbell F, Moore T, et al. Laser Doppler imaging—a new technique for quantifying microcirculatory flow in patients with primary Raynaud's phenomenon and systemic sclerosis. Microvasc Res 1999;57:284–91.

[70] Caglayan E, Huntegeburth M, Karasch T, et al. Phosphodiesterase type 5 inhibition is a novel therapeutic option in Raynaud disease. Arch Intern Med 2006;166:231–3.

[71] Murray AK, Moore TL, King TA, et al. Abnormal microvascular response is localized to the digits in patients with systemic sclerosis. Arthritis Rheum 2006;54:1952–60.

[72] Hummers LK, Wigley FM. Management of Raynaud's phenomenon and digital ischemic lesions in scleroderma. Rheum Dis Clin North Am 2003;29:293–313.

[73] Harrison BJ, Silman AJ, Hider SL, et al. Cigarette smoking as a significant risk factor for digital vascular disease in patients with systemic sclerosis. Arthritis Rheum 2002;46:3312–6.

[74] Thompson AE, Shea B, Welch V, et al. Calcium-channel blockers for Raynaud's phenomenon in systemic sclerosis. Arthritis Rheum 2001;44:1841–7.

[75] Malamet R, Wise RA, Ettinger WH, et al. Nifedipine in the treatment of Raynaud's phenomenon. Evidence for inhibition of platelet activation. Am J Med 1985;78:602–8.

[76] Allanore Y, Borderie D, Lemarechal H, et al. Acute and sustained effects of dihydropyridine-type calcium channel antagonists on oxidative stress in systemic sclerosis. Am J Med 2004;116:595–600.

[77] Kahan A, Bour B, Couturier D, et al. Nifedipine and esophageal dysfunction in progressive systemic sclerosis. A controlled manometric study. Arthritis Rheum 1985;28:490–5.

[78] Sturgill MG, Seibold JR. Rational use of calcium-channel antagonists in Raynaud's phenomenon. Curr Opin Rheumatol 1998;10:584–8.

[79] Mancini GB, Henry GC, Macaya C, et al. Angiotensin-converting enzyme inhibition with quinapril improves endothelial vasomotor dysfunction in patients with coronary artery disease. The TREND (Trial on Reversing ENdothelial Dysfunction) Study. Circulation 1996;94:258–65.

[80] Chrysant SG. Vascular remodeling: the role of angiotensin-converting enzyme inhibitors. Am Heart J 1998;135:S21–30.

[81] Gliddon AE, Doré CJ, Black CM, et al. Prevention of vascular damage in scleroderma and autoimmune Raynaud's phenomenon: a randomised controlled trial of the ACE-inhibitor quinapril. Arthritis Rheum 2007;56:3837–46.

[82] Dziadzio M, Denton CP, Smith R, et al. Losartan therapy for Raynaud's phenomenon and scleroderma: clinical and biochemical findings in a fifteen-week, randomized, parallel-group, controlled trial. Arthritis Rheum 1999;42:2646–55.

[83] Pope J, Fenlon D, Thompson A, et al. Prazosin for Raynaud's phenomenon in progressive systemic sclerosis. Cochrane Database of Syst Rev 1998;2:CD000956.

[84] Chotani MA, Flavahan S, Mitra S, et al. Silent α 2c-adrenergic receptors enable cold-induced vasoconstriction in cutaneous arteries. Am J Physiol Heart Circ Physiol 2000; 278:H1075–83.

[85] Wise RA, Wigley FM, White B, et al. Efficacy and tolerability of a selective α_{2C}-adrenergic receptor blocker in recovery from cold-induced vasospasm in scleroderma patients. A single-center, double-blind, placebo-controlled, randomized crossover study. Arthritis Rheum 2004;50:3994–4001.

[86] Fishman AP. Pulmonary hypertension—beyond vasodilator therapy. N Engl J Med 1998; 338:321–2.

[87] Stratton R, Shiwen X, Martini G, et al. Iloprost suppresses connective tissue growth factor production in fibroblasts and in the skin of scleroderma patients. J Clin Invest 2001;108: 241–50.

[88] Mittag M, Beckheinrich P, Haustein UF. Systemic sclerosis-related Raynaud's phenomenon: effects of iloprost infusion therapy on serum cytokine, growth factor and soluble adhesion molecule levels. Acta Derm Venereol 2001;81:294–7.

[89] Pope J, Fenlon D, Thompson A, et al. Iloprost and cisaprost for Raynaud's phenomenon in progressive systemic sclerosis. Cochrane Database of Syst Rev 1998;2:CD000953.

[90] Zulian F, Corona F, Gerloni V, et al. Safety and efficacy of iloprost for the treatment of ischaemic digits in paediatric connective tissue diseases. Rheumatology 2004;43:229–33.

[91] Rademaker M, Cooke ED, Almond NE, et al. Comparison of intravenous infusions of iloprost and oral nifedipine in treatment of Raynaud's phenomenon in patients with systemic sclerosis: a double blind randomised study. Br Med J 1989;298:561–4.

[92] Wigley FM, Wise RA, Seibold JR, et al. Intravenous iloprost infusion in patients with Raynaud phenomenon secondary to systemic sclerosis. A multicenter, placebo-controlled, double-blind study. Ann Intern Med 1994;120:199–206.

[93] Scorza R, Caronni M, Mascagni B, et al. Effects of long-term cyclic iloprost therapy in systemic sclerosis with Raynaud's phenomenon. A randomized, controlled study. Clin Exp Rheumatol 2001;19:503–8.

[94] Milio G, Corrado E, Genova C, et al. Iloprost treatment in patients with Raynaud's phenomenon secondary to systemic sclerosis and the quality of life: a new therapeutic protocol. Rheumatology 2006;45:999–1004.

[95] Wigley FM, Korn JH, Csuka ME, et al. Oral iloprost treatment in patients with Raynaud's phenomenon secondary to systemic sclerosis: a multi-center, placebo-controlled, double-blind study. Arthritis Rheum 1998;41:670–7.

[96] Vayssairat M. Preventative effect of an oral prostacyclin analog, beraprost sodium, on digital necrosis in systemic sclerosis. French microcirculation society multicentre group for the study of vascular acrosyndromes. J Rheumatol 1999;26:2173–8.

[97] Khan F, Belch JJF. Skin blood flow in patients with systemic sclerosis and Raynaud's phenomenon: effects of oral L-arginine supplementation. J Rheumatol 1999;26:2389–94.

[98] Freedman RR, Girgis R, Mayes MD. Acute effect of nitric oxide on Raynaud's phenomenon in scleroderma. Lancet 1999;354:739.

[99] Teh LS, Manning J, Moore T, et al. Sustained-release transdermal glyceryl trinitrate patches as a treatment for primary and secondary Raynaud's phenomenon. Br J Rheumatol 1995;34:636–41.

[100] Khan F, Greig IR, Newton DJ, et al. Skin blood flow after transdermal S-nitrosothioacetylglucose. Lancet 1997;350:410–1.

[101] Tucker AT, Pearson RM, Cooke ED, et al. Effect of nitric-oxide-generating system on microcirculatory blood flow in skin in patients with severe Raynaud's syndrome: a randomised trial. Lancet 1999;354:1670–5.

[102] Anderson ME, Moore TL, Hollis S, et al. Digital vascular response to topical glyceryl trinitrate, as measured by laser Doppler imaging, in primary Raynaud's phenomenon and systemic sclerosis. Rheumatology 2002;41:324–8.

[103] Kumana CR, Cheung GTY, Lau CS. Severe digital ischaemia treated with phosphodiesterase inhibitors. Ann Rheum Dis 2004;63:1522–4.

[104] Fries R, Shariat K, von Wilmowsky H, et al. Sildenafil in the treatment of Raynaud's phenomenon resistant to vasodilatory therapy. Circulation 2005;112:2980–5.

[105] Gore J, Silver R. Oral sildenafil for the treatment of Raynaud's phenomenon and digital ulcers secondary to systemic sclerosis. Ann Rheum Dis 2005;64:1387.

[106] Friedman EA, Harris PA, Wood AJJ, et al. The effects of tadalafil on cold-induced vasoconstriction in patients with Raynaud's phenomenon. Clin Pharmacol Ther 2007;81:503–9.

[107] Rajagopalan S, Pfenninger D, Somers E, et al. Effects of cilostazol in patients with Raynaud's syndrome. Am J Cardiol 2003;92:1310–5.

[108] Kirchengast M, Munter K. Endothelin-1 and endothelin receptor antagonists in cardiovascular remodeling. Proc Soc Exp Biol Med 1999;221:312–25.

[109] Mayes MD. Endothelin and endothelin receptor antagonists in systemic rheumatic disease. Arthritis Rheum 2003;48:1190–9.

[110] Vancheeswaran R, Azam A, Black C, et al. Localization of endothelin-1 and its binding sites in scleroderma skin. J Rheumatol 1994;21:1268–76.

[111] Korn JH, Mayes M, Matucci Cerinic M, et al, for the RAPIDS-1 Study Group. Digital ulcers in systemic sclerosis. Prevention by treatment with bosentan, an oral endothelin receptor antagonist. Arthritis Rheum 2004;50:3985–93.

[112] Seibold JR, Matucci-Cerinic M, Denton CP, et al. Bosentan reduces the number of new digital ulcers in patients with systemic sclerosis [abstract]. Ann Rheum Dis 2006;65(Suppl II):90.

[113] Pope J, Fenlon D, Thompson A, et al. Ketanserin for Raynaud's phenomenon in progressive systemic sclerosis. Cochrane Database of Syst Rev 1998;2:CD000954.

[114] Coleiro B, Marshall SE, Denton CP, et al. Treatment of Raynaud's phenomenon with the selective serotonin reuptake inhibitor fluoxetine. Rheumatology 2001;40:1038–43.

[115] Herrick AL, Matucci Cerinic M. The emerging problem of oxidative stress and the role of antioxidants in systemic sclerosis. Clin Exp Rheumatol 2001;19:4–8.

[116] Denton CP, Bunce TD, Dorado MB, et al. Probucol improves symptoms and reduces lipoprotein oxidation susceptibility in patients with Raynaud's phenomenon. Rheumatology 1999;38:309–15.

[117] Herrick AL, Hollis S, Schofield D, et al. A double-blind placebo-controlled trial of antioxidant therapy in limited cutaneous systemic sclerosis. Clin Exp Rheumatol 2000;18:349–56.

[118] Cracowski J-L, Girolet S, Imbert B, et al. Effects of short-term treatment with vitamin E in systemic sclerosis: a double-blind, randomized, controlled clinical trial of efficacy based on urinary isoprostane measurement. Free Radic Biol Med 2005;38:98–103.

[119] Beckett VL, Conn DL, Fuster V, et al. Trial of platelet-inhibiting drug in scleroderma. Arthritis Rheum 1984;27:1137–43.

[120] Denton CP, Howell K, Stratton RJ, et al. Long-term low molecular weight heparin therapy for severe Raynaud's phenomenon: a pilot study. Clin Exp Rheumatol 2000;18:499–502.

[121] Lakshminarayanan S, Maestrello SJ, Vazquez-Abad D, et al. Treatment of severe Raynaud's phenomenon and ischemic ulcerations with tissue plasminogen activator. Clin Exp Rheumatol 1999;17:260.

[122] Van Beek AL, Lim PK, Gear AJ, et al. Management of vasospastic disorders with botulinum toxin A. Plast Reconstr Surg 2007;119:217–26.

[123] Yee AMF, Hotchkiss RN, Paget SA. Adventitial stripping: a digit saving procedure in refractory Raynaud's phenomenon. J Rheumatol 1998;25:269–76.

[124] McCall TE, Petersen DP, Wong LB. The use of digital artery sympathectomy as a salvage procedure for severe ischemia of Raynaud's disease and phenomenon. J Hand Surg [Am] 1999;24:173–7.

[125] Tomaino MM, Goitz RJ, Medsger TA. Surgery for ischemic pain and Raynaud's phenomenon in scleroderma: a description of treatment protocol and evaluation of results. Micro-
surgery 2001;21:75–9.

[126] Kotsis SV, Chung KC. A systematic review of the outcomes of digital sympathectomy for
treatment of chronic digital ischemia. J Rheumatol 2003;30:1788–92.

[127] Bogoch ER, Gross DK. Surgery of the hand in patients with systemic sclerosis: outcomes
and considerations. J Rheumatol 2005;32:642–8.

[128] Klyscz T, Junger M, Meyer H, et al. Improvement of acral circulation in a patient with
systemic sclerosis with stellate blocks. Vasa 1998;27:39–42.

ELSEVIER
SAUNDERS

Rheum Dis Clin N Am
34 (2008) 115–143

RHEUMATIC
DISEASE CLINICS
OF NORTH AMERICA

Fibrosis in Systemic Sclerosis

John A. Varga, MD[a],*, Maria Trojanowska, PhD[b]

[a]*Division of Rheumatology, Northwestern University Feinberg School of Medicine,
McGaw 2300, 240 East Huron Street, Chicago IL 60611-2909, USA*
[b]*Division of Rheumatology, Medical University of South Carolina,
Charleston, SC 29425, USA*

Fibrosis is the pathological hallmark of systemic sclerosis (SSc). Uncontrolled production of collagens and other extracellular matrix (ECM) proteins by fibroblasts residing in the skin, lungs, and other vital organs leads to excess connective tissue accumulation. Over time, progressive buildup of connective tissue disrupts the normal tissue architecture of affected organs, causing their dysfunction and eventual failure (Fig. 1). Thus, the fibrotic process contributes significantly to the morbidity and mortality of SSc. New research challenges the traditional view that pathological fibrosis is always irreversible. This paradigm shift has profound implications for the design and development of novel treatments aimed directly at fibrosis. This article reviews current understanding of the pathophysiology of fibrosis in SSc, highlighting recent discoveries, insights, and emerging research, and potential opportunities for the development of targeted antifibrotic therapies.

Tissue fibrosis: the skin

Fibrosis of the skin is the clinical hallmark of SSc. Skin fibrosis causes marked expansion of the dermis and obliterates the hair follicles, sweat glands, and other skin appendages. Collagen fiber accumulation is most prominent in the reticular dermis. With progression, the subjacent adipose layer also becomes affected, with entrapment of fat cells. Skin biopsies from patients who have early SSc may reveal the presence of deep dermal inflammatory cell infiltrates, composed largely of T lymphocytes and monocytes [1]. Less prominently B cells, mast cells, and eosinophils also may be detected. The proportion of myofibroblasts, mesenchymal cells that are intermediate between fibroblasts and contractile smooth muscle cells and play a major

---

* Corresponding author.
E-mail address: j-varga@northwestern.edu (J.A. Varga).

doi:10.1016/j.rdc.2007.11.002   *rheumatic.theclinics.com*

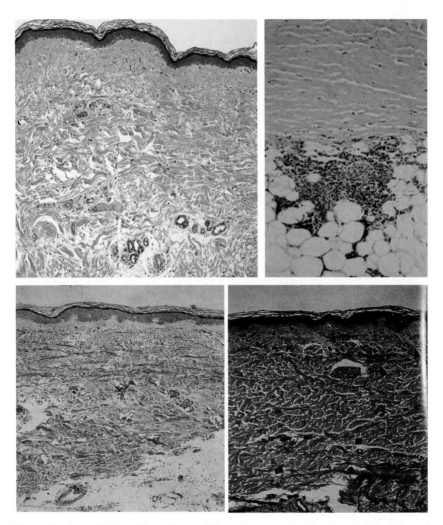

Fig. 1. Histology of skin and lung fibrosis: diffuse cutaneous systemic sclerosis. (*Top left panel*) Dense skin fibrosis with increased extracellular matrix deposition in the dermis. (*Top right panel*) Late stage disease. Secondary structures within the skin such as hair follicles and sweat glands are reduced, and rete pegs are flattened. H&E stain. (*Bottom panels*) Lung tissue from systemic sclerosis. Masson's trichrome staining shows progression of fibrosis.

role in fibrogenesis, is increased [2]. With time, the skin undergoes atrophy, with thinning of the epidermis and effacement of the rete pegs. The largely acellular sclerotic and homogeneous dermis is packed densely with thickened bundles of hyalinized collagen and other ECM proteins (see Fig. 1). Paucity of dermal capillaries contributes to tissue hypoxia. Chronic hypoxia in turn drives local production of vascular endothelial growth factor (VEGF) and other angiogenic factors. Evidence of tissue hypoxia even can be found in clinically uninvolved apparently normal skin of patients who have SSc [3].

Biochemical analysis shows that the collagens in the fibrotic dermis are normal, and relative proportions of the main fibrillar collagens (type 1 and type 3) are comparable to those of healthy skin. In contrast, type 7 collagen, a minor nonfibrillar collagen normally restricted to the dermal–epidermal basement membrane zone, is abundant throughout the lesional dermis [4]. In addition, lesional skin also shows elevated levels of enzymes mediating post-translational collagen modification, such as lysyl hydroxylase (PLOD2). Elevated PLOD2 may contribute to increased formation of aldehyde-derived collagen cross-links, which accounts for the densely sclerotic nature and increased stiffness of the fibrotic dermis [5].

Recent studies using DNA microarray technology to systematically analyze gene expression in skin biopsies have provided a better definition of cellular and molecular events that underlie fibrosis in SSc. Multiple studies reveal strikingly altered patterns of gene expression in skin from patients who have SSc compared with healthy controls. In particular, many genes whose products contribute to the ECM, or are involved in signaling by TGF-β, connective tissue growth factor (CTGF/CCN2), and Wnt ligands are elevated in SSc, pointing to important roles for these mediators in initiating or sustaining the fibrotic process in the skin [6,7]. Additional genes that have been shown to be overexpressed in SSc skin biopsies include a B cell signature and collagens, COMP1, and autoantigens. There appears to be substantial molecular heterogeneity among SSc patients, with some subsets of patients, for example, showing a strong TGF-β signature in DNA microarrays, and others showing little evidence of up-regulation of these genes. Of significance, the number of differentially expressed genes in SSc is much greater in skin samples than it is in explanted dermal fibroblasts, indicating an extinction of the activated pattern of gene expression in cultured fibroblasts over time. Remarkably, DNA microarray studies of SSc consistently have shown that clinically involved skin and uninvolved skin are indistinguishable in terms of their gene expression profiles [8,9]. The intriguing conundrum of scleroderma-like pattern of abnormal gene expression in skin that is clinically normal and appears uninvolved remains to be resolved.

Fibrosis in the lungs

Much less is known about the cellular and molecular events that underlie the development of lung fibrosis in SSc, and the potential role of alveolar epithelial cell injury in this process. In early stage lung disease, patchy infiltration of the alveolar walls with lymphocytes, plasma cells, macrophages, and eosinophils may be seen. At this stage, alveolar lavage fluid contains inflammatory leukocytes and evidence of a Th2-polarized immune response [10]. With progression, lung inflammation subsides and interstitial fibrosis and vascular damage tend to predominate, often coexisting within the same lesions. Pulmonary fibrosis is characterized by expansion of the alveolar interstitium caused by local accumulation of collagens and other connective tissue proteins (see Fig. 1). The most characteristic histologic pattern on lung biopsy is nonspecific interstitial pneumonitis (NSIP). This form of interstitial lung disease is characterized by mild-to-moderate interstitial inflammation, type 2 pneumocyte hyperplasia, and fairly uniform distribution of fibrosis. Less commonly, SSc-associated interstitial lung disease (ILD) shows a histological picture of usual interstitial pneumonia (UIP) characterized by scattered fibroblastic foci and patchy fibrosis. Compared with NSIP, UIP generally carries a worse prognosis [11,12]. Progressive thickening of the alveolar septae ultimately results in air space obliteration of the air spaces and honeycombing.

Fibrosis in other organs

Prominent pathological changes can occur in the gastrointestinal tract at any level from the mouth to the rectum. The esophagus is virtually always affected, with fibrosis in the lamina propria, submucosa, and muscular layers. Replacement of the normal intestinal architecture results in disordered peristaltic activity, gastroesophageal reflux and small bowel dysmotility, pseudo-obstruction, and bacterial overgrowth. In the kidneys, vascular lesions predominate, and glomerulonephritis is rare. Chronic renal ischemia is associated with shrunken glomeruli and other ischemic changes. Cardiac involvement is found at autopsy in up to 80% of patients who have SSc. The characteristic pathological finding is myocardial contraction band necrosis, thought to reflect repeated ischemia reperfusion injury. Significant interstitial and perivascular fibrosis are found, often in the absence of clinically evident heart involvement [13]. With progression, the process contributes to diastolic dysfunction.

Pathogenesis of fibrosis

Overview: molecular and cellular determinants

The pathogenesis of SSc is complex and incompletely understood. A holistic approach must integrate fibrosis with the two other cardinal features of SSc: vascular injury and autoimmunity [14]. As illustrated in Fig. 2, interplay among these distinct processes initiates and sustains progressive tissue damage in SSc. Fibrosis in any organ is characterized pathologically by replacement of normal tissue architecture with dense connective tissue. The ECM consists of a cellular compartment (both resident cells and circulation-derived infiltrating cells) and of connective tissue composed of a multiplicity of large and small structural molecules (including collagens, proteoglycans, elastins, fibrillins, and adhesion molecules) [15]. The ECM also serves as the major reservoir for secreted growth factors such as TGF-β and matricellular proteins such as CCN2/CTGF, which, together with the connective tissue compartment, provide the cues that control differentiation, proliferation, function, and survival of resident cells. Excessive accumulation of connective tissue results

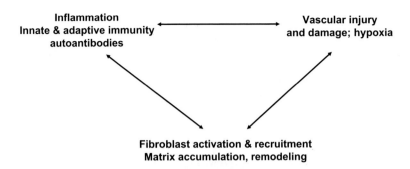

Fig. 2. The pathogenetic triad of systemic sclerosis. The pathogenesis of systemic sclerosis involves autoimmunity, vasculopathy, and fibrosis. Both autoimmunity and vasculopathy appear to precede the onset, and contribute to the progression of fibrosis. Vascular injury and fibrosis, in turn, enhance and sustain chronic autoimmunity and inflammation.

from overproduction by mesenchymal cells that have undergone autocrine/ paracrine activation in response to secreted molecules, the surrounding ECM, or by means of cell-cell interactions. In addition, impaired degradation and turnover of the ECM, and expansion of the pool of mesenchymal cells contributing to ECM accumulation also play a role.

Cellular determinants of fibrosis: fibroblasts

Under the influence of appropriate extracellular signals, fibroblasts or their progenitor cells are induced to synthesize collagens and other ECM macromolecules, adhere to and contract connective tissue, secrete growth factors, cytokines and chemokines, express surface receptors for these ligands, and undergo transdifferentiation into myofibroblasts. Together, these biosynthetic, proinflammatory, contractile, and adhesive properties enable fibroblasts to mediate effective wound healing. In contrast to physiologic conditions, where the fibroblast repair program is controlled tightly and self-limited, pathological fibrosis is characterized by sustained and amplified fibroblast activation, resulting in exaggerated ECM accumulation and remodeling. Inappropriate fibroblast activation is the fundamental pathogenetic alteration underlying fibrosis in SSc.

Cellular determinants of fibrosis: myofibroblasts and pericytes

In fibrosis, the tissue pool of activated mesenchymal cells contributing to ECM accumulation, and remodeling is expanded by local transdifferentiation of other cell lineage (Fig. 3) and the influx of bone marrow-derived mesenchymal progenitor cells from the circulation [16]. Myofibroblasts are specialized cells that arise from fibroblasts in response to TGF-β and express the cytoskeletal protein alpha smooth muscle actin, synthesize collagens, tissue inhibitors of metalloproteases, and other ECM components. They are a major source of TGF-β during the fibrotic response [17]. Their primary physiologic role is contraction of early granulation tissue during normal wound healing, where myofibroblasts are detected transiently and then disappear. Removal of

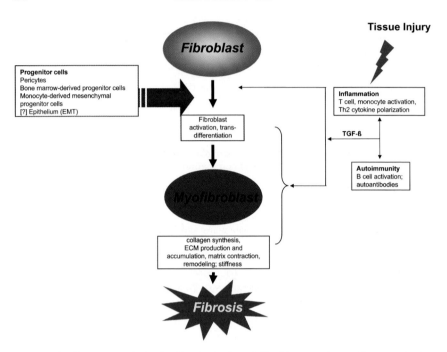

Fig. 3. Fibroblast accumulation in fibrosis. Activated fibroblasts produce collagen and other connective tissue molecules, and contract and remodel their extracellular matrix. Fibroblast accumulation in lesional fibrotic tissue reflects activation and proliferation of resident cells, transdifferentiation and persistence of myofibroblasts, and recruitment and differentiation of bone marrow-derived circulating fibrocytes and mesenchymal progenitor cells, and potentially, plasticity of epithelial cells. (*Data from* Varga J, Abraham DJ. Systemic sclerosis: paradigm multisystem fibrosing disorder. J Clin Invest 2007;117(3):557–67.)

myofibroblasts from the lesion by means of apoptosis is a crucial step in wound resolution. In contrast, in pathological fibrogenesis myofibroblasts persist in lesional tissue, resulting in excessively contracted ECM characteristic of chronic scar. The presence of alpha smooth muscle actin-positive myofibroblasts expressing Thy-1 is associated strongly with fibrotic disorders and SSc, but is absent from normal skin [18,19]. Pericytes are mesenchymal cells that normally reside in the walls of microvessels in intimate contact with the underlying endothelium. Pericytes play a role in maintaining vascular homeostasis. In SSc, the microvascular pericyte compartment shows marked hyperplasia and increased expression of PDGF receptors [19]. Activated pericytes can transdifferentiate into collagen-producing fibroblasts and myofibroblasts, thus linking microvascular injury and fibrosis.

Cellular determinants of fibrosis: the role of plasticity

Resident fibroblasts and pericytes can transdifferentiate to become myofibroblasts. The ability of a differentiated cell with specialized function to change or transition to a cell with a different function is termed cellular plasticity. Under certain conditions, epithelial cells can undergo transformation to fibroblasts, a process called epithelial–mesenchymal transition (EMT) that has a vital role during vertebrate embryonic development. Epithelial cell transition into mesenchymal cells can be induced by TGF-β; the process is suppressed by bone morphogenetic protein (BMP)-7. Pathological EMT occurs in cancer, renal fibrosis, and idiopathic pulmonary fibrosis [20]. To date, the role of epithelial cells and EMT in fibrosis in the skin and lungs in SSc has not been examined.

Cellular determinants of fibrosis: bone marrow-derived mesenchymal progenitor cells

Fibrocytes are CD34+ bone marrow-derived mesenchymal cells normally present in small numbers in the peripheral blood. These cells express CD14+ (a monocyte marker), and chemokine receptors (CCR3, CCR5, and CXCR4) that allow them to traffic into and accumulate in specific tissues. Significantly, fibrocytes can synthesize collagen and present antigen [21]. It has been suggested that fibrocytes originating from bone marrow traffic into fibrotic lesional tissue, where they undergo specialization into fibroblasts and myofibroblasts, losing the CD14 and CD34 markers in the process [22]. Other studies have identified multipotent monocyte-derived mesenchymal progenitor cells in peripheral blood [23]. The role of pericytes, fibrocytes and other monocyte-derived fibroblast progenitor cells in fibrosis in SSc is the subject of intense research [24].

Molecular determinants of fibrosis

Intrinsic regulation of collagen synthesis

The regulation of collagen gene expression and ECM accumulation is controlled tightly. The process is modulated by paracrine/autocrine mediators, cell–cell contact, hypoxia, and contact with the surrounding ECM. Fibroblasts are the cells primarily responsible for collagen production. In normal fibroblasts, type 1 collagen synthesis is regulated by cytokines and other secreted molecules (Table 1) and cell–cell and cell–matrix contact and tissue hypoxia. These environmental cues allow fibroblast to respond to dynamic tissue requirements during development and tissue repair [25]. The collagen genes harbor cis-acting regulatory elements with conserved nucleotide sequences that are recognized specifically by DNA-binding transcription factors. In response to extracellular cues, Sp1, Ets1, Smad3, Egr-1, and CCAAT-binding factor (CBF) stimulate collagen transcription, whereas Sp3, C/EBP, YB1, c-Krox, and Fli1 suppress it [26]. Transcription factors interact with one another, and with non-DNA-binding cofactors, scaffold proteins, and chromatin-modifying enzymes such as p300/CBP,

Table 1
Mediators implicated in fibrosis in systemic sclerosis

Growth factor	Cellular source	Elevated in systemic sclerosis
TGF-β	Inflammatory cells, platelets, fibroblasts, macrophages	+
PDGF	Platelets, macrophages, fibroblasts, endothelial cells	+
CTGF/CCN2	Fibroblasts	+
Insulin-like growth factor-1	Fibroblasts	+
Interleukin (IL)-4, IL-13	Th2 lymphocytes, mast cells	+
IL-6	Macrophages, B cells, T cells, fibroblasts	+
Th17 cytokines (IL-17, IL-23)	T lymphocytes	+
Chemokines (MCP-1, MCP-3)	Neutrophils, epithelial cells, endothelial cells, fibroblasts	+
Fibroblast growth factor	Fibroblasts	+
Endothelin-1	Endothelial cells	+

PCAF, and histone deacetylases. The intracellular trafficking, activities, and interactions among transcription factors and cofactors are regulated by extracellular mediators. Enzymes that modify chromatin structure at target gene promoters facilitate access by DNA-binding factors to their corresponding cis-acting regulatory sequences, inducing transcription. Therefore, chromatin-modifying enzymes such as p300/CBP have emerged as important elements of the regulatory network that provide a novel framework for epigenetic control of collagen transcription [27]. Alterations in the expression levels, activities, or interactions among the various transcription factors and cofactors contribute to persistent fibroblast activation in SSc.

Intrinsic negative regulation of collagen synthesis

To prevent excessive matrix accumulation and scarring, multiple redundant biological mechanisms exist for controlling ECM synthesis and fibroblast activation. Fibroblasts are equipped with endogenous molecules that repress ECM gene expression and TGF-β stimulation. For example, an inhibitory member of the Smad family Smad7 blocks Smad-mediated TGF-β signal transduction by inducing ubiquitin-mediated degradation of the TGF-β receptor. Functional impairment of Smad7 was demonstrated in SSc fibroblasts [28,29]. Other molecules that appear to function as cell-intrinsic endogenous repressors of collagen synthesis include the transcription factors Fli-1, p53, Ras, and the nuclear hormone receptor peroxisome proliferator-activated receptor (PPAR)-γ [30–32]. Recent studies indicate that in SSc, the expression, regulation, or function of these endogenous inhibitors may be impaired. The resultant defect in suppression of fibrogenic responses may contribute to failure to limit fibroblast activation, thereby contributing to ECM up-regulation and fibrosis.

Modulation of collagen synthesis and extracellular matrix accumulation: TGF-β

TGF-β is considered to be the master regulator of physiologic fibrogenesis (wound healing and tissue repair) and pathological fibrosis, and it is emerging as an important therapeutic target in fibrotic diseases [33]. Selective inhibition of TGF-β function (using small molecule inhibitors, soluble TGF-0β receptors, natural TGF-β binding proteins or ligand-specific neutralizing antibodies) would be highly desirable as pharmacotherapy (Table 2). A member of a large cytokine superfamily that also includes activin and bone morphogenetic proteins, TGF-β (three isoforms: TGFβ1, TGF-β2 and TGF-β3) is produced by platelets, monocytes/macrophages, T cells, and fibroblasts. Most cell types secrete TGF-β as latent molecules that are sequestered within the ECM complexed to structural proteins such as fibrillin-1 and latent TGF-β binding protein (LTBP). Latent TGF-β is converted to its biologically active form by thrombospondins and proteolytic enzymes such as plasmin. In addition, various cell surface

Table 2
Potential strategies toward pharmacological TGF-β inhibition in fibrosis

Approach to inhibiting TGF-β	Comment
Drugs in development	
Anti-TGF-β neutralizing antibodies	Extensive preclinical animal experience
Soluble TGF-β receptors (TβRII)	Extensive preclinical animal experience
Natural TGF-β binding proteins (decorin)	Animal experience
Antisense oligonucleotides	Clinical experience (glioma)
ALK5 receptor kinase inhibitors (numerous)	Extensive preclinical animal experience
Smad-specific aptamers	In vitro studies
Existing drugs	
Pirfenidone	Blocks TGF-β activation; efficacy in clinical trial of idiopathic pulmonary fibrosis
Tranilast	Blocks TGF-β production; in clinical use for allergic diseases in Japan; well-tolerated
Angiotensin receptor blockers (losartan)	In clinical use for hypertension, Raynaud phenomenon; well-tolerated; decreased TGF-β production
Statins	In clinical use as cholesterol-lowering drugs; well-tolerated; antagonizes TGF-β stimulation of collagen, CTGF
Thiazolidenediones (rosiglitazone)	In clinical use as insulin-sensitizing antidiabetic drugs; well-tolerated; antagonizes TGF-β stimulation of collagen, CTGF
Imatinib mesylate (Gleevec)	In clinical use in chronic myelogenous leukemia; well-tolerated; antagonizes TGF-β stimulation of collagen, myofibroblast transdifferentiation

Data from Prud'homme GJ. Pathobiology of transforming growth factor beta in cancer, fibrosis and immunologic disease, and therapeutic considerations. Lab Invest 2007;87(11):1077–91.

integrins (alpha 5, beta 3, beta 5, beta 6, and beta 8) also can mediate latent TGF-β activation by means of distinct mechanisms. TGF-β shows functional pleiotropism, and its biological responses are specific for target cell lineage and are highly context-dependent. In mesenchymal cells, TGF-β acts as a potent inducer of fibrillar collagen synthesis, enhances ECM stiffness, stimulates fibroblast proliferation, migration, adhesion and trans-differentiation into myofibroblasts, and suppresses the production of matrix-degrading metalloproteinases (Box 1).

Each of the three TGF-β isoforms binds to the type 2 TGF-β receptor, triggering an evolutionarily conserved intracellular signal transduction cascade that leads to the induction of target genes [34]. The canonical TGF-β signal transduction pathway involves sequential phosphorylation of the activin-like kinase 5 (ALK5) type 1 TGF-β receptor (TβR1), and a group of intracellular signaling proteins called Smads (Fig. 4, left panel). Ligand-induced phosphorylation of Smad2/3 allows them to form heterocomplexes with Smad4 and translocate from the cytoplasm into the nucleus. Within the nucleus, the activated Smad complex specifically binds to a cis-acting DNA sequence (CAGAC) that defines the consensus Smad-binding element (SBE). Upon binding to the SBE, activated Smad recruits transcriptional cofactors to the DNA. In the case of type 1 collagen gene, an important target regulated by TGF-β/Smad3, recruitment of p300 to the SBE by activated Smad3 is essential for robust stimulation of transcription [35]. Signal transduction through the Smad pathway is tightly controlled by endogenous inhibitors such as Smad7, whose expression is itself regulated by TGF-β. Pharmacological blockade of ALK5 kinase activity with small molecules such as SB431542 or SD208 results in normalization of selected profibrotic features of SSc fibroblast in vitro [36–38]. Therefore, ALK5 blockade represents a promising novel therapeutic approach to fibrosis in SSc. In light of the multiple and diverse physiological functions of TGF-β, there is concern that inhibiting its activity may be associated with adverse effects, such as

---

Box 1. Fibrogenic TGF-ß activities with potential relevance to fibrosis in systemic sclerosis

Stimulates synthesis of collagens, fibronectin, proteoglycans, elastin, TIMPs; inhibits matrix metalloproteinases
Stimulates fibroblast proliferation, chemotaxis
Induces CTGF and endothelin-1 production
Stimulates expression of surface receptors for TGF-β, PDGF
Promotes fibroblast-myofibroblast differentiation, monocyte-fibrocyte differentiation; epithelial–mesenchymal transition
Inhibits fibroblast apoptosis
Enhances ECM stiffness

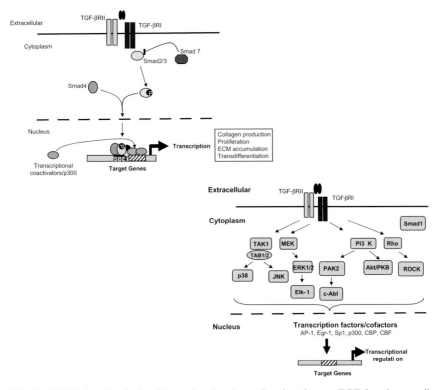

Fig. 4. TGF-β signaling in fibroblasts: Smad and non-Smad pathways. TGF-β activates cell surface TGF-β receptors TβR1 and TβR2, resulting in phosphorylation of downstream targets, such as Smads. Activated Smad2 and Smad3 form a complex with Smad4, and transit from the cytoplasm into the nucleus, bind to conserved DNA sequences and activate (or repress) transcription. Transcriptional cofactors provide tissue and gene specificity (*top panel*). In addition to this canonical TGF-β signal transduction mechanism, TGF-β also can activate complex Smad-independent intracellular kinase cascades that are involved in specific TGF-β responses (*bottom panel*). (*Data from* Varga J, Abraham DJ. Systemic sclerosis: paradigm multisystem fibrosing disorder. J Clin Invest 2007;117(3):557–67.)

autoimmunity or cellular dysplasia and progression to cancer. Surprisingly however, no such adverse effects have been observed in preclinical studies of TGF-β blockade, possibly because of the inability of current anti-TGF-β therapies to achieve complete TGF-β blockade [39].

Cellular signaling by TGF-β: noncanonical pathways and fresh insights

Although the Smad pathway is the central intracellular mediator of signals from the TGF-β receptors, recent evidence indicates that alternative non-Smad pathways exist that also mediate TGF-β responses [40]. As shown in Fig. 4 (right panel) non-Smad signal transduction cascades involve protein kinases (MAP kinases p38 and JNK, focal adhesion kinase FAK, and TGF-β activated kinase TAK1), lipid kinases such as PI3 kinase and its downstream target Akt, the calcium-dependent phosphatase calcineurin, and the nonreceptor tyrosine kinase c-Abl [41–44]. These non-Smad pathways interact with one another and with Smads, creating complex intracellular signaling networks. Their relative importance in mediating specific TGF-β responses and their role in physiologic and pathological fibrosis remain to be elucidated.

Smad1

Although earlier studies highlighted the important role of canonical Smad TGF-β signaling pathways in fibrosis in SSc, new findings also implicate noncanonical pathways such as Smad1. Normally, Smad1, along with Smad 5 and Smad8, serves as substrate for the BMP and anti-Mullerian substance receptors. A recent study, however, provided evidence for the role of Smad1, in addition to Smad3, in TGF-β dependent stimulation of collagen and CTGF/CCN2 genes [45]. Activation of Smad1 in dermal fibroblasts by TGF-β may require cooperation between ALK5 and ALK1 receptors as shown in endothelial cells [46]. The role of the ALK1/Smad1 pathway in fibrosis is supported by the observations of activation of this pathway in liver and kidney fibrosis [47–49]. Smad1 may be activated in SSc fibroblasts as a result of the altered ratio of the type I and type 2 TGF-β receptors, and may contribute directly to profibrotic gene expression in SSc [50,51].

Egr-1

Egr-1 is a DNA-binding transcription factor that is rapidly and transiently induced at sites of acute injury and implicated in cell proliferation, differentiation, and survival. TGF-β was shown also to induce Egr-1 expression in normal dermal fibroblasts [52]. The response was transient and occurred by means of an MEK1–ERK1/2-dependent and Smad-independent mechanism. Additional observations highlight the potential significance of Egr-1 as a novel mediator of the fibrotic process. For example, Egr-1 not only causes direct stimulation of collagen gene expression, but also induces the production of TGF-β and TGF-β receptors, and enhances cellular accumulation of the co-activator p300, thereby amplifying TGF-β induced cellular responses [53]. Egr-1 expression is elevated in lesional SSc skin and lung, and in the bleomycin-induced mouse model of scleroderma. Significantly, mice lacking Egr-1 show markedly attenuated fibrotic response to bleomycin in vivo (Wu M, Varga J, unpublished data, 2008). Furthermore, transgenic mice that overexpress TGF-β or interleukin (IL)-13 on an Egr-1-deficient genetic background fail to develop lung fibrosis [54]. These findings indicate a role for Egr-1 in fibrosis in SSc, and identify this transcription factor as a novel target for therapy. The role of other Egr-1 family members in mediating TGF-β responses and fibrosis has not been evaluated.

Fli1

Several recent studies have highlighted the important role of endogenous repressors of TGF-β signaling in regulating collagen synthesis. One of the best characterized is the transcription factor Fli1 (Friend leukemia integration-1), a member of the Ets (E26 transformation-specific) family [55]. Reducing Fli1 in normal fibroblasts results in induction of a TGF-β dependent profibrotic gene program, including increased synthesis of CTGF/CCN2 and type I collagen [56]. Conversely, forced expression of Fli1 completely prevented TGF-β induced profibrotic gene expression [32]. TGF-β abrogates the repressor function of Fli1 by means of PCAF-dependent acetylation, which results in Fli1 dissociation from the collagen promoter and subsequent degradation [8]. Because Fli1 is markedly down-regulated in SSc fibroblasts and in lesional tissue [32], the absence of Fli1 may contribute to the process of cutaneous fibrosis. Epigenetic mechanisms may be in part responsible for low Fli1 gene expression in SSc [9].

Peroxisome proliferator-activated receptor-γ: endogenous
repressor of fibrotic responses

Peroxisome proliferator-activated receptor gamma (PPAR-γ) is a nuclear steroid hormone receptor and ligand-activated transcription factor with a well-recognized role in adipogenesis. The thiazolidenedione class of insulin-sensitizing drugs used in the treatment of type 2 diabetes (such as rosiglitazone or pioglitazone) activates the PPAR-γ receptor. Recent studies implicate PPAR-γ in inflammation, atherosclerosis, and cancer. An entirely novel function for PPAR-γ as an endogenous anti-fibrotic has emerged recently. In normal fibroblasts, activation of PPAR-γ by either natural (15d-prostaglandin J_2) or synthetic (rosiglitazone) agonist ligands resulted in abrogation of TGF-β–induced collagen stimulation [57]. In addition, PPAR-γ ligands block the transcriptional activity of Egr-1 [58] and induce phosphate and tensin homologue (PTEN), a negative regulator of myofibroblast activation and collagen synthesis. Significantly, rosiglitazone treatment in normal mice markedly attenuated dermal fibrosis induced by bleomycin (M Wu and J Varga, unpublished data, 2007). Of interest, the expression of PPAR-γ is reduced in lesional skin biopsies from SSc patients, and in the lungs. These observations indicate that the PPAR-γ axis is a potent endogenous antagonist of TGF-β signaling, and further suggest that PPAR-γ has a physiologic role in preventing excessive fibrosis. In light of its novel function as an endogenous antifibrotic, it will be interesting to determine if fibrosis in SSc and other disorders is associated with reduced expression or impaired function of PPAR-γ. Furthermore, these findings raise the possibility that agonists of PPAR-γ may be useful as antifibrotic agents. Such a therapeutic approach to SSc is particularly intriguing in light of the availability of numerous PPAR-γ agonists, such as the glitazone type antidiabetic drugs that have been characterized extensively and are in wide clinical use already.

c-Abelson: novel mediator of TGF-β response in fibroblasts

In normal fibroblasts, TGF-β induces activation of c-Abelson (c-Abl), a member of the Src family of nonreceptor tyrosine kinases [44]. c-Abl is involved in regulating cell proliferation and survival, and is constitutively activated in hematopoietic cells in chronic myelogenous leukemia (CML) because of a chromosomal translocation, resulting in the fusion protein bcr-Abl (the Philadelphia chromosome). Activation of c-Abl by TGF-β was independent of Smad2/3, and endogenous c-Abl was required for pro-fibrotic responses induced by TGF-β (Ishida W and Varga J, unpublished data, 2007) [44]. These and similar findings therefore identify c-Abl as a pre-viously unrecognized component of the fibroblast response to TGF-β. Ima-tinib mesylate (Gleevec) is a potent pharmacologic inhibitor of c-Abl kinase that is highly effective in the treatment of CML. In vitro, imatinib blocked the TGF-β induced stimulation of collagen synthesis and fibroblast prolifer-ation, and down-regulated collagen gene expression in SSc fibroblasts (Ishida W, Varga J, unpublished data, 2007). Imatinib also was shown to prevent skin fibrosis induced by bleomycin in mice [59]. In light of the fundamental role of TGF-β in fibrosis in SSc, along with recent findings im-plicating autoantibody-mediated activation of the PDGF receptor, imatinib as a dual inhibitor of both TGF-βR and PDGF receptors may be effective as a therapy for fibrosis in SSc. Results from ongoing clinical trials of imatinib therefore will be of great interest.

MAP kinases ERK1/2 implicated in fibrosis

Earlier studies have linked activation of the ERK1/2 MAP kinase path-way by PDGF to up-regulation of MMP1, a key enzyme involved in col-lagen degradation [60]. More recently, ERK1/2 was shown to be activated by TGF-β in many cell types and to be required for CTGF and collagen gene stimulation [61]. ERK1/2 is activated constitutively in SSc lung and skin fibroblasts [31,62]. A recent study linked ERK1/2 activation to PDGF receptor signaling [31]. Sera from patients who had SSc were shown to contain autoantibodies directed against PDGF receptors. These autoan-tibodies triggered activation of the PDGF-ROS-ERK1/2 signaling cascade in normal fibroblasts, with consequent up-regulation of collagen gene ex-pression. These intriguing results suggest the possibility that autoanti-bodies may be directly responsible for fibroblast activation and fibrosis in SSc [63].

Integrin-mediated regulation of fibroblast biology

In addition to growth factors, chemokines and other soluble mediators, fibroblasts are influenced strongly by interaction with the surrounding ECM by means of integrin receptors [64]. The αvβ5 and αvβ3 integrins are elevated significantly in SSc fibroblasts [65,66]. The functional significance of elevated integrin expression was established using cultured fibroblasts. These studies showed that integrin receptors contribute to elevated collagen synthesis and myofibroblast transdifferentiation [67]. Both integrins exert their profibrotic ef-fects by activating latent TGF-β and establishing autocrine TGF-β stimulatory loops. Together with previous studies [68] that demonstrated elevated thrombo-spondin, another activator of latent TGF-β, in SSc fibroblasts, these studies point to the multiple mechanisms involved in TGF-β activation and autocrine stimulation in SSc (the autocrine TGF-β hypothesis).

Molecular effectors of fibrosis: growth factors and chemokines

Multiple growth factors, chemokines, and eicosanoids regulate collagen production, ECM accumulation, and mesenchymal cell function, and are expressed abnormally in SSc. These mediators, most prominently CTGF/CCN2, PDGF, IL-4, IL-6, IL-13, and endothelin-1, interact with TGF-β and directly contribute to the pathogenesis of fibrosis, and represent potential targets for antifibrotic therapy.

Connective tissue growth factor

Connective tissue growth factor or CCN2, a cysteine-rich 40 kDa member of the CCN early-response gene family, is a matricellular growth factor with important functional roles in angiogenesis, wound healing, and development. Expression of CTGF/CCN2 is generally undetectable in most tissues in normal adults, but is markedly elevated SSc and other fibrotic conditions. Serum levels of CTGF/CCN2 in SSc correlate with the extent of skin and pulmonary fibrosis [69,70]. A recent study of 500 patients (representing some 10% of all SSc patients in the United Kingdom) identified a single nucleotide polymorphism (G945C) in the CTGF/CCN2 gene promoter that was significantly associated with susceptibility to SSc and with ILD [71]. In normal fibroblasts, CTGF/CCN2 expression can be induced by TGF-β, as well as IL-4 and VEGF, whereas tumor necrosis factor α and iloprost blocked stimulation [72]. In vivo, CTGF/CCN2 induces a transient fibrotic response in mice, and markedly enhances the TGF-β response [73]. In vitro, CTGF/CCN2 stimulates fibroblast proliferation, chemotaxis and adhesion, and enhances the synthesis of collagen and fibronectin. Because many of the affects of CTGF/CCN2 closely parallel those induced by TGF-β, it has been proposed that TGF-β responses are mediated through endogenous CTGF/CCN2 [74]; however, fibroblasts from CCN2-null mouse embryos show normal responses to TGF-β in vitro [75]. The fibroblast receptors for CTGF/CCN2 and the mechanism of action underlying CTGF /CCN2 profibrotic responses remain incompletely characterized.

Platelet-derived growth factor

Platelet-derived growth factors are heterodimeric proteins consisting of an A and a B chain that act mainly on stromal cells and regulate the wound healing process. Originally isolated from platelets, PDGF isoforms also are produced by macrophages, endothelial cells, and fibroblasts. PDGF is a potent fibroblast mitogen and chemoattractant. It induces the synthesis of collagen, fibronectin, and proteoglycans and stimulates the secretion of TGF-β1, MCP-1, and IL-6. Fibroblasts from patients who have SSc show elevated expression of PDGF and PDGF-β receptor [76], and PDGF levels are increased in bronchoalveolar lavage fluid [77]. Serum autoantibodies directed against the PDGF receptor are detectable in patients with SSc, and are capable of inducing fibroblast activation in vitro [78]. Stimulatory autoantibodies directed against the PDGF receptor are not specific for SSc, and have also been detected in patients who have graft-versus-host disease [79].

Other cytokines and chemokines with potential roles in fibrosis in systemic sclerosis

The Th2 cytokine IL-4 stimulates fibroblast proliferation, chemotaxis, and collagen synthesis and production of TGF-β, CTGF/CCN2 and TIMP [80]. Serum levels of IL-4 are elevated in SSc patients [81], and the number of IL-4-producing T lymphocytes is increased in peripheral blood [82]. Expression of IL-4 and its mRNA is elevated markedly in SSc lesional skin and cultured fibroblasts [83]. IL-6, produced by monocytes, T lymphocytes, fibroblasts, and endothelial cells, stimulates collagen and TIMP-1 synthesis, and promotes a Th2-polarized immune response. The biological activities of IL-6 are mediated by means of the common Jak–Stat intracellular signaling pathway shared with other cytokines. Serum IL-6 levels are elevated in SSc and correlate with skin involvement [81]. IL-13 is implicated in asthma and other fibrotic conditions. The profibrotic effects of IL-13 involve both indirect mechanisms because of stimulation of TGF-β production by macrophages, and direct stimulation of fibroblast proliferation and collagen synthesis [84,85]. Serum levels of IL-13 are elevated in patients who have SSc. Recent studies indicate a role for Th17 cytokines, such as IL-17 and IL-23, in the pathogenesis of fibrosis in SSc.

Chemokines represent a superfamily of over 40 low molecular weight soluble mediators originally characterized by their chemotactic effects on leukocytes, but now recognized to have a broad range of cellular targets and biological activities, and to play important roles in angiogenesis, wound healing, and fibrosis. The CC chemokine MCP-1 stimulates collagen production directly and through induction of endogenous TGF-β. Serum levels of MCP-1, along with those of MIP-1 alpha, IL-8, CXCL8, and CCL18, are elevated in SSc, and correlate with the severity of skin fibrosis [86–88]. Mononuclear cells and dermal fibroblasts from patients who have SSc spontaneously produce these chemokines, and lesional SSc fibroblasts show constitutive up-regulation of the MCP-1 receptor CCR2 [89]. The MCP-1-CCR2 axis is thought to play a major role in the pathogenesis of SSc by amplifying collagen stimulation and promoting Th2 cytokine polarization. Significantly, MCP-1 null mice are resistant to induction of fibrosis by bleomycin [90]. Strong expression of MCP-1 and MCP-3 was noted in lesional skin in SSc, particularly in early disease [91]. The levels of MIP-1alpha, CXCL8, and CCL18 also are elevated in SSc bronchoalveolar lavage fluid. Elevated CCL18 levels identified SSc patients who had pulmonary fibrosis [92]. Additional chemokines overexpressed in SSc, or in animal models of scleroderma, included the CC chemokines RANTES and PARC, and the CXC chemokines IL-8, MIP-2, and fractalkine. The insulin-like growth factor binding protein-1 (IGFBP-1) stimulates collagen synthesis and fibroblast proliferation and induces TGF-β [93]. Patients who have SSc have elevated levels of IGF-1 in bronchoalveolar lavage fluids [94]. Expression of IGFBP-3 is elevated markedly in SSc fibroblasts [95]. Adenovirally mediated overexpression of IGFBP-5 resulted in the induction of chronic scleroderma-like fibrosis in mice [96].

Interferon-gamma

Interferon-γ, produced primarily by Th1 lymphocytes, is a major negative regulator of fibroblast activation. Interferon-γ represses collagen gene expression and abrogates stimulation induced by TGF-β [97–100]. Interferon-γ also inhibits fibroblast proliferation, fibroblast-mediated matrix contraction, and myofibroblast transdifferentiation. Significantly, some studies have shown that fibroblasts from patients who have SSc are relatively resistant to the inhibitory effects of interferon-γ [101]. Open-label clinical trials of IFN-γ in SSc have demonstrated modest improvement in skin fibrosis [102–104].

In vitro and in vivo experimental models of scleroderma

The scleroderma fibroblast: autocrine TGF-β hypothesis

Fibroblasts explanted from lesional skin or fibrotic lungs of patients who have SSc display an abnormal activated phenotype that persists during their serial passage in vitro, indicating autonomous alteration in cell function [105]. The SSc phenotype is characterized by the following: enhanced ECM synthesis, secretion of profibrotic cytokines and chemokines and increased expression of their cell surface receptors, and resistance to interferon-gamma and other inhibitory signals. Moreover, SSc fibroblasts show features of myofibroblastic transdifferentiation, attributed in part to constitutive activation of the FAK focal adhesion kinase [106]. It remains unsettled whether the activated phenotype of SSc fibroblasts represents an abnormality intrinsic to these cells, or reflects their activation elicited by exogenous stimuli.

Numerous molecules involved in intracellular signal transduction and transcriptional regulation are elevated or activated in SSc fibroblasts. The list includes protein kinase C, Smad3, Egr-1, p300/CBP, and c-Abl (Table 3). Elevated expression of the prosurvival factors Bcl-2 and Akt in SSc fibroblasts may play a role in their relative resistance to apoptosis [107]. Because most of the characteristics of SSc fibroblast can be induced by TGF-β in normal

Table 3
Intracellular signaling molecules implicated in the pathogenesis of fibrosis in systemic sclerosis

Molecule	Change in systemic sclerosis	Effect on collagen production
ERK1/2	Increased phosphorylation	Stimulation
PKCδ	Increased phosphorylation	Stimulation
c-Abl	Increased phosphorylation	Stimulation
Smad3	Increased phosphorylation	Stimulation
Smad1	Increased expression	Stimulation
Egr1	Increased expression	Stimulation
c-Myb	Increased expression	Stimulation
Fli1	Decreased expression	Inhibition
PPAR-γ	Decreased expression	Inhibition
PTEN	Decreased expression	Inhibition
Caveolin1 (?)	Decreased expression	Inhibition

fibroblasts, it has been suggested that the SSc phenotype is caused by auto-crine TGF-β signaling [108]. The levels of TGF-β receptors are elevated on SSc fibroblasts, enabling these cells to mount a robust response to endogenously produced TGF-β or to low levels of environmental TGF-β [109–111]. Furthermore, SSc fibroblasts express thrombospondin and integrins that mediate latent TGF-β activation at the cell surface [68]. Consistent with the autocrine TGF-β hypothesis, SSc fibroblasts show constitutive activation of intracellular TGF-β signaling, with elevated expression and nuclear accumulation of activated Smad3 [112–114] and constitutive Smad3 interaction with the transcriptional coactivator p300/CBP [35,115]. Other studies demonstrate defective expression or function of endogenous suppressors of TGF-β signaling and ECM production (such as Fli-1, PPAR-γ and Smad7), suggesting that failure to terminate fibroblast activation may represent a fundamental defect in SSc. The autocrine TGF-β hypothesis cannot fully account for all of the phenotypic hallmarks of SSc fibroblasts such as constitutive CTGF/CCN2 production, implicating both Smad-independent TGF-β signaling, and non-TGF-β-mediated activation events in the induction or maintenance of the SSc phenotype. The autonomous SSc phenotype also could result from integrin-mediated signaling from the surrounding ECM. Moreover, recent evidence indicates that epigenetic alterations in SSc fibroblasts are associated with heritable fibroblast dysfunction. For example, silencing the inhibitory Fli-1 gene by means of DNA methylation or histone deacetylation resulted in reduced Fli-1 expression in SSc fibroblasts, accompanied by concomitant increase in collagen synthesis [9].

In vitro model of scleroderma: altered ratio of type 1
and type 2 TGF-β receptors

Although cultured SSc fibroblasts constitute a principal experimental model to investigate SSc fibrosis, this model has several limitations including limited material because of the finite life span of human fibroblasts, inconsistency of findings because of the heterogeneity of cultured fibroblasts, and progressive loss of the phenotype with the serial passage. Recent gene array studies, which demonstrated a disproportionately higher number of differentially expressed genes in biopsies versus cultured fibroblasts, highlighted the need for better experimental models of SSc suitable for mechanistic studies [6,7]. Based on the findings that TGF-βRI protein levels are elevated in SSc skin in vivo and that most SSc fibroblasts exhibit an elevated ratio of TGF-β type 1 to type 2 receptors, an experimental model that mimics this condition has been established in normal fibroblasts by titrating the dose of an adenoviral vector expressing TGF-βRI [50]. Comprehensive gene expression analysis indicated that this model recapitulates major features of activated SSc phenotype. This model will be helpful in uncovering novel signaling pathways, such as Smad1, that are relevant to SSc fibrosis.

Animal models of scleroderma

Unfortunately, there are no animal models that reproduce all three cardinal features of SSc (obliterative/proliferative vasculopathy, autoimmunity, and fibrosis). Nonetheless, particular models are useful for studying the fibrotic process [116]. Such mouse models can be naturally occurring, caused by spontaneous mutations such as tight skin (Tsk1/+ mouse), or induced where the scleroderma phenotype is elicited by chemical exposures or manipulation of the immune system (bleomycin-induced skin and lung fibrosis, transplantation of HLA-mismatched bone marrow cells resulting in chronic sclerodermatous graft-versus-host disease) and genetic manipulations giving rise to novel mouse strains with heritable scleroderma-like traits (Table 4).

Heritable mouse models of fibrosis

The tight skin mouse (Tsk1/+), originally described 30 years ago, shows diffuse thickening and tethering of the skin as a result of a spontaneously arising mutation [117]. Although mice homozygous for the Tsk1 mutation die in utero at 8 to 10 days of gestation, heterozygous mice (Tsk1/+) survive to develop thickened skin that is bound firmly to the underlying subcutaneous tissue. Anaylsis of lesional skin has shown evidence for up-regulation of the Wnt-γ catenin pathways [118]. In contrast to human SSc (where fibrosis of the dermis is the pathological hallmark), Tsk1/+ mice have subcutaneous hyperplasia, with relatively normal-appearing dermis [119]. The skin phenotype in Tsk1/+ is caused by tethering and thickening of the hypodermal tissue rather than the dermal fibrosis characteristic of SSc, raising questions regarding the relevance of the Tsk1/+ mouse as a bona fide model for human disease [120]. Further distinguishing the Tsk phenotype from human SSc, the lungs of Tsk1/+ mice show emphysematous changes rather than fibrosis, and vasculopathy does not occur. Although skin inflammation is uncommon, Tsk1/+ mice display autoimmunity associated with serum autoantibodies directed against topoisomerase-I. The mutation responsible for

Table 4
Selected mouse models of scleroderma

Model	Features of the systemic sclerosis pathological triad that are reproduced				
	Vasculopathy, vascular activation	Inflammation	Autoimmunity	Fibrosis	Key aspects
Naturally occurring					
Tsk-1	–	–	✓	✓	Duplication mutation in fibrillin-1 gene associated with skin tethering
Tsk-2	–	✓	✓	✓	Unknown genetic defect; dermal fibrosis
Induced					
Bleomycin (s.c.)	–	✓	–	✓	Early monocytic inflammation; skin, lung, and renal fibrosis.
GVHD (B10.D2 versus Rag-2–/–)	✓	✓	✓	✓	Transfer of spleen cells into RAG-2 null mice results in systemic fibrosis, inflammation, autoantibodies
Transgenic					
TGFβRII DN	–	✓	–	✓	Mice expressing a dominant negative TGFβRII paradoxically develop tissue fibrosis.
MRL/lpr/ IFNγR–/–	–	✓	✓	✓	MRL/lpr mouse strain lacking IFN-gamma receptors develop spontaneous fibrosis.
Conditional TβRI[ca]	✓	–	–	✓	Conditional expression of constitutively-active type I TGF-β receptor in fibroblasts induces widespread skin fibrosis.

the Tsk1 phenotype has been localized to mouse chromosome 2, subsequently identified as an intragenic tandem duplication in the gene encoding fibrillin-1 [121]. Fibrillin, an ECM protein that interacts with elastin fibers, contains structural domains with TGF-β binding activity.

Another inherited model of fibrosis with potential relevance to SSc is the Tsk2 mouse, originally described in 1995. Mice heterozygous for the Tsk2 mutation spontaneously develop scleroderma-like dense dermal fibrosis by age 3 to 4 weeks [122]. The Tsk2 mutation, originally induced in normal mice by ethylnitrosurea, is located on mouse chromosome 1 and is inherited as an autosomal-dominant trait. The underlying molecular defect responsible for the tight skin phenotype in these mice has not been identified.

Inducible mouse models of fibrosis with potential relevance to systemic sclerosis

Chronic skin and lung fibrosis can be induced in normal BALB/c or C57 mice by repeated subcutaneous injections of the chemotherapeutic agent bleomycin [123]. The sequence of histopathological changes elicited by bleomycin injection in the lesional skin closely resembles that seen in SSc. There is early and self-limited infiltration with blood-derived mononuclear cells and elevated local levels of cytokines and chemokines such as TGF-β and MCP-1. This initial inflammatory stage is succeeded by the development of dermal fibrosis [124,125]. The involved skin shows excessive collagen deposition and accumulation of alpha smooth muscle actin-positive myofibroblasts in the dermis. In contrast to SSc, bleomycin-induced scleroderma in the mouse is not associated with either vascular changes or autoantibodies, and skin fibrosis is limited in its extent and its duration, regressing after bleomycin is stopped. Nonetheless, in light of its reproducibility, relative murine strain independence and ease of induction, this mouse model now is used widely for investigating the pathogenic roles of specific gene products in fibrosis and for evaluating antifibrotic interventions [126,127]. Transplantation of HLA-mismatched bone marrow or spleen cells into sublethally irradiated recipient mice results in sclerodermatous graft-versus-host disease, characterized by chronic fibrosis of the skin and lung, perivascular fibrosis, and autoimmunity [128,129]. In this model, skin fibrosis is preceded by mononuclear cell infiltration and elevation of TGF-β and chemokines.

Genetic manipulations giving rise to scleroderma-like mouse phenotypes

Recent studies have focused on the generation of novel genetically engineered mouse strains with spontaneous development of scleroderma-like fibrotic phenotypes (see Table 4). These gain-of-function (transgenic) and loss-of-function (knockout) mice undergoing intensive study may provide robust novel experimental tools for understanding the pathophysiology of fibrosis. Particularly valuable are mouse strains with constitutive or inducible expression of genes of interest restricted to fibroblasts. For example, modulation of intracellular TGF-β signaling in fibroblasts (as, for example, by expression of a constitutively active TβR1), results in mouse phenotypes that recapitulate key clinical histological and biochemical aspects of SSc in the absence of antecedent inflammation [130,131].

Summary

Fibrosis is the pathological hallmark of SSc. Progressive damage to the skin, blood vessels, and internal organs resulting from the fibrotic process is responsible for major clinical manifestations and mortality of SSc. Fibrosis in SSc shares multiple pathophysiologic aspects of fibrosis in other diseases; examples of partial overlap include idiopathic pulmonary fibrosis, glomerulosclerosis, and myocardial fibrosis [132]. Although traditionally viewed as an irreversible and end-stage process, recent insights from animal models indicate that fibrosis is dynamic and in fact may be reversible, and thus is potentially amenable to treatment. Therefore it is becoming imperative to gain a precise understanding of the pathogenesis of fibrosis, and to identify the distinct cellular and molecular players and their interactions. A growing body of research indicates that mesenchymal cell plasticity and bone marrow-derived progenitor cell trafficking and differentiation, intracellular signaling pathways regulating normal and aberrant collagen gene expression and ECM accumulation, and extracellular signals such as TGF-β, CTGF/CCN2, Wnt PDGF, angiotensin, and endothelins are all potential drug targets in fibrosis. Drugs that modulate the expression or function of these molecules are either under development, or are already available by virtue of the known off-target activities of currently used drugs; examples include mycophenolate, imatinib mesylate, traniPast, losentan, losartan, statins, or thiazolidenediones. The main contemporary challenge for the development of fibrosis treatments is the assessment of their safety and efficacy in the proper clinical setting. Successfully overcoming this challenge will require intense focused preclinical research, the development and validation of biomarkers and imaging techniques for monitoring progression or regression of tissue fibrosis, selection of the appropriate patient populations, and the design and execution of robust multicenter clinical trials with clearly defined endpoints.

References

[1] Kraling BM, Maul GG, Jimenez SA. Mononuclear cellular infiltrates in clinically involved skin from patients with systemic sclerosis of recent onset predominantly consist of monocytes/macrophages. Pathobiology 1995;63(1):48–56.
[2] Jelaska A, Korn JH. Role of apoptosis and transforming growth factor beta1 in fibroblast selection and activation in systemic sclerosis. Arthritis Rheum 2000;43(10):2230–9.

[3] Davies CA, Jeziorska M, Freemont AJ, et al. The differential expression of VEGF, VEGFR-2, and GLUT-1 proteins in disease subtypes of systemic sclerosis. Hum Pathol 2006;37(2):190–7 [Epub 2005 Dec 15].

[4] Rudnicka L, Varga J, Christiano AM, et al. Elevated expression of type VII collagen in the skin of patients with systemic sclerosis. Regulation by TGF-ß. J Clin Invest 1994;93(4):1709–15.

[5] van der Slot AJ, Zuurmond AM, Bardoel AF, et al. Identification of PLOD2 as telopeptide lysyl hydroxylase, an important enzyme in fibrosis. J Biol Chem 2003;278(42):40967–72 [Epub 2003 Jul 24].

[6] Gardner H, Shearstone JR, Bandaru R, et al. Gene profiling of scleroderma skin reveals robust signatures of disease that are imperfectly reflected in the transcript profiles of explanted fibroblasts. Arthritis Rheum 2006;54(6):1961–73.

[7] Whitfield ML, Finlay DR, Murray JI, et al. Systemic and cell type-specific gene expression patterns in scleroderma skin. Proc Natl Acad Sci U S A 2003;100(21):12319–24.

[8] Asano Y, Czuwara-Ladykowska J, Trojanowska M. TGF-beta regulates DNA-binding activity of transcription factor Fli1 by PCAF-dependent acetylation. J Biol Chem 2007; 282(48):34672–83.

[9] Wang Y, Fan PS, Kahaleh B. Association between enhanced type I collagen expression and epigenetic repression of the FLI1 gene in scleroderma fibroblasts. Arthritis Rheum 2006; 54(7):2271–9.

[10] Atamas SP, Yurovsky VV, Wise R, et al. Production of type 2 cytokines by CD8+ lung cells is associated with greater decline in pulmonary function in patients with systemic sclerosis. Arthritis Rheum 1999;42(6):1168–78.

[11] Bouros D, Wells AU, Nicholson AG, et al. Histopathologic subsets of fibrosing alveolitis in patients with systemic sclerosis and their relationship to outcome. Am J Respir Crit Care Med 2002;165(12):1581–6.

[12] Veeraraghavan S, Nicholson AG, Wells AU. Lung fibrosis: new classifications and therapy. Curr Opin Rheumatol 2001;13(6):500–4.

[13] Fernandes F, Ramires FJ, Arteaga E, et al. Cardiac remodeling in patients with systemic sclerosis with no signs or symptoms of heart failure: an endomyocardial biopsy study. J Card Fail 2003;9(4):311–7.

[14] Varga J, Abraham DJ. Systemic sclerosis: paradigm multisystem fibrosing disorder. J Clin Invest 2007;117(3):557–67.

[15] Varga J, Bashey RI. Regulation of connective tissue synthesis in systemic sclerosis. Int Rev Immunol 1995;12(2–4):187–99.

[16] Abraham DJ, Eckes B, Rajkumar V, et al. New developments in fibroblast and myofibroblast biology: implications for fibrosis and scleroderma. Curr Rheumatol Rep 2007;9(2):136–43.

[17] Tomasek JJ, Gabbiani G, Hinz B, et al. Myofibroblasts and mechanoregulation of connective tissue remodeling. Nat Rev Mol Cell Biol 2002;3(5):349–63.

[18] Rajkumar VS, Howell K, Csiszar K, et al. Shared expression of phenotypic markers in systemic sclerosis indicates a convergence of pericytes and fibroblasts to a myofibroblast lineage in fibrosis. Arthritis Res Ther 2005;7(5):R1113–23 [Epub 2005 Jul 21].

[19] Helmbold P, Fiedler E, Fischer M, et al. Hyperplasia of dermal microvascular pericytes in scleroderma. J Cutan Pathol 2004;31(6):431–40.

[20] Kalluri R, Neilson EG. Epithelial–mesenchymal transition and its implications for fibrosis. J Clin Invest 2003;112(12):1776–84.

[21] Abe R, Donnelly SC, Peng T, et al. Peripheral blood fibrocytes: differentiation pathway and migration to wound sites. J Immunol 2001;166(12):7556–62.

[22] Quan TE, Cowper S, Wu SP, et al. Circulating fibrocytes: collagen-secreting cells of the peripheral blood. Int J Biochem Cell Biol 2004;36(4):598–606.

[23] Kuwana M, Okazaki Y, Kodama H, et al. Human circulating CD14+ monocytes as a source of progenitors that exhibit mesenchymal cell differentiation. J Leukoc Biol 2003; 74(5):833–45.

[24] Bellini A, Mattoli S. The role of the fibrocyte, a bone marrow-derived mesenchymal progenitor, in reactive and reparative fibroses. Lab Invest 2007;87(9):858–70 [Epub 2007 Jul 2].

[25] Abraham DJ, Varga J. Scleroderma: from cell and molecular mechanisms to disease models. Trends Immunol 2005;26(11):587–95.

[26] Varga J, Trojanowska M. Molecular pathways as novel therapeutic targets in systemic sclerosis. Current Opin Rheumatol 2007;19(6):568–73.

[27] Ghosh AK, Varga J. The transcriptional coactivator and acetyltransferase p300 in fibroblast biology and fibrosis. J Cell Physiol 2007;213(3):663–71.

[28] Dong C, Zhu S, Wang T, et al. Deficient Smad7 expression: a putative molecular defect in scleroderma. Proc Natl Acad Sci U S A 2002;99(6):3908–13.

[29] Asano Y, Ihn H, Yamane K, et al. Impaired Smad7-Smurf-mediated negative regulation of TGF-beta signaling in scleroderma fibroblasts. J Clin Invest 2004;113(2):253–64.

[30] Ghosh AK, Bhattacharyya S, Varga J. The tumor suppressor p53 abrogates Smad-dependent collagen gene induction in mesenchymal cells. J Biol Chem 2004;279(46):47455–63 [Epub 2004 Sep 1].

[31] Svegliati S, Cancello R, Sambo P, et al. Platelet-derived growth factor and reactive oxygen species (ROS) regulate Ras protein levels in primary human fibroblasts via ERK1/2. Amplification of ROS and Ras in systemic sclerosis fibroblasts. J Biol Chem 2005;280(43):36474–82 [Epub 2005 Aug 4].

[32] Kubo M, Czuwara-Ladykowska J, Moussa O, et al. Persistent down-regulation of Fli1, a suppressor of collagen transcription, in fibrotic scleroderma skin. Am J Pathol 2003;163(2):571–81.

[33] Mauviel A. Transforming growth factor-beta: a key mediator of fibrosis. Methods Mol Med 2005;117:69–80.

[34] Massague J, Seoane J, Wotton D. Smad transcription factors. Genes Dev 2005;19(23):2783–810.

[35] Bhattacharyya S, Ghosh AK, Pannu J, et al. Fibroblast expression of the coactivator p300 governs the intensity of profibrotic response to transforming growth factor beta. Arthritis Rheum 2005;52(4):1248–58.

[36] Ishida W, Mori Y, Lakos G, et al. Intracellular TGF-beta receptor blockade abrogates Smad-dependent fibroblast activation in vitro and in vivo. J Invest Dermatol 2006;126(8):1733–44 [Epub 2006 Jun 1].

[37] Mori Y, Ishida W, Bhattacharyya S, et al. Selective inhibition of activin receptor-like kinase 5 signaling blocks profibrotic transforming growth factor beta responses in skin fibroblasts. Arthritis Rheum 2004;50(12):4008–21.

[38] Chen Y, Shi-wen X, Eastwood M, et al. Contribution of activin receptor-like kinase 5 (transforming growth factor beta receptor type I) signaling to the fibrotic phenotype of scleroderma fibroblasts. Arthritis Rheum 2006;54(4):1309–16.

[39] Prud'homme GJ. Pathobiology of transforming growth factor beta in cancer, fibrosis and immunologic disease, and therapeutic considerations. Lab Invest 2007;87(11):1077–91.

[40] Moustakas A, Heldin CH. Non-Smad TGF-beta signals. J Cell Sci 2005;118:3573–84.

[41] Sato M, Shegogue D, Gore EA, et al. Role of p38 MAPK in transforming growth factor beta stimulation of collagen production by scleroderma and healthy dermal fibroblasts. J Invest Dermatol 2002;118(4):704–11.

[42] Hayashida T, Decaestecker M, Schnaper HW. Cross-talk between ERK MAP kinase and Smad signaling pathways enhances TGF-beta dependent responses in human mesangial cells. FASEB J 2003;17(11):1576–8 [Epub 2003 Jun 17].

[43] Hayashida T, Wu M, Pierce A, et al. MAP kinase activity necessary for TGF-ß stimulated mesangial cell type I collagen expression requires adhesion-dependent phosphorylation of FAK tyrosine 397. J Cell Sci 2007;120(Pt 23):4230–40.

[44] Daniels CE, Wilkes MC, Edens M, et al. Imatinib mesylate inhibits the profibrogenic activity of TGF-beta and prevents bleomycin-mediated lung fibrosis. J Clin Invest 2004;114:1308–16.

[45] Pannu J, Nakerakanti S, Smith E, et al. Transforming growth factor-beta receptor type I-dependent fibrogenic gene program is mediated via activation of Smad1 and ERK1/2 pathways. J Biol Chem 2007;282:10405–13.

[46] Goumans MJ, Valdimarsdottir G, Itoh S, et al. Activin receptor-like kinase (ALK)1 is an antagonistic mediator of lateral TGFbeta/ALK5 signaling. Mol Cell 2003;12:817–28.

[47] Abe H, Matsubara T, Iehara N, et al. Type IV collagen is transcriptionally regulated by Smad1 under advanced glycation end product (AGE) stimulation. J Biol Chem 2004;279: 14201–6.

[48] Matsubara T, Abe H, Arai H, et al. Expression of Smad1 is directly associated with mesangial matrix expansion in rat diabetic nephropathy. Lab Invest 2006;86:357–68.

[49] Takahashi T, Abe H, Arai H, et al. Activation of STAT3/Smad1 is a key signaling pathway for progression to glomerulosclerosis in experimental glomerulonephritis. J Biol Chem 2005;280:7100–6.

[50] Pannu J, Gardner H, Shearstone JR, et al. Increased levels of transforming growth factor beta receptor type I and up-regulation of matrix gene program: a model of scleroderma-Arthritis Rheum 2006;54:3011–21.

[51] Holmes A, Abraham DJ, Chen Y, et al. Constitutive connective tissue growth factor expression in scleroderma fibroblasts is dependent on Sp1. J Biol Chem 2003;278:41728–33.

[52] Chen SJ, Ning H, Ishida W, et al. The early-immediate gene EGR-1 is induced by transforming growth factor-beta and mediates stimulation of collagen gene expression. J Biol Chem 2006;281:21183–97.

[53] Yu J, de Belle I, Liang H, et al. Coactivating factors p300 and CBP are transcriptionally cross-regulated by Egr1 in prostate cells, leading to divergent responses. Mol Cell 2004; 15:83–94.

[54] Cho SJ, Kang MJ, Homer RJ, et al. Role of early growth response-1 (Egr-1) in interleukin-13 induced inflammation and remodeling. J Biol Chem 2006;281:8161–8.

[55] Czuwara-Ladykowska J, Shirasaki F, Jackers P, et al. Fli-1 inhibits collagen type I production in dermal fibroblasts via an Sp1-dependent pathway. J Biol Chem 2001;276: 20839–48.

[56] Nakerakanti SS, Kapanadze B, Yamasaki M, et al. Fli1 and Ets1 have distinct roles in connective tissue growth factor/CCN2 gene regulation and induction of the profibrotic gene program. J Biol Chem 2006;281:25259–69.

[57] Ghosh AK, Bhattacharyya S, Lakos G, et al. Disruption of transforming growth factor beta signaling and profibrotic responses in normal skin fibroblasts by peroxisome proliferator-activated receptor gamma. Arthritis Rheum 2004;50:1305–18.

[58] Cheng S, Afif H, Martel-Pelletier J, et al. Activation of peroxisome proliferator-activated receptor gamma inhibits interleukin-1beta induced membrane-associated prostaglandin E2 synthase-1 expression in human synovial fibroblasts by interfering with Egr-1. J Biol Chem 2004;279:22057–65.

[59] Distler JH, Jungel A, Huber LC, et al. Imatinib mesylate reduces production of extracellular matrix and prevents development of experimental dermal fibrosis. Arthritis Rheum 2007;56(1):311–22.

[60] Kolch W. Coordinating ERK/MAPK signaling through scaffolds and inhibitors. Nat Rev Mol Cell Biol 2005;6:827–37.

[61] Hayashida T, Poncelet AC, Hubchak SC, et al. TGF-beta1 activates MAP kinase in human mesangial cells: a possible role in collagen expression. Kidney Int 1999;56(5):1710–20.

[62] Tourkina E, Gooz P, Pannu J, et al. Opposing effects of protein kinase C-alpha and protein kinase C-epsilon on collagen expression by human lung fibroblasts are mediated via MEK/ERK and caveolin-1 signaling. J Biol Chem 2005;280:13879–87.

[63] Tan FK. Autoantibodies against PDGF receptor in scleroderma. N Engl J Med 2006; 354(25):2709–11.

[64] Eckes B, Zigrino P, Kessler D, et al. Fibroblast-matrix interactions in wound healing and fibrosis. Matrix Biol 2000;19:325–32.

[65] Asano Y, Ihn H, Yamane K, et al. Increased expression of integrin alpha(v)beta3 contributes to the establishment of autocrine TGF-beta signaling in scleroderma fibroblasts. J Immunol 2005;175:7708–18.

[66] Asano Y, Ihn H, Yamane K, et al. Increased expression levels of integrin alphavbeta5 on scleroderma fibroblasts. Am J Pathol 2004;164:1275–92.

[67] Asano Y, Ihn H, Yamane K, et al. Increased expression of integrin alphavbeta5 induces the myofibroblastic differentiation of dermal fibroblasts. Am J Pathol 2006; 168:499–510.

[68] Mimura Y, Ihn H, Jinnin M, et al. Constitutive thrombospondin-1 overexpression contributes to autocrine transforming growth factor-beta signaling in cultured scleroderma fibroblasts. Am J Pathol 2005;166:1451–63.

[69] Sato S, Nagaoka T, Hasegawa M, et al. Serum levels of connective tissue growth factor are elevated in patients with systemic sclerosis: association with extent of skin sclerosis and severity of pulmonary fibrosis. J Rheumatol 2000;27(1):149–54.

[70] Igarashi A, Nashiro K, Kikuchi K, et al. Significant correlation between connective tissue growth factor gene expression and skin sclerosis in tissue sections from patients with systemic sclerosis. J Invest Dermatol 1995;105(2):280–4.

[71] Fonseca C, Lindahl GE, Ponticos M, et al. A polymorphism in the CTGF promoter region associated with systemic sclerosis. N Engl J Med 2007;357(12):1210–20.

[72] Leask A, Abraham DJ. The role of connective tissue growth factor, a multifunctional matricellular protein, in fibroblast biology. Biochem Cell Biol 2003;81(6):355–63.

[73] Chujo S, Shirasaki F, Kawara S, et al. Connective tissue growth factor causes persistent proalpha2(I) collagen gene expression induced by transforming growth factor-beta in a mouse fibrosis model. J Cell Physiol 2005;203(2):447–56.

[74] Grotendorst GR. Connective tissue growth factor: a mediator of TGF-beta action on fibroblasts. Cytokine Growth Factor Rev 1997;8(3):171–9.

[75] Mori Y, Hinchcliff M, Wu M, et al. Connective tissue growth factor/CCN2-null mouse embryonic fibroblasts retain intact transforming growth factor-beta responsiveness. Exp Cell Res 2008, in press.

[76] Klareskog L, Gustafsson R, Scheynius A, et al. Increased expression of platelet-derived growth factor type B receptors in the skin of patients with systemic sclerosis. Arthritis Rheum 1990;33(10):1534–41.

[77] Ludwicka A, Ohba T, Trojanowska M, et al. Elevated levels of platelet derived growth factor and transforming growth factor-beta 1 in bronchoalveolar lavage fluid from patients with scleroderma. J Rheumatol 1995;22(10):1876–83.

[78] Baroni SS, Santillo M, Bevilacqua F, et al. Stimulatory autoantibodies to the PDGF receptor in systemic sclerosis. N Engl J Med 2006;354:2667–76.

[79] Svegliati S, Olivieri A, Campelli N, et al. Stimulatory autoantibodies to PDGF receptor in patients with extensive chronic graft-versus-host disease. Blood 2007;110(1):237–41 [Eppub 2007 Mar 15].

[80] Postlethwaite AE, Holness MA, Katai H, et al. Human fibroblasts synthesize elevated levels of extracellular matrix proteins in response to interleukin 4. J Clin Invest 1992;90(4): 1479–85.

[81] Hasegawa M, Fujimoto M, Kikuchi K, et al. Elevated serum levels of interleukin 4 (IL-4), IL-10, and IL-13 in patients with systemic sclerosis. J Rheumatol 1997;24:328–32.

[82] Sakkas LI, Tourtellotte C, Berney S, et al. Increased levels of alternatively spliced interleukin 4 (IL-4delta2) transcripts in peripheral blood mononuclear cells from patients with systemic sclerosis. Clin Diagn Lab Immunol 1999;6(5):660–4.

[83] Salmon-Ehr V, Serpier H, Nawrocki B, et al. Expression of interleukin-4 in scleroderma skin specimens and scleroderma fibroblast cultures. Potential role in fibrosis. Arch Dermatol 1996;132(7):802–6.

[84] Fichtner-Feigl S, Fuss IJ, Young CA, et al. Induction of IL-13 triggers TGF-beta1 dependent tissue fibrosis in chronic 2,4,6-trinitrobenzene sulfonic acid colitis. J Immunol 2007; 178(9):5859–70.

[85] Jinnin M, Ihn H, Yamane K, et al. Interleukin-13 stimulates the transcription of the human alpha2(I) collagen gene in human dermal fibroblasts. J Biol Chem 2004;279(40):41783–91.

[86] Yamamoto T. Chemokines and chemokine receptors in scleroderma. Int Arch Allergy Immunol 2006;140(4):345–56.

[87] Yanaba K, Komura K, Kodera M, et al. Serum levels of monocyte chemotactic protein-3/CCL7 are raised in patients with systemic sclerosis: association with extent of skin sclerosis and severity of pulmonary fibrosis. Ann Rheum Dis 2006;65(1):124–6.

[88] Reitamo S, Remitz A, Varga J, et al. Demonstration of interleukin-8 and autoantibodies to interleukin-8 in the serum of patients with systemic sclerosis and related disorders. Arch Dermatol 1993;129(2):189–93.

[89] Carulli MT, Ong VH, Ponticos M, et al. Chemokine receptor CCR2 expression by systemic sclerosis fibroblasts: evidence for autocrine regulation of myofibroblast differentiation. Arthritis Rheum 2005;52(12):3772–82.

[90] Ferreira AM, Takagawa S, Fresco R, et al. Diminished induction of skin fibrosis in mice with MCP-1 deficiency. J Invest Dermatol 2006;126(8):1900–8.

[91] Ong VH, Evans LA, Shiwen X, et al. Monocyte chemoattractant protein 3 as a mediator of fibrosis: overexpression in systemic sclerosis and the type 1 tight-skin mouse. Arthritis Rheum 2003;48(7):1979–91.

[92] Prasse A, Pechkovsky DV, Toews GB, et al. CCL18 as an indicator of pulmonary fibrotic activity in idiopathic interstitial pneumonias and systemic sclerosis. Arthritis Rheum 2007; 56(5):1685–93.

[93] Pilewski JM, Liu L, Henry AC, et al. Insulin-like growth factor binding proteins 3 and 5 are overexpressed in idiopathic pulmonary fibrosis and contribute to extracellular matrix deposition. Am J Pathol 2005;166(2):399–407.

[94] Harrison NK, Cambrey AD, Myers AR, et al. Insulin-like growth factor-I is partially responsible for fibroblast proliferation induced by bronchoalveolar lavage fluid from patients with systemic sclerosis. Clin Sci (Lond) 1994;86(2):141–8.

[95] Feghali CA, Wright TM. Identification of multiple, differentially expressed messenger RNAs in dermal fibroblasts from patients with systemic sclerosis. Arthritis Rheum 1999; 42(7):1451–7.

[96] Yasuoka H, Zhou Z, Pilewski JM, et al. Insulin-like growth factor-binding protein-5 induces pulmonary fibrosis and triggers mononuclear cellular infiltration. Am J Pathol 2006;169(5):1633–42.

[97] Jimenez SA, Freundlich B, Rosenbloom J. Selective inhibition of human diploid fibroblast collagen synthesis by interferons. J Clin Invest 1984;74(3):1112–6.

[98] Duncan MR, Berman B. Gamma interferon is the lymphokine and beta interferon the monokine responsible for inhibition of fibroblast collagen production and late but not early fibroblast proliferation. J Exp Med 1985;162(2):516–27.

[99] Jaffe HA, Gao Z, Mori Y, et al. Selective inhibition of collagen gene expression in fibroblasts by an interferon-gamma transgene. Exp Lung Res 1999;25(3):199–215.

[100] Ghosh AK, Yuan W, Mori Y, et al. Antagonistic regulation of type I collagen gene expression by interferon-gamma and transforming growth factor-beta. Integration at the level of p300/CBP transcriptional coactivators. J Biol Chem 2001;276(14):11041–8.

[101] Chizzolini C, Rezzonico R, Ribbens C, et al. Inhibition of type I collagen production by dermal fibroblasts upon contact with activated T cells: different sensitivity to inhibition between systemic sclerosis and control fibroblasts. Arthritis Rheum 1998;41(11):2039–47.

[102] Freundlich B, Jimenez SA, Steen VD, et al. Treatment of systemic sclerosis with recombinant interferon-gamma. A phase I/II clinical trial. Arthritis Rheum 1992;35(10):1134–42.

[103] Grassegger A, Schuler G, Hessenberger G, et al. Interferon-gamma in the treatment of systemic sclerosis: a randomized controlled multicentre trial. Br J Dermatol 1998;139(4): 639–48.

[104] Hunzelmann N, Anders S, Fierlbeck G, et al. Systemic scleroderma. Multicenter trial of 1 year of treatment with recombinant interferon gamma. Arch Dermatol 1997;133(5):609–13.

[105] Trojanowska M. What did we learn by studying scleroderma fibroblasts? Clin Exp Rheumatol 2004;22(3 Suppl 33):S59–63.

[106] Mimura Y, Ihn H, Jinnin M, et al. Constitutive phosphorylation of focal adhesion kinase is involved in the myofibroblast differentiation of scleroderma fibroblasts. J Invest Dermatol 2005;124(5):886–92.

[107] Jun JB, Kuechle M, Min J, et al. Scleroderma fibroblasts demonstrate enhanced activation of Akt (protein kinase B) in situ. J Invest Dermatol 2005;124(2):298–303.

[108] Ihn H. Autocrine TGF-beta signaling in the pathogenesis of systemic sclerosis. J Dermatol Sci 2008;49(2):103–13.

[109] Yamane K, Ihn H, Kubo M, et al. Increased transcriptional activities of transforming growth factor beta receptors in scleroderma fibroblasts. Arthritis Rheum 2002;46(9):2421–8.

[110] Kawakami T, Ihn H, Xu W, et al. Increased expression of TGF-beta receptors by scleroderma fibroblasts: evidence for contribution of autocrine TGF-beta signaling to scleroderma phenotype. J Invest Dermatol 1998;110(1):47–51.

[111] Kubo M, Ihn H, Yamane K, et al. Up-regulated expression of transforming growth factor-beta receptors in dermal fibroblasts of skin sections from patients with systemic sclerosis. J Rheumatol 2002;29(12):2558–64.

[112] Mori Y, Chen SJ, Varga J. Expression and regulation of intracellular SMAD signaling in scleroderma skin fibroblasts. Arthritis Rheum 2003;48(7):1964–78.

[113] Varga J. SSc and Smads: dysfunctional Smad family dynamics culminating in fibrosis. Arthritis Rheum 2002;46(7):1703–13.

[114] Verrecchia F, Laboureau J, Verola O, et al. Skin involvement in scleroderma—where histological and clinical scores meet. Rheumatology (Oxford) 2007;46(5):833–41 [Epub 2007 Jan 25].

[115] Ihn H, Yamane K, Asano Y, et al. Constitutively phosphorylated Smad3 interacts with Sp1 and p300 in scleroderma fibroblasts. Rheumatology (Oxford) 2006;45(2):157–65 [Epub 2005 Nov 30].

[116] Clark SH. Animal models in scleroderma. Curr Rheumatol Rep 2005;7(2):150–5.

[117] Green MC, Sweet HO, Bunker LE. Tight-skin, a new mutation of the mouse causing excessive growth of connective tissue and skeleton. Am J Pathol 1976;82(3):493–512.

[118] Bayle J, Fitch J, Jacobsen K, et al. Increased expression of Wnt2 and SFRP4 in Tsk mouse skin: role of Wnt signaling in altered dermal fibrillin deposition and systemic sclerosis. J Invest Dermatol 2007 [epub ahead of print].

[119] Jimenez SA, Millan A, Bashey RI. Scleroderma-like alterations in collagen metabolism occurring in the TSK (tight skin) mouse. Arthritis Rheum 1984;27(2):180–5.

[120] Baxter RM, Crowell TP, McCrann ME, et al. Analysis of the tight skin (Tsk1/+) mouse as a model for testing antifibrotic agents. Lab Invest 2005;85(10):1199–209.

[121] Siracusa LD, McGrath R, Ma Q, et al. A tandem duplication within the fibrillin 1 gene is associated with the mouse tight skin mutation. Genome Res 1996;6(4):300–13.

[122] Christner PJ, Peters J, Hawkins D, et al. The tight skin 2 mouse. An animal model of scleroderma displaying cutaneous fibrosis and mononuclear cell infiltration. Arthritis Rheum 1995;38(12):1791–8.

[123] Yamamoto T, Takagawa S, Katayama I, et al. Animal model of sclerotic skin. I: local injections of bleomycin induce sclerotic skin mimicking scleroderma. J Invest Dermatol 1999; 112(4):456–62.

[124] Lakos G, Melichian D, Wu M, et al. Increased bleomycin-induced skin fibrosis in mice lacking the Th1-specific transcription factor T-bet. Pathobiology 2006;73(5):224–37.

[125] Lakos G, Takagawa S, Chen SJ, et al. Targeted disruption of TGF-beta/Smad3 signaling modulates skin fibrosis in a mouse model of scleroderma. Am J Pathol 2004;165(1):203–17.

[126] Lakos G, Takagawa S, Varga J. Animal models of SSc. Methods Mol Med 2004;102: 377–93.

[127] Zhang Y, Gilliam AC. Animal models for scleroderma: an update. Curr Rheumatol Rep 2002;4(2):150–62.

[128] Zhang Y, McCormick LL, Desai SR, et al. Murine sclerodermatous graft-versus-host disease, a model for human scleroderma: cutaneous cytokines, chemokines, and immune cell activation. J Immunol 2002;168(6):3088–98.

[129] Ruzek MC, Jha S, Ledbetter S, et al. A modified model of graft-versus-host-induced systemic sclerosis (scleroderma) exhibits all major aspects of the human disease. Arthritis Rheum 2004;50(4):1319–31.

[130] Sonnylal S, Denton CP, Zheng B, et al. Postnatal induction of transforming growth factor beta signaling in fibroblasts of mice recapitulates clinical, histologic, and biochemical features of scleroderma. Arthritis Rheum 2007;56:334–44.

[131] Denton CP, Lindahl GE, Khan K, et al. Activation of key profibrotic mechanisms in transgenic fibroblasts expressing kinase-deficient type II TGF-ß receptor. J Biol Chem 2005; 280(16):16053–65.

[132] Wynne T. Cellular and molecular mechanisms of fibrosis. J Pathol 2008;214(2):199–210.

ELSEVIER
SAUNDERS

Rheum Dis Clin N Am
34 (2008) 145–159

RHEUMATIC
DISEASE CLINICS
OF NORTH AMERICA

Novel Treatment Approaches to Fibrosis in Scleroderma

Jörg Distler, MD[a], Oliver Distler, MD[b],*

[a]*Department of Internal Medicine III and Institute for Clinical Immunology, University of Erlangen-Nuremberg, Krankenhausstrasse 12, 91054 Erlangen, Germany*
[b]*Department of Rheumatology, Center of Experimental Rheumatology, University Hospital Zurich, 8091 Zurich, Switzerland*

The accumulation of extracellular matrix proteins is one of the hallmarks in the pathogenesis of systemic sclerosis (SSc). However, the molecular mechanisms leading to tissue fibrosis were only poorly understood in the past and even today, in times of rapidly advancing molecular techniques, the cause or trigger of SSc is still unknown. However, remarkable breakthrough findings have been obtained regarding the identification of key molecules, key cellular mechanisms, and key intracellular signaling cascades, which mediate the perpetuation of fibrosis rather than trigger it. These findings have true translational implications, because modifiers of these key mediators and key mechanisms are often in clinical use in other disease indications, such as cancer. This article summarizes the clinical and preclinical evidence of examples of these novel antifibrotic treatment approaches in SSc, including stem cell transplantation, modifiers of transforming growth factor-β1 signaling, intravenous immunoglobulins, tyrosine kinase inhibitors, and histone deacetylase inhibitors.

High-dose immunosuppressive therapy and autologous hematopoietic stem cell transplantation

The first results from a multicenter phase I and II trial of high-dose immunosuppressive therapy (HDIT) and autologous hematopoietic stem cell transplantation (HSCT) in patients with SSc were reported in 2001 [1]. Forty-one subjects were included in the study, including 37 subjects with diffuse SSc and 4 with limited disease. All of the subjects with limited disease

---

* Corresponding author.
E-mail address: oliver.distler@usz.ch (O. Distler).

suffered from life-threatening pulmonary fibrosis or pulmonary hypertension. Sixty-one percent of the patients had a modified Rodnan skin score (mRSS) of greater than or equal to 26. Scleroderma lung disease was detectable in 76% of the subjects, with a mean forced vital capcity (FVC) of less than or equal to 70% in 50% of the subjects. Pulmonary hypertension was present in 19% and renal disease in 14%. Regimens for mobilization and conditioning were not uniform in this study. For mobilization, cyclophosphamide and granulocyte colony stimulating factor (G-CSF) were used. For conditioning, seven different protocols were tested, including six regimens with hemoablative doses of cyclophosphamide or anti-thymocyte globulin or total body irradiation. After a mean follow-up of 12 months, 11 subjects had died, with seven deaths related to the procedure. Of the remaining subjects, 29 were evaluated. Of those subjects, 69% experienced an improvement of the mRSS of more than 25%. Lung function did not change and pulmonary hypertension remained stable. Renal disease worsened in one out of five subjects, but no new cases of renal disease occurred during follow-up. Disease progression occurred in 19% of the subjects after HDIT and HSCT.

Similar results regarding initial responses were reported from a French multicenter phase I and II trial [2]. In this study, 12 subjects with progressive and refractory SSc, a disease duration of less than 4 years, and involvement of at least one major organ system were included. In contrast to the first study, uniform protocols were used for mobilization and conditioning. Peripheral blood mononuclear cells (PBMCs) were mobilized using cyclophosphamide (2×2 g/m^2) and G-CSF (5 µg/kg per day). The collected PBMCs were selected for CD34 positive cells and reinfused after conditioning with cyclophosphamide (200 mg/kg) or melphalan (140 mg/m^2). In this trial, failure of mobilization, selection, or enrichment occurred in three out twelve subjects. Eleven subjects were finally transplanted, ten with autologous PBMCs and one with autologous bone marrow. The median time to hematopoietic reconstitution of neutrophils and platelets were 12 and 10 days, respectively. Major responses were defined as a performance status of 0 and a scleroderma health assessment questionnaire (SHAQ) of less than 0.5, plus a decrease of the mRSS by more than 50% and a decrease of the forced expiratory volume in the first second of expiration (FEV$_1$) by more than 30%. Partial responses were defined as a performance status of less than or equal to 1 or a SHAQ of 0.6 to 1, plus a decrease of the mRSS by less than 50% and a decrease of the FEV$_1$ between 15% and 30%. Significant improvements fulfilling the criteria for major response were observed in eight out of eleven subjects. In addition, partial responses were noticed in two subjects. However, a high rate of relapses was noted in this cohort. Of the eight subjects with initial responses, five relapsed within 12 months.

The results of two single-arm studies of HDIT and HSCT in SSc with long-term follow-up results have recently been published. In a phase II single-arm study of HDIT and HSCT in SSc from several centers in the United

States, 34 subjects with diffuse SSc were included [3]. All subjects were 65 years of age or younger. The subjects included into the study belong to one of the following two groups.

The first group was characterized by a disease duration of less than 4 years and an mRSS of greater than or equal to16, plus significant visceral organ involvement with a diffusion capacity for carbon monoxide (DLCO) or an FVC of less than 70%, myocardial disease, proteinuria less than 500 mg every 24 hours, or an elevated serum creatinine.

The second group of subjects included in the study suffered from progressive pulmonary disease with a decrease of the FVC or the DLCO of greater than or equal to 15% in the previous 6 months, or new onset of alveolitis on HRCT, or a bronchoalveolar lavage with greater than or equal to 3% polymononuclear cells plus eosinophils. In this study, peripheral blood stem cells were mobilized with G-CSF (16 µg/kg per day) and collected and selected for CD34 positive cells after 4 days. The HDIT regimen consisted of fractioned total body irradiation (800 cGy), cyclophosphamide (120 mg/kg), and equine antithymocyte globulin (90 mg/kg). Methylprednisolone at a dose of 1 mg/kg was given intravenously with each dose of antithymocyte globulin. Total body irradiation without shielding was used for the first eight subjects included in the study, but in all other subjects the lungs were shielded to a total dose of 200 cGy. Prednisone was given at a dose of 0.5 mg/kg per day from the start of conditioning until 30 days after transplantation, and then tapered over a month in most subjects. G-CSF (5 µg/kg per day) was given intravenously from day 0 until the absolute neutrophil count was greater than 0.5×10^9/l. Infection prophylaxes included trimethoprim-sulfamethoxazole, acyclovir, and fluconazole. Of the 34 subjects enrolled in the study, 27 survived the first year. In these subjects, the mean mRSS decreased strongly from 30.1 to 8 (70.3%). A significant reduction of the accumulation of collagen in the dermis was observed histologically in eight out of ten subjects for whom biopsies were taken before and after HDIT and HSCT. The strongest decrease of the mRSS of 58.3% was observed in the first year. Between the third year and the final evaluation after up to eight years, the mean mRSS remained stable. A significant decrease was also noted for the HAQ score; however, modest but significant worsening of renal and myocardial function was observed. The serum creatinine concentration increased by 0.25 mg/dL and the ejection fraction decreased by 2.37%. Furthermore, the DLCO tended to decrease by 6% at the final evaluation.

The estimated progression free survival was 64% at 5 years. In total, 12 subjects died during the study, eight because of transplantation related complications and four because of SSc. Fatal pulmonary toxicities occurred in two of the eight subjects without lung shielding, but in none of the subjects with lung shielding. Renal crisis or dysfunction occurred in six subjects, all within the first 2 months after HDIT and HSCT. Two subjects developed myelodysplastic syndromes and a stage I non-small-cell lung carcinoma was detected in one subject with a longstanding history of smoking cigarettes, who had lung shielding, after 5 years. A fatal Epstein-Barr virus associated lymphoproliferative disorder occurred. A case of gastrointestinal cytomega- lovirus disease resolved with antiviral therapy. Bacteremia occurred in 11 subjects. Reactivation of varicella zoster virus occurred in six subjects not receiving prophylaxis with acyclovir. The investigators suggested that toxicity might be reduced further by shielding the lungs and the kidneys in future studies.

Long-term follow-up results on 26 SSc subjects treated with HDIT and HSCT from two of the leading centers of the European Autologous Stem cell Transplantation International Scleroderma (ASTIS) trial also suggested beneficial responses [4]. All but three subjects had received treatment with various disease-modifying antirheumatic drugs (DMARDs). The mean mRSS was 32, pulmonary involvement was present in 17 subjects and 5 sub- jects had a creatinine clearance below 70 mL per minute. After a median fol- low-up of 5.3 years, 21 out of 26 subjects demonstrated a clinically beneficial response. A decrease of the mRSS of more than 25% was observed in 19 out of 26 subjects after 1 year, and in 15 out of 16 subjects after 5 years. The reduction of the mRSS was most pronounced after 1 year, with a mean decrease of 11.6 units, and decreased further by 2.6 units in the following years. The mean vital capacity, the FEV_1, and the DLCO did not improve. Cardiac and renal function remained stable. Relapses occurred in six sub- jects, two of whom had initial major response and four of whom had partial response within 2 to 4 years after transplantation. The Kaplan-Meier estimated survival at 5 years was 96.2% (95% confidence interval or CI, 70.2%–100.0%). The event-free survival, defined as absence of mortality, re- lapse, or progression of SSc was 64.3% (95% CI, 47.9%–86.0%) at 5 years. Infectious complications with herpes zoster reactivation or atypical myco- bacteria occurred in five subjects. One subject had persistent pancytopenia that required several transfusions and recovered suboptimal blood counts. One subject developed a basal carcinoma 4 years after transplantation.

The outcome of HDIT and HSCT in patients with SSc is currently being studied further in two randomized controlled trials in the Europe and in the United States. The European ASTIS trial was launched in 2001 to compare the safety and efficacy of HDIT and HSCT with 12 monthly pulses of intra- venous cyclophosphamide at doses of 750 mg/m^2. A medium intensity was chosen for immunoablation in the ASTIS protocol, consisting of cyclophos- phamide (2×2 g/m^2) plus G-CSF (10 µg/kg), and selection of the apheresis product for CD34 positive cells, and conditioning with cyclophosphamide (200 mg/kg) and rabbit antithymocyte globulin (7.5 mg/kg), followed by HSCT. The primary endpoint is event-free survival, defined as the time in days from the day of randomization until the occurrence of death or the development of persistent major organ failure (heart, lung, and kidney) dur- ing the study period of 2 years. It is intended to enroll 200 subjects in total with diffuse SSc and a disease duration of 4 years or less from the onset of skin thickening. Subjects must be between 16 and 60 years old and have an mRSS of greater than or equal to 15, plus major organ involvement with documented evidence of onset or clinically significant worsening in the previous 6 months, or diffuse scleroderma with disease duration of 2 years since development of the first sign of skin thickening, plus an mRSS greater than or equal to 20 plus involvement of trunk, plus an erythrocyte sedimentation rate of greater than 25 mm or hemoglobin less than 11 g/dL, not explained by other causes than active scleroderma. Subjects with previous treatment with alkylating agents, including cyclophosphamide, are excluded from the study. Currently, approximately 140 subjects have been assigned to the ASTIS trial.

The North American counterpart of the ASTIS trial, the SCOT (Scleroderma: Cyclophosphamide or Transplantation) trial, also compares the safety and efficacy of HDIT and HSCT, with high-dose intravenous cyclophosphamide. The primary objective is to evaluate differences in the rates of death and significant organ damage between the HDIT/HSCT group and the cyclophosphamide group 44 months after enrolment. It is planned to enroll 226 subjects between 18 and 65 years of age with severe SSc and a poor prognosis. Inclusion criteria include an mRSS of greater than or equal to 16, a disease duration of 4 years or less from the onset of the first non-Raynaud's symptom, presence of SSc-related pulmonary disease with FVC or a DLCO of less than 70%, plus evidence of alveolitis by high-resolution chest CT scan or bronchoalveolar lavage, or a history of SSc-related renal crisis or disease, not active at the time of screening.

In addition to autologous stem cell transplantation, the outcomes of two SSc patients with allogeneic transplantation have been reported [5]. Both patients received a myeloablative regimen consisting of busulfan (700 ng/mL), cyclophosphamide (120 mg/kg), and equine antithymocyte globulin (90 mg/kg). The graft bone marrow was derived from HLA-identical siblings. Cyclosporine and methotrexate were administered for prophylaxes of graft versus host disease (GvHD). Trimethoprim/sulfamethoxazole, fluconazole, and acyclovir were used to prevent infectious complications. Both patients had early disease of less than 3 years and diffuse disease. The first patient had an mRSS of 36 and progressive lung involvement with active alveolitis, a DLCO of 43%, and a FVC of 68%. In addition, she suffered from severe Raynaud's phenomenon and digital ulcers. Five years after transplantation, her mRSS had decreased to 2 to 4 and her alveolitis had resolved. The FVC had improved to 96%, whereas the DLCO had not changed substantially. Her HAQ score improved from 1.35 to 0, and the Raynaud's phenomenon improved, with complete resolution of her digital ulcers. Apart from a BK virus infection and a bacterial pneumonia within the first 2 months after transplantation, no other complications occurred in this patient.

The second patient had an mRSS of 40 and suffered from Raynaud's syndrome without ulcers and arthralgias resistant to multiple DMARDs. Furthermore, she had abnormal lung function tests, with a DLCO of 63% and a FVC of 64%. CT scans did not demonstrate any pathologic findings, but bronchoalveolar lavage (BAL) fluid analysis demonstrated 48% lymphocytes and 3% neutrophils. This patient developed acute GvHD of the skin, which was treated with prednisone at a dose of 2 mg/kg per day. Shortly after initiation of prednisone, she developed severe renal crisis, which could be controlled with antihypertensive therapy. The dose of prednisone was decreased to 1 mg/kg per day and mycophenolate mofetil was initiated. The acute GvHD resolved at day 80, so prednisone and mycophenolate mofetil were discontinued. On day 100 after transplantation, the patient developed chronic GvHD and prednisone and mycophenolate mofetil were restarted. In this patient, the mRSS was reduced from 40 to 11 and the percentage of lymphocytes in the BAL had decreased to 9% without eosinophils at 16 months. Furthermore, the patient's arthralgias and Raynaud's syndrome had resolved. However, at 18 months, she died from overwhelming sepsis with *Pseudomonas aeruginosa*.

It has to be emphasized that final conclusions cannot be drawn until the two randomized controlled trials are finished. However, the data presented so far suggest impressive effects of HDIT and HSCT for the treatment of SSc with profound regression of skin fibrosis and also of microvascular disease. Still, the first reports indicate a substantial rate of treatment-related mortality of greater 20%. Although the rate of acute treatment-related mortality might be improved by a better selection of subjects and development of less toxic treatment protocols, there might be substantial long-term toxicity with an increased rate of neoplasias because of the drugs used for myeloablation. Thus, HDIT and HSCT will probably be reserved for patients with progressive, life threatening disease that does not respond to other therapies. Challenges for the future regarding this treatment include the identification of patients with an acceptable risk or benefit profile and the molecular and cellular mechanism mediating the clinical effects.

The indications and relevance of allogeneic stem cell transplantation are completely unclear. It is not known, whether allogeneic transplantation is more effective than autologous HSCT in inducing remission and event-free survival. If allogeneic transplantation is more effective than HDIT and autologous HSCT, allogeneic stem cell transplantation might be a potential option for patients in whom HDIT and autologous HSCT were not effective. Based on the findings in the second SSc patient reported, and the longstanding experience of patients with hematologic neoplasias, there seems to be a high rate of treatment-related death. It is unclear whether allogeneic stem cell transplantation has improved survival of SSc patients with progressive diffuse disease.

Recombinant human antitransforming growth factor-β1 antibodies

The safety, tolerability, and pharmacokinetics of a neutralizing human antitransforming growth factor-β1 (TGFβ1) antibody, called CAT-192, was recently evaluated in a phase I and II trial for the treatment of early diffuse SSc [6]. Forty-five SSc subjects fulfilling the American College of Rheumatology (ACR) criteria for SSc, with a disease duration of less than 18 months from the onset of first non-Raynaud's phenomenon manifestation, were enrolled into the study. All subjects had an mRSS between 10 and 28 and progressive disease. The subjects were assigned to either one of the three groups receiving CAT-192 or to the placebo group. Infusions of CAT-192 were given in doses of 0.5 mg/kg, 5 mg/kg, or 10 mg/kg on day 0 and after 6, 12 and 18 weeks. Four subjects died during the study, one in the group receiving 0.5 mg/kg of CAT-192 and three in the group receiving 10 mg/kg of CAT-192. Adverse events and serious adverse events were two to six times more common in patients receiving CAT-192, but there was no increase in the number of adverse events in the groups receiving higher doses. After 24 weeks, there was no evidence of a treatment effect of CAT-192. Neither the mRSS, nor the SHAQ, nor the assessment of organ based disease or the levels of the N terminal propeptide of type I and type III collagen differed significantly between the treatment groups and the placebo group. Similarly, the levels of col 1a1, col 3a1, TGFβ1, and TGFβ2 did not change during treatment.

A potential reason for the lack of efficacy of CAT-192, despite the beneficial effects of inhibitors of TGFβ signaling in several preclinical models, is the specificity of CAT-192 for TGFβ1. In most animal model of SSc, strategies were used that targeted all isoforms of TGFβ instead of a single isoform. Thus, effective prevention of fibrosis might require simultaneous blockade of TGFβ1, TGFβ2, and TGFβ3, for example, by panspecific antibodies, soluble receptors or recombinant latency associated peptide. Moreover, this trial was not designed as an efficacy study and larger studies with a different population might have led to different results. Taken together, this study clearly does not exclude that TGFβ-targeted therapies could be effective in SSc.

Intravenous immunoglobulins

Intravenous immunoglobulins (IVIG) have also been suggested to be beneficial for the treatment of SSc. In the tight-skin 1 mouse model of SSc, treatment with IVIG, starting at an age of 4 weeks for a total of 8 weeks, decreased the mRNA levels of type I collagen and accumulation of collagen in the skin [7]. Furthermore, the production of profibrotic cytokines, such as TGFβ and interleukin-4, by splenocytes was reduced in mice treated with IVIG.

A retrospective study investigated the effects of the administration of IVIG on patients with tissue fibrosis in the setting of different diseases, including three patients with SSc [8]. All three SSc patients had diffuse disease with progressive skin fibrosis that had not responded to conservative treatment. The duration of their illness ranged from less than 1 year to 20 years.

Six cycles of 120 g IVIG were given to two patients, resulting in an impressive decrease in the mRSS from 26 before IVIG treatment to 16 after treatment in one patient, and from 34 to 20 in the other. The third patient responded favorably to three cycles of IVIG treatment, with a decrease of the mRSS from 32 to 20. In addition, an increase of the pulmonary DLCO from 70% to 84% was noted in this patient.

Based on this retrospective study, the efficacy of IVIG for the treatment of fibrosis in patients with SSc was evaluated in two additional open-label uncontrolled studies [9,10]. In the first of these studies, 15 subjects with SSc were treated with IVIG, including ten subjects with diffuse SSc and five subjects with limited SSc [9]. The mean disease duration was 4.7 plus or minus 4.8 years, with the onset of the disease defined as the time at which the ACR criteria were met. All subjects received monthly infusions of IVIG at doses of 2 g/kg over a 5-day period for each course. Eleven subjects received six courses, three subjects received four courses and one subject received only three courses. The extent of skin fibrosis was evaluated with the mRSS before and after the last infusion and the quality of life was assessed with the HAQ score. The mRSS decreased in all but one patient after treatment with IVIG, with a mean decrease of 35%. Interestingly, the decrease of the mRSS was more pronounced in subjects with later disease than in those with earlier disease (44% versus 21%). Furthermore, the HAQ score fell from 2.7 at the beginning of the study to 1.3 after the last course. Pretreatment or side effects of IVIG were not reported in this study.

Similar results were also obtained in a more recent study on seven subjects with SSc with refractory joint pain [10]. Five subjects with limited SSc and two subjects with diffuse SSc and a mean disease duration of 3.6 plus or minus 2.5 years since the onset of Raynaud's syndrome were enrolled in the study. Joint space reduction, erosions, and juxta-articular osteoporosis was detected by x-ray in all subjects, particularly at the wrists, the metacarpophalangeal joints, the proximal interphalangeal joints, and the knees. Four subjects were pretreated with methotrexate and three with cyclophosphamide. Neither treatment with nonsteroidal anti-inflammatory drugs nor with methotrexate or cyclophosphamide was effective in controlling the joint pain. Subjects were treated with six monthly courses of IVIG at a dosage of 2 g/kg over 4 days. A moderate decrease of the mean mRSS by 28% was assessed after six courses of IVIG. The number of swollen joints decreased from 10 to 7 and the number of tender joints from 19 to 10. Furthermore, the HAQ was reduced from 2.3 to 1.

All three studies suggested that IVIG might be beneficial for the treatment of dermal fibrosis in SSc. However, the number of subjects is very small and control groups are lacking. Thus, the moderate decreases of the mRSS of 35% and 28% might just reflect the natural course of the disease. Because of resolution of inflammation and edema and atrophy of the involved skin, the mRSS tends to decrease in the course of SSc, with mean reductions of about 25% reported in patients in early stages of the disease [11]. Thus, randomized controlled trials with sufficient power for statistical analyses are needed to further evaluate the efficacy of IVIG for the treatment of fibrosis before IVIG can be recommended. This is particularly true because the mechanisms of action of intravenous immunoglobulins in SSc are incompletely understood. Possible mechanisms include interactions with Fc receptors, activation of idiotype-anti-idiotype reaction, inhibition of the synthesis of autoantibodies, and reduction of chemokines and complement activation [12].

Tyrosine kinase inhibitors

Imatinib mesylate (STI571, Gleevec/Glivec) is a small molecule tyrosine kinase inhibitor that binds to the adenosine triphosphate-binding pocket of abelson kinase (c-abl) and blocks efficiently its tyrosine kinase activity; c-abl is an important downstream signaling molecule of TGFβ [13–16]. In cells deficient for c-abl, the induction of extracellular matrix proteins by TGFβ is strongly decreased. In addition to its effects on c-abl, imatinib mesylate interferes also with platelet derived growth factor (PDGF) signaling by blocking the tyrosine kinase activity of PDGF receptors. Besides c-abl and PDGF-receptors, imatinib also inhibits the tyrosine kinase activity of the gene product of the protooncogene c-kit, a transmembrane receptor for stem cell factor and c-fms. Other tyrosine kinases are not affected in physiologic concentrations, highlighting the specificity of imatinib mesylate [17,18]. Thus, imatinib mesylate targets simultaneously and selectively two major profibrotic pathways activated in SSc.

Imatinib mesylate is an orally administered drug, which is currently widely used for the treatment of bcr-abl positive chronic myelogenous leukemia and gastrointestinal stromal tumors, with more 100,000 patients treated so far. Imatinib mesylate possesses favorable pharmacokinetic properties. It is readily absorbed after oral administration and has to be taken only once daily because of its long half-life of 13 to 16 hours [18].

The authors have demonstratee that imatinib mesylate inhibited strongly the synthesis of the major extracellular matrix proteins col 1a1, col 1a2, and fibronectin-1 by dermal fibroblasts from SSc subjects and healthy controls on the mRNA, as well as protein level by up to 90% at concentrations of 1 μg/ml [19]. No changes of the expression of tissue inhibitors of metalloproteinase (TIMPs) and matrix metalloproteinase (MMPs) were observed that might have counterbalanced the decreased production of extracellular matrix proteins. Furthermore, treatment with imatinib mesylate efficiently reduced the development of fibrosis in the mouse model of bleomycin-induced dermal fibrosis. Treatment of mice with imatinib at doses of 50 mg/kg per day and 150 mg/kg per day had strong antifibrotic effects without toxic side effects. Imatinib prevented the differentiation of resting fibroblasts into myofibroblasts and reduced dose-dependently the synthesis and accumulation of extracellular matrix in lesional skin. Of note, the concentrations used in the authors' study for the treatment of mice produce serum levels of imatinib similar to those observed in human beings, with standard doses of 400 mg to 800 mg imatinib per day by mouth, because of a faster metabolization of imatinib in mice. Similarly, the concentration of 1 μg/ml imatinib is below the mean serum through concentrations observed in human beings [18,20].

Smaller clinical studies also suggested also that treatment of patients with chronic myelogenous leukemia (CML) might lead to a regression of concomitant bone marrow fibrosis [21,22]. Of note, the antifibrotic effect did not correlate with the cytogenetic response, suggesting an effect independent from the suppression of Philadelphia chromosome-positive cancer cells [22]. Although it is clear that the mechanisms of bone marrow fibrosis associated with CML are different from skin and organ fibrosis in SSc, imatinib mesylate might not only prevent the progression of fibrosis in SSc patients, but might also be effective for the treatment of established fibrosis.

Previous clinical trials on subjects with CML suggested that imatinib mesylate is well tolerated, with severe adverse side effects leading to the discontinuation of the drug in less than 1% of subjects [23]. However, mild side effects are common, and outside of clinical trials up to 30% of patients discontinue imatinib because of adverse effects [24]. The major adverse events responsible for discontinuation are dose-dependent and include severe edema, muscle cramps, uncontrollable diarrhea, and bone marrow toxicity [23,24]. Furthermore, abl-kinase inhibitors might induce congestive heart failure. So far, ten patients have been reported who developed congestive heart failure while on imatinib mesylate [25]. Histologic evaluation of cardiac sections suggested a toxic cardiomyopathy. A potential causal role of the inhibition of c-abl in the pathogenesis of congestive heart failure was suggested by experimental data. However, the interpretation of this report is complicated by the fact that the majority of patients reported with congestive heart failure while on imatinib had pre-existing cardiac disease or cardiovascular risk factors. One also has to keep in mind that more than 100,000 patients have been treated with imatinib and only ten patients from one center have been reported to develop congestive heart failure. Nevertheless, because cardiac involvement with fibrosis is frequent in SSc patients, this potential side effects needs particular attention in clinical trials with SSc patients.

Because of the potent antifibrotic effects in-vitro and in-vivo in several animal models for tissue fibrosis, the favorable pharmacokinetics, and the good clinical experience in other diseases, imatinib mesylate is currently investigated in clinical trials as an antifibrotic drug for the treatment of SSc. It needs to be emphasized that this treatment cannot be recommended for routine use in patients with SSc, as long as its safety, pharmacokinetics, and efficacy have been analyzed in these trials. Moreover, costs of this treatment are high.

Most recently, dasatinib (Spyrcel) and nilotinib (Tasigna), two novel inhibitors of abl-kinases and PDGF receptors, have been approved for the treatment of bcr-abl-positive CML with resistance or intolerance to imatinib. Dasatinib and nilotinib are also highly selective small molecule tyrosine kinase inhibitors that can be administered orally [26–30]. Like imatinib, nilotinib selectively inhibits the tyrosine kinase activity of abl-kinases, PDGF receptor and c-kit. Additionally, dasatinib inhibits the structurally related family of src-kinases [28]. Both, dasatinib and nilotinib inhibit the activity of abl-kinases much more potent than imatinib and are effective in most cell lines resistant to imatinib [31]. The spectra of adverse effects of dasatinib and nilotinib differ from that of imatinib, and patients with intolerance to imatinib can often be switched safely to nilotinib or dasatinib [27,32–34]. Thus, dasatinib and nilotinib might be interesting candidates for the treatment of patients that cannot tolerate imatinib.

This might be particularly because of dasatinib, which also inhibits src kinases, because src kinases have recently been shown to play an important role in the production of extracellular matrix proteins in dermal fibroblasts [35]. Src kinases are activated by profibrotic cytokines, such as TGFβ or PDGF, in SSc fibroblasts. Inhibition of src kinases by chemical inhibitors, or overexpression of a dominant negative mutant of src and the endogenous antagonist csk, reduced strongly the synthesis of col 1a1, col 1a2 and fibronectin-1 by SSc and healthy dermal fibroblasts on the mRNA, as well as the protein level. Inhibition of src did not induce counter regulatory changes of TIMPs and MMPs. Furthermore, treatment of mice with a specific inhibitor of src kinases reduced dose-dependently the devolvement of dermal fibrosis in the mouse model of bleomycin-induced dermal fibrosis, with reduced dermal thickness and collagen content in the skin. Thus, in addition to c-abl, src kinases might also represent interesting novel targets for antifibrotic therapeutic approaches in SSc.

Histone deacetylase inhibitors

Epigenetic modifications are defined as heritable alterations of the DNA without changes in the nucleotide sequence. Unlike alterations of the genome, epigenetic changes are reversible and offer the potential opportunity to modify the epigenetic pattern through therapeutic interventions [36]. Modifications of histones, histone acetylation or deacetylation in particular, are among the principal mechanisms that have been described as epigenetic changes. In resting cells, DNA is normally highly organized within nucleosomes, in an octomeric core unit of chromatin and in DNA-binding nucleoproteins, the histones. Modifications of the packaging of chromatin regulate the extent of gene transcription. Hyperacetylation of histones leads to a loosened state of the chromatin packaging and an increased rate of gene transcription. On the other hand, deacetylation of histones causes tighter packaging of the DNA and decreases gene transcription by preventing the binding of transcription factors and RNA polymerase II [37]. The degree of acetylation of histones is regulated by histone deacetylases (HDACs) and histone acetylases. HDACs are enzyme complexes consisting of multiple subunits that remove the acetyl group from the histones via a charge-relay system, using zinc ions as prosthetic groups [38]. HDAC inhibitors dislodge the zinc ion, thus turning off the charge-relay system.

During recent years, HDAC inhibitors have been evaluated in clinical trials as a novel therapeutic strategy for various malignancies [39]. In these studies, HDAC inhibitors have been shown to potently induce cell cycle arrest, cell differentiation, and apoptotic cell death in tumor cells.

Besides a potential role as a novel therapeutic strategy against cancer, HDAC inhibitors might also be beneficial for the treatment of fibrotic disorders. Trichostatin A (TSA) is a potent inhibitor of HDACs. TSA has been shown to exert antifibrotic effects on cultured hepatic stellate cells in vitro [40]. At a concentration of 100 nmol/L, TSA reduced the expression of α-smooth muscle actin, suggesting an inhibition of the differentiation of stellate cells into myofibroblasts. Furthermore, TSA inhibited the synthesis of collagen types I and III. TSA also strongly inhibited the proliferation of hepatic stellate cells.

Inhibitors of HDACs have recently been shown to prevent fibrosis in a murine model of SSc [41]. TSA prevented the induction of col 1a1 and fibronectin in dermal fibroblasts from SSc subjects and healthy controls upon stimulation with TGFβ, PDGF, and interleukin-4 on the mRNA and the protein level. Potent antifibrotic effects of TSA were also observed in the mouse model of bleomycin-induced dermal fibrosis. In concentrations of 0.5 mg/kg per day and 1 mg/kg per day, TSA reduced the accumulation of collagen and the atrophy of the subcutis to levels comparable with those of control mice not receiving bleomycin. Consistent with the low rate of side effects reported in first preliminary reports about the clinical trials in human beings, no obvious toxic side effects were observed in mice treated with TSA, suggesting that TSA might be well tolerated, despite its broad mechanism of action, with alteration of the expression of many different genes.

Different mechanisms of action have been proposed for the antifibrotic effects of TSA. TSA inhibits directly TGFβ signaling in dermal fibroblasts by preventing the nuclear translocation and the DNA binding of Smad 3 and Smad 4 complexes upon stimulation of dermal fibroblasts with TGFβ. In addition, inhibition of proliferation of fibroblasts might contribute to the antifibrotic effects of TSA, as TSA up-regulates of cell cycle inhibitor p21.

Based on the promising results in this preclinical model of dermal fibrosis and its good tolerability in first clinical trials in subjects with malignancies, clinical trials in SSc subjects with HDAC inhibitors are expected to be launched within the next few years.

Summary

Mortality has significantly increased in SSc. Despite extensive research, therapeutic options for antifibrotic treatment are very limited. So far, a significant antifibrotic effect has only been demonstrated for cyclophosphamide. However, several promising approaches are currently being evaluated. First results from uncontrolled trials suggest that HDIT with autologous HSCT might be very effective and become established as an important option for selected SSc patients with severe, progressive SSc. Preliminary data of a limited number of patients indicate that IVIG might be a candidate for randomized controlled trials in SSc. Most promising appear to be treatment strategies that target specific key molecules in the pathogenesis of the disease. Among these are blocking strategies of TGFβ signaling; however, a first small clinical trial did not indicate clinical efficacy of a TGFβ antibody. Furthermore, preclinical data suggest that the small molecule inhibitor imatinib, and related drugs such as dasatinib and nilotinib that selectively and simultaneously target TGFβ and PDGF signaling, have potent antifibrotic effects, and the results of ongoing clinical trials are expected with eagerness. Finally, src kinases and HDACs might also be interesting targets, and clinical trials with inhibitors of src and HDACs are expected to be launched soon.

References

[1] Binks M, Passweg JR, Furst D, et al. Phase I/II trial of autologous stem cell transplantation in systemic sclerosis: procedure related mortality and impact on skin disease. Ann Rheum Dis 2001;60(6):577–84.

[2] Farge D, Marolleau JP, Zohar S, et al. Autologous bone marrow transplantation in the treatment of refractory systemic sclerosis: early results from a French multicentre phase I-II study. Br J Haematol 2002;119(3):726–39.

[3] Nash RA, McSweeney PA, Crofford LJ, et al. High-dose immunosuppressive therapy and autologous hematopoietic cell transplantation for severe systemic sclerosis: long-term follow-up of the US multicenter pilot study. Blood 2007;110(4):1388–96.

[4] Vonk MC, Marjanovic Z, van den Hoogen FH, et al. Long-term follow-up results after autologous haematopoietic stem cell transplantation for severe systemic sclerosis. Ann Rheum Dis 2008;67(1):98–104.

[5] Nash RA, McSweeney PA, Nelson JL, et al. Allogeneic marrow transplantation in patients with severe systemic sclerosis: resolution of dermal fibrosis. Arthritis Rheum 2006;54(6): 1982–6.

[6] Sonnylal S, Denton CP, Zheng B, et al. Postnatal induction of transforming growth factor beta signaling in fibroblasts of mice recapitulates clinical, histologic, and biochemical features of scleroderma. Arthritis Rheum 2007;56(1):334–44.

[7] Demetri GD, von Mehren M, Blanke CD, et al. Efficacy and safety of imatinib mesylate in advanced gastrointestinal stromal tumors. N Engl J Med 2002;347(7):472–80.

[8] Amital H, Rewald E, Levy Y, et al. Fibrosis regression induced by intravenous gammaglobulin treatment. Ann Rheum Dis 2003;62(2):175–7.

[9] Levy Y, Amital H, Langevitz P, et al. Intravenous immunoglobulin modulates cutaneous involvement and reduces skin fibrosis in systemic sclerosis: an open-label study. Arthritis Rheum 2004;50(3):1005–7.

[10] Nacci F, Righi A, Conforti ML, et al. Intravenous immunoglobulins improve the function and ameliorate joint involvement in systemic sclerosis: a pilot study. Ann Rheum Dis 2007;66(7):977–9.

[11] Seibold JR, Furst DE, Clements PJ. Why everything (or nothing) seems to work in the treatment of scleroderma. J Rheumatol 1992;19(5):673–6.

[12] Sapir T, Shoenfeld Y. Facing the enigma of immunomodulatory effects of intravenous immunoglobulin. Clin Rev Allergy Immunol 2005;29(3):185–99.

[13] Abdollahi A, Li M, Ping G, et al. Inhibition of platelet-derived growth factor signaling attenuates pulmonary fibrosis. J Exp Med 2005;201(6):925–35.

[14] D'Angelo WA, Fries JF, Masi AT, et al. Pathologic observations in systemic sclerosis (scleroderma). A study of fifty-eight autopsy cases and fifty-eight matched controls. Am J Med 1969;46(3):428–40.

[15] Wang S, Wilkes MC, Leof EB, et al. Imatinib mesylate blocks a non-Smad TGF-beta pathway and reduces renal fibrogenesis in vivo. FASEB J 2005;19(1):1–11.

[16] Yoshiji H, Noguchi R, Kuriyama S, et al. Imatinib mesylate (STI-571) attenuates liver fibrosis development in rats. Am J Physiol Gastrointest Liver Physiol 2005;288(5):G907–13.

[17] Druker BJ, Lydon NB. Lessons learned from the development of an abl tyrosine kinase inhibitor for chronic myelogenous leukemia. J Clin Invest 2000;105(1):3–7.

[18] Savage DG, Antman KH. Imatinib mesylate—a new oral targeted therapy. N Engl J Med 2002;346(9):683–93.

[19] Distler JH, Jungel A, Huber LC, et al. Imatinib mesylate reduces production of extracellular matrix and prevents development of experimental dermal fibrosis. Arthritis Rheum 2007; 56(1):311–22.

[20] Daniels CE, Wilkes MC, Edens M, et al. Imatinib mesylate inhibits the profibrogenic activity of TGF-beta and prevents bleomycin-mediated lung fibrosis. J Clin Invest 2004;114(9): 1308–16.

[21] Beham-Schmid C, Apfelbeck U, Sill H, et al. Treatment of chronic myelogenous leukemia with the tyrosine kinase inhibitor STI571 results in marked regression of bone marrow fibrosis. Blood 2002;99(1):381–3.

[22] Bueso-Ramos CE, Cortes J, Talpaz M, et al. Imatinib mesylate therapy reduces bone marrow fibrosis in patients with chronic myelogenous leukemia. Cancer 2004;101(2):332–6.

[23] Druker BJ, Guilhot F, O'Brien SG, et al. Five-year follow-up of patients receiving imatinib for chronic myeloid leukemia. N Engl J Med 2006;355(23):2408–17.

[24] Atallah E, Kantarjian H, Cortes J. Emerging safety issues with imatinib and other Abl tyrosine kinase inhibitors. Clin Lymphoma Myeloma 2007;7(Suppl 3):S105–12.

[25] Kerkela R, Grazette L, Yacobi R, et al. Cardiotoxicity of the cancer therapeutic agent imatinib mesylate. Nat Med 2006;12(8):908–16.

[26] Cannell E. Dasatinib is effective in imatinib-resistant CML. Lancet Oncol 2007;8(4):286.

[27] Kantarjian H, Giles F, Wunderle L, et al. Nilotinib in imatinib-resistant CML and Philadelphia chromosome-positive ALL. N Engl J Med 2006;354(24):2542–51.

[28] Kantarjian H, Jabbour E, Grimley J, et al. Dasatinib. Nat Rev Drug Discov 2006;5(9):717–8.

[29] Nygren P, Larsson R. Overview of the clinical efficacy of investigational anticancer drugs. J Intern Med 2003;253(1):46–75.

[30] Weisberg E, Manley P, Mestan J, et al. AMN107 (nilotinib): a novel and selective inhibitor of BCR-ABL. Br J Cancer 2006;94(12):1765–9.

[31] O'Hare T, Walters DK, Stoffregen EP, et al. Combined Abl inhibitor therapy for minimizing drug resistance in chronic myeloid leukemia: Src/Abl inhibitors are compatible with imatinib. Clin Cancer Res 2005;11(19 Pt 1):6987–93.

[32] Cortes J, Rousselot P, Kim DW, et al. Dasatinib induces complete hematologic and cytogenetic responses in patients with imatinib-resistant or -intolerant chronic myeloid leukemia in blast crisis. Blood 2007;109(8):3207–13.

[33] Guilhot F, Apperley J, Kim DW, et al. Dasatinib induces significant hematologic and cytogenetic responses in patients with imatinib-resistant or -intolerant chronic myeloid leukemia in accelerated phase. Blood 2007;109(10):4143–50.

[34] Talpaz M, Shah NP, Kantarjian H, et al. Dasatinib in imatinib-resistant Philadelphia chromosome-positive leukemias. N Engl J Med 2006;354(24):2531–41.

[35] Skhirtladze C, Distler O, Dees C, et al. Src kinases in systemic sclerosis: central roles in fibroblast activation and in skin fibrosis. Arthritis Rheum 2008, in press.

[36] Sigalotti L, Fratta E, Coral S, et al. Epigenetic drugs as pleiotropic agents in cancer treatment: biomolecular aspects and clinical applications. J Cell Physiol 2007;212(2):330–44.

[37] Wade PA. Transcriptional control at regulatory checkpoints by histone deacetylases: molecular connections between cancer and chromatin. Hum Mol Genet 2001;10(7):693–8.

[38] de Ruijter AJ, van Gennip AH, Caron HN, et al. Histone deacetylases (HDACs): characterization of the classical HDAC family. Biochem J 2003;370(Pt 3):737–49.

[39] Monneret C. Histone deacetylase inhibitors. Eur J Med Chem 2005;40(1):1–13.

[40] Niki T, Rombouts K, De Bleser P, et al. A histone deacetylase inhibitor, trichostatin A, suppresses myofibroblastic differentiation of rat hepatic stellate cells in primary culture. Hepatology 1999;29(3):858–67.

[41] Huber LC, Distler JH, Moritz F, et al. Trichostatin A prevents the accumulation of extracellular matrix in a mouse model of bleomycin-induced skin fibrosis. Arthritis Rheum 2007; 56(8):2755–64.

ELSEVIER
SAUNDERS

Rheum Dis Clin N Am
34 (2008) 161–179

RHEUMATIC
DISEASE CLINICS
OF NORTH AMERICA

Current Approaches to the Management of Early Active Diffuse Scleroderma Skin Disease

Svetlana I. Nihtyanova, MBBS,
Christopher P. Denton, PhD, FRCP*

Centre for Rheumatology, Royal Free Hospital, Pond Street, London NW3 2QG, UK

Skin fibrosis is a hallmark feature of systemic sclerosis (SSc). Depending on the extent of skin sclerosis, the disease is classified into two major subsets: *limited cutaneous SSc* (lcSSc) when only skin distal to the elbows and knees is affected and *diffuse cutaneous SSc* (dcSSc) when the skin thickening spreads proximally.

Although skin involvement, particularly in the diffuse pattern, can be related to severe disability, it is well appreciated that frequency and degree of internal organ involvement is the major contributor to mortality and morbidity. Therefore, treatment of SSc is largely focused on management of specific internal organ complications. The success of that strategy is well illustrated by the significantly reduced mortality among patients who have SSc-related renal crisis since the advent of angiotensin-converting enzyme (ACE) inhibitors, and the significantly improved survival of patients who have SSc-related pulmonary arterial hypertension (PAH) since new therapies targeting specific pathophysiological pathways underlying this condition became available and started being used in combination [1,2]. Important advancements have also been made in the treatment of SSc-associated pulmonary fibrosis (SSc-PF) with two overall positive double-blind, placebo-controlled trials of oral and intravenous cyclophosphamide [3,4].

Before presenting the evidence for efficacy of the different agents in treatment of scleroderma skin disease, it is important to discuss several points about skin tightness evolution in the disease course and its relation to internal organ involvement in patients who have SSc.

---

* Corresponding author.
E-mail address: c.denton@medsch.ucl.ac.uk (C.P. Denton).

0889-857X/08/$ - see front matter © 2008 Elsevier Inc. All rights reserved.
doi:10.1016/j.rdc.2007.11.005
rheumatic.theclinics.com

Firstly, the skin score generally tends to improve for a large proportion of patients who have dcSSc, irrespective of treatment, and this improvement correlates strongly with disease duration [5–8]. Assuming that at disease onset the skin score is 0, initial worsening of skin tightness occurs, with patients who have disease duration of less than 18 months being much more likely to show modified Rodnan skin score (MRSS) worsening compared with those who have longer disease duration [9]. Analysis of the MRSS changes over time in 635 patients who had dcSSc participating in seven different clinical trials showed that skin score peaks on average at 40 months from disease onset [9]. In the authors' center, longitudinal analysis of the dcSSc cases reviewed suggested that peak skin score occurs within 24 months of disease onset in more than half the cases (Fig. 1). This finding has implications for clinical trial recruitment and the likelihood of showing treatment effect in placebo-controlled trials that recruit cases within the first 3 years of disease.

Conversely, skin score improvement does not necessarily indicate disease improvement/stability, because internal organ complications can still develop [8]. Although good correlation exists between skin score change and survival [8,10], the relationship between skin score change and internal organ involvement is not straightforward and skin should not be used as a surrogate marker for disease activity. Therefore, skin score change is a poor primary outcome in trials assessing overall treatment efficacy in SSc [8].

To properly assess drug efficacy for treatment of skin sclerosis, clinical trials should be placebo-controlled and ideally involve patients at the same disease stage. Trials involving patients who have early SSc (<18 months) and a short follow-up period (<1 year) are more likely to show worsening skin tightness, whereas trials involving patients who have had SSc for 2 to 3 years are more likely to show skin score improvement. Patients who have late-stage SSc (>5 years) and who have entered the plateau phase of the disease may show very little change in skin thickness over time.

The various currently used treatment strategies for skin disease in scleroderma address mainly two aspects of SSc pathogenesis: inflammation and

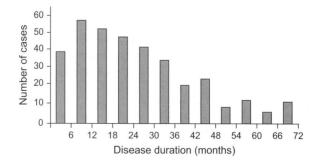

Fig. 1. Disease duration at peak skin score of the patients who had dcSSc from the Royal Free Hospital scleroderma database. More than half of cases show their peak skin score within the first 24 months of disease defined by time from the first non-Raynaud's manifestation.

fibrosis. The link between these processes is evidenced by histologic examination of SSc skin (Fig. 2). Distinguishing potential immunologic or anti-inflammatory mechanisms from antifibrotic strategies is often difficult because of the complex biologic networks interlocking these processes.

Broad spectrum immunomodulatory therapies

Mycophenolate mofetil

Mycophenolate mofetil (MMF) is an antiproliferative immunosuppressant that is metabolized to mycophenolic acid, which is an inosine-

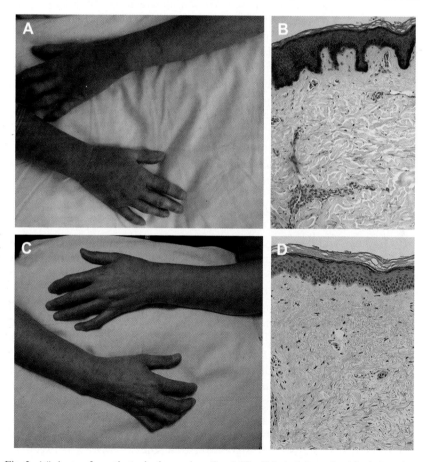

Fig. 2. (*A*) Arms of a patient who has early active dcSSc. Skin is tightened, with pitting edema and early flexion contractures of the fingers are present. (*B*) Hematoxylin/eosin staining of a patient who has early active dcSSc. Perivascular inflammatory infiltration is present; dermal papillae are preserved. (*C*) Arms of a patient who has late-stage dcSSc. Skin is less tight with atrophic changes; more prominent flexion contractures of the fingers and multiple telangiectasia are present. (*D*) Hematoxylin/eosin staining of a patient who has longstanding dcSSc. Dermis is avascular with increased extracellular matrix; loss of dermal papillae has occurred.

5'monophosphate dehydrogenase inhibitor. It inhibits the de novo synthesis of purines, thereby suppressing T- and B-lymphocyte proliferation [11]. Although MMF is currently licensed only for prophylaxis of solid-organ transplant rejection, over the past decade it has been used to treat various autoimmune conditions, most widely in patients who have lupus nephritis.

Stratton and colleagues [12] initially showed the benefit of MMF in treating skin sclerosis in patients who had early dcSSc. In an open-label study, it was given as maintenance treatment after induction of immunosuppression with antithymocyte globulin (ATG), and statistically significant improvement in MRSS was seen compared with baseline after 12 months of treatment (see also ATG section).

The results of a much larger retrospective analysis of 172 patients who had SSc (109 treated with MMF and 63 treated with other immunosuppressants) suggested some benefit in survival and prevention of serious lung involvement, but no difference in skin sclerosis change [5]. Skin score improved similarly in both groups, suggesting that MMF is noninferior to the other currently used immunosuppressants in terms of its effect on the skin. It was well tolerated and the few side effects were not life-threatening, making it a safe therapeutic option in patients who have SSc and active skin disease. Nevertheless, further evaluation with placebo-controlled trials is needed to establish the role of MMF in SSc treatment.

Cyclophosphamide

Cyclophosphamide is a cytotoxic drug used to treat malignancies and as a disease-modifying treatment of rheumatic diseases, such as systemic lupus erythematosus and vasculitis. It has been widely studied in the treatment of SSc-PF. Two randomized, double-blind, placebo-controlled trials showed that oral (Scleroderma Lung Study [3]) and intravenous (FAST trial [4]) cyclophosphamide have beneficial effects on lung function in patients who have SSc-PF, and currently cyclophosphamide is the most frequently used treatment for this serious scleroderma complication.

The patients in the Scleroderma Lung Study had MRSS measurements performed at baseline and 12 and 24 months. The Scleroderma Lung Study involved treatment with either oral cyclophosphamide at a dosage of up to 2 mg/kg per day or matching placebo for 12 months and a further 12-month follow-up period off the treatment medication. Analysis of the 12-month data showed that statistically significant difference in MRSS between the groups was seen only among the patients who had dcSSc. The mean ± standard deviation MRSS in the actively treated group fell from 21.7 ± 10.1 to 15.9 ± 11.0, whereas it showed very little change in the placebo group, for whom it was 20.2 ± 9.3 at baseline and 19.1 ± 11.2 at 12 months ($P < .01$). Nevertheless, further analysis at 18 and 24 months showed that the treatment advantage disappeared and the difference in skin score was no longer statistically significant ($P = .23$), suggesting that longer-term immunosuppressive treatment may be required to maintain treatment benefit [13].

Skin score assessment was not performed in the FAST trial, but few open-label uncontrolled studies have assessed the use of intravenous cyclophosphamide in scleroderma-related interstitial lung disease which have used skin score as a secondary endpoint. Pakas and colleagues [14] treated 28 patients who had dcSSc or lcSSc and interstitial lung disease with monthly intravenous pulses of cyclophosphamide for 6 months and bimonthly pulses for another 6 months. Sixteen patients received a high dosage of oral prednisolone (1 mg/kg per day for 4 weeks, then reduced by 5 mg/d on alternating days each 2 weeks) and the remaining 12 received a low dosage (< 10 mg/d). At the end of the 12 months, no significant difference was seen in MRSS compared with baseline in the group treated with a low dosage of prednisolone, whereas a significant decline occurred in skin score compared with baseline ($P = .01$) in those treated with a high dosage of prednisolone. Comparison of skin score change between the two groups was not presented. Griffiths and colleagues [15] investigated the use of intravenous cyclophosphamide in combination with intravenous methylprednisolone given at three weekly intervals for the first three pulses, and at four weekly intervals for a further three pulses. Comparison of MRSS pre- and posttreatment showed a 35% improvement from median score of 17 at baseline to 13 after completion of treatment ($P = .0058$). The results of both trials suggest that intravenous cyclophosphamide may be useful in treating skin disease in SSc, although firm conclusions cannot be made until more robust data are available and the role of corticosteroids is investigated.

Methotrexate

Methotrexate is a folate analog that competitively binds the enzyme dihydrofolate reductase and thus inhibits the de novo synthesis of purines, leading to inhibition of DNA synthesis. It was initially used to treat malignant diseases, although currently it is a standard therapy for autoimmune conditions such as Crohn's disease, psoriasis, and inflammatory arthritis. Controlled trials have explored its efficacy in scleroderma, and the two largest studies are discussed.

In the first trial, van den Hoogen and colleagues [16] treated 29 patients who had SSc with 15 mg weekly of intramuscular methotrexate or matching placebo for 24 weeks in a double-blind trial, followed by another 24 weeks of an observational trial. The analysis at 24 weeks showed a trend toward statistical significance in the difference between the total skin score in the groups, with skin score reduction seen in the actively treated group and worsening of the skin tightness in the patients treated with placebo ($P = .06$). However, this study included patients who had both limited and diffuse subsets of SSc, and the disease duration varied in the groups from less than a year to more than 10 years.

In a more recent larger study ,Pope and colleagues treated 71 patients with 15 mg weekly of methotrexate or placebo for 12 months [17]. The inclusion criteria were much more rigorous and all patients had dcSSc for less than 3 years. Initially, only patients who completed the 12-month study were included in the data analysis, showing no difference in skin score between patients treated with methotrexate and placebo. When analysis was repeated on an intent-to-treat basis, the results showed a trend favoring methotrexate, with a statistically significant difference in the skin scores when using University of California, Los Angeles (UCLA) skin scoring method, but only a trend toward statistical significance when using MRSS ($P = .04$ and $P = .09$, respectively). Methotrexate is currently the preferred treatment for patients who have scleroderma/myositis or scleroderma/inflammatory arthritis overlap syndromes.

Rapamycin (sirolimus)

Rapamycin is a macrolide antibiotic with antifungal and antitumor properties that inhibits the interleukin 2–dependent T-cell proliferation and thus also has immunosuppressive action. It is currently used for prophylaxis of renal transplant rejection. In a small, randomized, single-blind study of 18 patients who had dcSSc lasting less than 5 years, it was compared with methotrexate [18]. The patients received either methotrexate, 15 mg weekly, or rapamycin at a dosage of 1 to 11 mg/d (blood levels of 10–15 mg/mL). Of these patients, 16 completed at least 8 weeks of treatment and 11 completed all 48 weeks. At the last completed visit, comparison of the patients showed similar degree of change in the MRSS, although rapamycin exhibited significant toxicity and two patients had to discontinue treatment because of uncontrollable hyperlipidemia.

Cyclosporin A

Cyclosporin A is a calcineurin inhibitor that suppresses T-cell activation. It is used to prevent organ or tissue transplant rejection, prophylaxis, and treatment of graft-versus-host disease and severe rheumatoid arthritis, eczema, and psoriasis. The use of cyclosporin A for treating SSc was evaluated in a 48-week open-label study of 10 patients (dcSSc, 9; lcSSc, 1) who had disease duration up to 60 months who were treated with up to 5 mg/kg per day of cyclosporin A [19]. For comparison, the investigators used the placebo-treated patients who had dcSSc and disease duration up to 60 months from a previous trial of chlorambucil versus placebo for treating SSc [20]. The change in skin score of the patients treated with cyclosporin A was significantly greater than that of the comparison group ($P < .004$). Adverse reactions to the treatment drug were very common, with 8 of 10 patients developing a 30% or more increase of serum creatinine, 2 of whom also experienced increased blood pressure. Cyclosporin A is nephrotoxic, and the development of hypertensive renal crisis in patients who have SSc has been well described [21]. Therefore, it is generally avoided in patients who have scleroderma.

Intravenous immunoglobulin

Human normal immunoglobulin is prepared from pooled plasma of a large number of healthy donors. It contains human polyclonal IgG consisting of antibodies against pathogens and foreign antigens and antibodies against several autoantigens through which it exerts its immunoregulatory effects [22]. In low doses (300–500 mg/kg every 3–4 weeks) it is used as replacement therapy in primary and secondary immunodeficiencies. Much higher dosage (2 g/kg given over 5 days) is used as an immunomodulatory therapy in several hematologic, neurologic, and dermatologic autoimmune conditions. It is a well-established treatment in several rheumatic diseases, including Kawasaki disease, polymyositis, and dermatomyositis.

Although no controlled trials have been performed of intravenous immunoglobulin treatment in patients who have SSc, a few open-label studies have shown encouraging results. These studies included subjects who had lcSSc or dcSSc with variable disease duration (≤20 years) who received 2 g/kg of intravenous immunoglobulin given over 4 or 5 days every month for up to 6 months [23–25]. Significant improvement in MRSS was seen in most patients, which in many cases could not be attributed to the natural course of the disease because of the comparatively long disease duration. Prospective placebo-controlled studies are needed to confirm the role of intravenous immunoglobulin as a therapeutic option in SSc.

High-dose immunosuppression with autologous hematopoietic stem cell transplantation

High-dose immunosuppression followed by hematopoietic stem cell transplantation (HSCT) emerged as a potential treatment for rheumatic diseases in the early 1990s based on anecdotal reports of patients who had autoimmune diseases experiencing remission after undergoing bone marrow transplantation for coexisting oncohematologic conditions, and observed disease improvement in animal models after HSCT [26]. This therapy is based on the concept that autoimmune diseases are mediated by autoantibodies and autoreactive lymphocytes [27]. The procedure involves three stages: (1) priming, or mobilization of autologous hematopoietic stem cells (AHSC); (2) conditioning of the immune system; and (3) AHSC treatment [28,29]. During the priming stage, the patient receives an infusion of cyclophosphamide and/or subcutaneous granulocyte colony–stimulating factor (G-CSF) and peripheral blood AHSC are collected through leukapheresis. At the second stage, peripheral autoreactive lymphocytes are eliminated through conditioning with immunosuppressive regimens that vary and can involve most often cyclophosphamide, ATG, and total body irradiation. Reinfusion of the harvested AHSC during the third stage leads to the development of a new generation of self-tolerant lymphocytes with immune reconstitution.

The first reported data on the use of HSCT for the treatment of SSc included 41 patients from a centralized database of the European Group for Blood and Marrow Transplantation and the European League Against Rheumatism (EBMT/EULAR International Stem Cell Project database) [30]. Three priming and seven conditioning regimens were used in the different centers. Serial MRSS data were available for 29 patients who had dcSSc. In 20 patients (69%), a significant improvement was seen in MRSS (>25% of baseline or >10% of the maximum skin score), and at 30, 90, and 180 days the mean MRSS was significantly lower than the baseline ($P < .005$). Two of the subjects who initially showed improvement in MRSS subsequently died. Mortality among treated patients was significant (11 patients [27%] after median follow-up of 12 months) with four disease-related and seven procedure-related deaths.

Another report 3 years later from the EBMT/EULAR International Stem Cell Project database included 32 of the original patients who underwent shorter follow-up and 25 newly registered subjects who had undergone HSCT and at least 6 months of follow-up [31]. Skin score measurements were available for 47 patients at 6 to 36 months after the procedure and showed significant improvement at 24 and 36 months compared with baseline. This report showed improved survival compared with the previous series, with total mortality of 23% (13 of the participating 57 patients) after a median follow-up of 20 months. The treatment-related mortality was 8.7% (n = 5), with only two cases from the newly enrolled 25 patients.

Most recently, long-term follow-up results were published from two similar phase 1/2 trials from the Netherlands and France using unified inclusion criteria and treatment protocol [32]. The included 26 patients had active dcSSc. Cyclophosphamide, 4 g/m^2, and G-CSF were used for priming and cyclophosphamide, 200 mg/kg, was used for conditioning followed by stem cell reinfusion after positive CD34 selection. A significant fall in MRSS was observed in most treated patients and was maintained for up to 7 years after the procedure. More rapid decrease occurred during the first year, with 73% of the subjects experiencing more than a 25%reduction in MRSS. Of 28 treated patients, 2 were excluded from the analysis because of death within the first 6 months of the study, and the survival of the remaining 26 patients was 96.2% and 84.8% at 5 and 7 years, respectively.

Parallel to the European trials, McSweeney and colleagues [33] used G-CSF alone for mobilization and a combination of cyclophosphamide, ATG, and total body irradiation for conditioning in 19 patients in an open-label study in the United States. Median MRSS decreased by 39% at 12 months and this trend continued for up to 3 years. These findings were confirmed by a larger, phase 2 trial of 34 patients followed up for up to 8 years [34].

Based on evidence that cyclophosphamide does not kill multipotent stem cells, Tehlirian and colleagues [35] used high doses of cyclophosphamide

(200 mg/kg given over four consecutive days) followed by G-CSF without stem cell rescue to treat six patients who had active dcSSc. One patient died early in the study and the remaining five experienced improvement in MRSS 3 months after the procedure. Three patients experienced a sustained improvement after 12 months of follow-up, whereas the remaining two showed worsening skin score.

Whether the treatment effect of HSCT is due to immune reconstitution or the immunosuppressive effect achieved during conditioning is unclear. Two large randomized controlled trials are currently underway: ASTIS Trial (Autologous Stem cell Transplantation International Scleroderma Trial) in Europe and SCOT (Scleroderma: Cyclophosphamide or Transplant) in the United States, both comparing high-dose immunosuppressive treatment followed by HSCT with standard therapy of monthly intravenous pulses of cyclophosphamide.

Targeted immunosuppression

Antithymocyte globulin

ATG is a polyclonal IgG derived from animals immunized with human thy-mocytes. Administration of ATG leads to T-lymphocyte depletion, with more recent evidence suggesting that it also affects adhesion molecules and surface chemokine receptor expression and B lymphocytes and natural killer cells [36]. It is used for prevention or treatment of acute graft rejection, for treatment of graft-versus-host disease, and aplastic anemia, and as a conditioning regimen for stem cell transplantation.

Anecdotal evidence initially suggested that ATG may be useful for treating SSc [37]. An open-label study of 10 patients who had early progressive SSc and were treated with ATG at a dosage of 10 mg/kg per day for 5 days and followed up for 12 months, showed no clinical benefit for skin and lung fibrosis [38]. Of the 10 patients, 3 developed treatment-related serious adverse events, includ-ing serum sickness, and 2 died of SSc-related complications.

Subsequently, another small open-label study of 13 patients used a lower dose of ATG, starting with 3 mg/kg on day one, followed by 4 mg/kg on day 2 and 5 mg/kg on days 3, 4, and 5 to treat patients who had early dcSSc for induction of immunosuppression [12]. This regimen was followed by main-tenance treatment with oral MMF, started 4 weeks after the ATG treatment and aiming for a standard dosage of 2 g/d for 12 months. Significant im-provement in MRSS was seen at 12 months (mean MRSS, 17) compared with baseline (mean MRSS, 28). One patient died of SSc-related renal crisis after the ATG treatment but before initiation of MMF. Despite the lower doses of ATG used and the prophylaxis with prednisolone, 5 of 13 patients developed serum sickness.

The frequency of adverse events (particularly serum sickness) associated with ATG treatment limits the use of ATG to cases with very severe early dcSSc. As the two studies showed, ATG alone does not confer long-term clinical benefit and must be followed by maintenance immunosuppressive treatment.

Tolerance to human type I collagen

Several authors have shown that patients who have SSc have immunity to type 1 collagen (CI) and that it is significantly more frequent than in control cohorts [39,40]. Because of the great similarities between human and bovine CI (92% homology at amino acid level), McKown and colleagues [41] used oral bovine CI to induce immune tolerance to human CI. In an open-label trial, 17 patients who had lcSSc or dcSSc with mean ± standard deviation disease duration of 9.1 ± 2.0 years were treated with solubilized bovine CI, 0.1 mg/d, for 1 month, followed by 0.5 mg/d for 11 months. At the end of the 12 months, MRSS decreased by 23% (from 26.35 ± 2.35 at baseline to 20.29 ± 2.53 at 12 months; $P = .005$), with greater improvement (26.6%) among subjects in the diffuse subset (baseline MRSS of 28.6 ± 2.5 compared with 21.0 ± 2.7 at 12 months; $P = .005$). Significant reduction in T-cell immunity to CI was shown with evidence of decreased T-cell activation. No side effects were observed.

Based on the encouraging results of this open-label study, a larger placebo-controlled trial of 168 patients who had early and late SSc investigated the effect of 0.5 mg/d of oral bovine CI compared with placebo over 12 months [42]. Although no significant difference in MRSS change was seen between the actively treated patients and the controls, subgroup analysis showed that patients who had late-stage SSc were more likely to benefit from oral tolerance induction. Compared with the patients treated with placebo, those treated with CI showed a trend toward statistical significance in MRSS improvement at 12 months, which became statistically significant at 15 months. MRSS decreased by 7.9 points in the CI-treated group, whereas it declined by 2.9 points ($P = .009$ by Wilcoxon rank sum and $P = .006$ by student t test) among the patients treated with placebo. These findings suggest that the effect on skin sclerosis of CI oral tolerance induction is delayed, warranting further studies with longer treatment and patient follow-up. The lack of efficacy of this treatment in early SSc may be caused by the fact that T cells play greater role in fibrogenesis in the later stages of the disease course. However, the treatment effect early in the disease may be masked by the natural tendency to reduction of MRSS in patients who have SSc.

Biologic therapies

Biologic agents have revolutionized the treatment of rheumatoid arthritis and are now becoming more widely used in other rheumatic diseases. Few studies have explored the use of different biologic agents in SSc, and all have been uncontrolled.

Anti–tumor necrosis factor α

Infliximab is a chimeric tumor necrosis factor (TNF)-α–specific antibody, consisting of a human Fc region and murine antigen-binding site. An open-label study of 16 patients who had early dcSSc with evidence of active skin disease assessed its efficacy and safety in the treatment of scleroderma [43]. The trial subjects received infliximab, 5 mg/kg, at weeks 0, 2, 6, 14, and 22. Although an overall decrease was seen in mean MRSS among the treated patients, the difference between the baseline and 26th-week MRSS did not reach statistical significance. Frequent MRSS assessments during the trial showed initial progression at week 6, followed by considerable reduction at week 22, which almost reached statistical significance. Given that only 66% of the patients actually completed the infliximab infusion at week 22 and a significant number of the subjects were positive for anti-infliximab antibodies, it could be argued that the treatment had some short-lived benefit. Almost half of the study cohort (44%) developed infusion reactions and had to discontinue the treatment.

Etanercept is a soluble TNF receptor that binds specifically to both TNF-α and TNF-β. It inhibits TNF binding to cell surface TNF receptors, thus inhibiting immune response mediated by TNF. In a retrospective analysis of 18 patients who had SSc treated with etanercept for inflammatory joint disease, a good response was generally seen with reduction in joint inflammation and pain [44]. Although MRSS improvement was observed, it was not statistically significant.

Anti-CD20

Rituximab is a monoclonal anti-CD20 antibody that depletes CD-20–expressing B lymphocytes. In an open-label study, 13 patients who had dcSSc of up to 18 months duration were treated with two1-g pulses of rituximab given 2 weeks apart [45]. Little change in skin score was seen at 6 and 12 months after treatment. No patients experienced serious adverse events.

The role of biologic agents in the treatment of SSc is still unclear and more prospective controlled trials are needed to elicit their efficacy.

Extracorporeal photopheresis

Extracorporeal photopheresis (ECP) is a process of exposure of 8-methoxypsoralen–treated lymphocytes to irradiation with ultraviolet-A light ex vivo with subsequent reinfusion into the patient. It is an established therapy for advanced cutaneous T-cell lymphoma and strong evidence suggests its usefulness in prophylaxis and treatment of solid organ transplant rejection and treatment of graft-versus-host disease. Several small uncontrolled studies have shown skin sclerosis improvement in patients who had SSc after treatment with ECP [46]. Nevertheless, most recently a randomized, double-blind, placebo-controlled trial of 64 patients who had recent onset (<2 years) of dcSSc who received either active or sham ECP on two consecutive days every 4 weeks for 12 months did not show any significant difference in the skin score change of the two treatment groups, although a trend was seen favoring active treatment [47].

Antifibrotic therapies

D-penicillamine

D-penicillamine (D-Pen) is a chelating agent that blocks the intra- and intermolecular cross-linking of collagen, making it a good candidate for antifibrotic treatment in patients who had SSc. Multiple uncontrolled studies and retrospective cohort comparison suggest D-Pen treatment improves skin sclerosis and reduces frequency of SSc-related renal crisis. In a 24-month, randomized, double-blind, controlled trial, treatment with high-dose D-Pen (750–1000 mg/d) was compared to treatment with low-dose D-Pen (125 mg every other day) in patients with dcSSc of up to 18 months duration [6]. Both intent-to-treat analysis and analysis of only the patients who completed the whole 24-month trial did not show any difference in skin score change in both patient groups. Because the dose of 125 mg on alternative days of D-Pen is considered too low to have any pharmacologic effect, D-Pen is generally considered ineffective in the treatment of skin sclerosis.

Minocycline

Some evidence shows that minocycline can be useful in treating calcinosis in patients who have lcSSc [48]. However, an open-label trial of 31 SSc patients treated with minocycline, using subjects from the D-Pen study as controls, did not show any statistically significant difference in the change in skin scores of both groups after 1 year of treatment, suggesting no benefit from minocycline treatment [49].

Interferons

Interferon-γ

An open-label, controlled trial of 44 patients (27 actively treated with 100 μg recombinant interferon-γ subcutaneously three times a week for 12 months and followed up for another 6 months, and 17 controls) investigated interferon-γ in the treatment of skin sclerosis [50]. Although interferon-γ was found to have mild beneficial effect on skin sclerosis, all enrolled patients had mild skin disease (skin sclerosis excluding the trunk), disease duration varied between 4 months and 34 years, and the mean baseline skin scores of the two treatment groups were significantly different. Therefore, conclusions cannot be made about the superiority of interferon-γ over placebo.

Interferon-α

A randomized, double-blind, placebo-controlled trial of 36 patients who had early dcSSc who were treated with subcutaneous injections of either interferon-α or indistinguishable placebo showed that treatment with Interferon-α has no benefit in the treatment of skin sclerosis and that it even may have a detrimental effect [51].

Relaxin

Relaxin is a peptide hormone secreted by corpus luteum and the uterus during pregnancy and its physiologic role is considered to be related to re-modeling of the uterus and loosening of the pelvic ligaments before birth. More recently it was also shown to target nonreproductive organs and have anti-inflammatory and antifibrotic action [52].

Its safety and efficacy in early (disease duration <5 years) dcSSc was assessed in a randomized, double-blind, placebo-controlled trial of 68 patients treated with recombinant human relaxin, 25 μg/kg per day or 100 μg/kg per day, or placebo for 24 weeks through continuous subcutaneous infusion [53]. MRSS was compared among the three treatment groups at 4, 12, and 24 weeks and was found to be significantly lower in the low-dose relaxin group compared with placebo at all assessments, whereas the MRSS of the patients treated with high-dose relaxin did not differ from that of the placebo group. The most frequent side effects were menorrhagia (11% of patients receiving placebo, 35% of patients receiving 25 μg/kg per day of relaxin, and 19% of patients receiving 100 μg/kg per day of relaxin) and metrorrhagia (5% of patients receiving placebo, 9% of patients receiving 25 μg/kg per day of relaxin, and 27% of patients receiving 100 μg/kg per day of relaxin). Unfortunately, a phase 3 trial of 239 patients treated with placebo or 10 or 25 μg/kg per day of relaxin showed no benefit of relaxin versus placebo and dampened the initial enthusiasm for this treatment.

Anti–transforming growth factor β1 antibody (CAT-192)

Transforming growth factor (TGF)-β is considered a key player in the fibrogenesis in SSc that promotes fibroblast activation and stimulates collagen synthesis [54]. Multiple studies have shown raised levels of TGF-β and increased TGB-β receptor expression in the skin of patients who have SSc [55,56]. CAT-192 is a recombinant human monoclonal antibody against active human TGF-β1, and a randomized, placebo-controlled trial of 45 patients who had early active SSc evaluated its potential role in the treatment of SSc [7]. The study subjects were treated with either placebo or CAT-192 at 0.5 mg/kg, 5 mg/kg, or 10 mg/kg, administered on day 0 and week 6, 12, and 18. Although the MRSS improved during the study, no statistically significant difference was seen among the treatment groups.

Potential biomarkers of skin disease

Great interest has been shown in finding laboratory markers that can be used to assess activity and severity of SSc. Multiple candidate markers are being evaluated, based on sensitivity and specificity for the different underlying pathophysiologic processes, and some of them have shown good correlation with skin disease in SSc.

Of the many mediators of fibrogenesis, TGF-β is believed to play a central role. Comparison of expression levels of mRNA for TGF-β1 and TGF-β2 in the subjects of the CAT-192 trial with those of healthy controls showed that the patients who had dcSSc had significantly higher expression of mRNA for both TGF-β1 and TGF-β2 in lesional skin biopsy tissue [7]. However, Dziadzio and colleagues [57] showed that patients who have dcSSc have significantly lower serum levels of active TGF-β1, with significant negative correlation between TGF-β1 levels and skin score and significant positive correlation between active TGF-β1 and disease duration. These data suggest that TGF-β may be sequestered in active skin. Connective tissue growth factor (CTGF) is another profibrotic factor that potentially can be used as a marker of disease activity. Although CTGF plasma and dermal interstitial fluid levels were shown to be comparable in patients who had SSc and healthy controls, its N-terminal cleavage product (N-terminal CTGF) was found to be significantly elevated in the plasma and dermal interstitial fluid of patients who had SSc, with highest levels seen in patients who had dcSSc [58].

Serum amino-terminal propeptides of type 3 and type 1 collagen are extracellular matrix molecules found in much higher levels in serum of patients who have SSc compared with healthy controls. Type 1 collagen levels also showed statistically significant correlation with MRSS changes (r = 0.37, $P = .027$) [7]. Other candidate molecules that may reflect skin disease in SSc are also being explored, including cartilage oligomeric matrix protein and other potential mediators, such as endothelin and chemokines [59,60].

Noninvasive assessment of skin disease

Although the MRSS is widely used as a clinical and research tool for assessing skin disease in SSc, attempts have been made to develop new tools and correlate these novel approaches with skin score and structure and histology of skin as observed on biopsy specimens. Assessment of biomechanical properties has shown promise, including the assessment of skin elasticity using BTC-2000 suction device [61]. Similarly, changes in skin score have been shown to correlate well with durometer measurements [62]. These devices may provide a simple way to assess skin hardness while having the advantage of potentially less variability between observers and the development of a continuous variable rather than the categorical skin score [63].

High-frequency ultrasound provides a tool to measure skin thickness and has been shown to reflect skin score [64,65] while providing potential information about biochemical composition of skin and the degree of edema [66]. These tools are likely to be more applicable to clinical trials than routine practice.

Current approach to management of skin disease in early diffuse cutaneous systemic sclerosis

Although the treatment of skin disease in early dcSSc remains a major challenge, the authors developed an operational approach to the treatment of cases attending their center. This approach is aligned with an observational study comparing outcome of dcSSc skin disease treated with various standardized protocols that form part of the normal clinical practice of SSc centers within the United Kingdom. However, no treatment has been shown to be unequivocally safe and effective for treating skin disease in dcSSc and controlled clinical trials should be a priority. Disease heterogeneity and the relative rarity of dcSSc mandate that, wherever possible, these should be multicenter trials to ensure adequate statistical power. Vigorous internationally collaborative groups are working together to develop and undertake these studies and up-to-date information about trials can be found on the Scleroderma Clinical Trials Consortium and EULAR Scleroderma Trials and Research group Web sites (www.sctc-online.org and www.eustar.org, respectively). Readers are encouraged to visit these sites and consider referring cases that may be eligible for participation in clinical studies.

In the authors' center, current practice is summarized in the flow diagram in Fig. 3. Once diagnosis is secure, the disease subset of the patients is considered. In most cases, skin disease in lcSSc is primarily managed by local measures. In dcSSc, the pattern of internal organ disease is considered

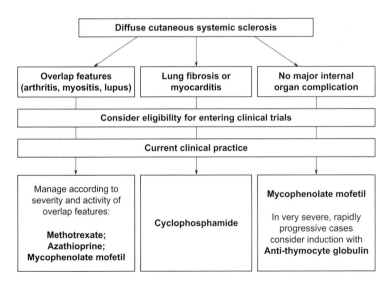

Fig. 3. Algorithm for management of skin disease in early dcSSc Current practice in the authors' center is summarized, with all patients being considered for treatment of skin disease. If ineligible for a clinical trial, immunosuppression is used and choice of agent based largely on clinical judgment and the presence of extracutaneous disease manifestations.

and, if significant or progressive lung fibrosis is present, intravenous cyclophosphamide with low-dose prednisolone is recommended. Significant overlap features of arthritis or myositis prompt use of MTX. When no evidence of internal organ involvement exists and no overlap features of connective tissue disease are present, MMF is used. In cases with active skin involvement that is rapidly progressive and severe, therapy is often initiated with ATG. All cases are systematically observed in line with the United Kingdom observational study of dcSSc for cases of less than 3 years duration. If possible, cases are enrolled into clinical trials.

Summary of key points

- Skin score change is a valuable parameter for classification and stratification of SSc;
- Skin score generally peaks around 18 months from disease onset and overall improves, making evaluation in clinical trials problematic;
- All patients who have dcSSc should undergo active treatment, and current evidence supports immunosuppressive strategies;
- Organ-based complications should always be considered because they may dictate the preferred therapy in patients who have active skin disease;
- More prospective, randomized, placebo-controlled clinical trials are needed with end points that are valid, clinically meaningful, and tailored to the patient cohort and duration of study.

Acknowledgments

The authors are grateful to Korsa Khan for preparation of the skin histology figures.

References

[1] Steen VD, Medsger TA. Changes in causes of death in systemic sclerosis, 1972–2002. Ann Rheum Dis 2007;66(7):940–4.
[2] Williams MH, Das C, Handler CE, et al. Systemic sclerosis associated pulmonary hypertension: improved survival in the current era. Heart 2006;92(7):926–32.
[3] Tashkin DP, Elashoff R, Clements PJ, et al. Cyclophosphamide versus placebo in scleroderma lung disease. N Engl J Med 2006;354(25):2655–66.
[4] Hoyles RK, Ellis RW, Wellsbury J, et al. A multicenter, prospective, randomized, double-blind, placebo-controlled trial of corticosteroids and intravenous cyclophosphamide followed by oral azathioprine for the treatment of pulmonary fibrosis in scleroderma. Arthritis Rheum 2006;54(12):3962–70.
[5] Nihtyanova SI, Brough GM, Black CM, et al. Mycophenolate mofetil in diffuse cutaneous systemic sclerosis–a retrospective analysis. Rheumatology 2007;46(3):442–5.
[6] Clements PJ, Furst DE, Wong WK, et al. High-dose versus low-dose D-penicillamine in early diffuse systemic sclerosis: analysis of a two-year, double-blind, randomized, controlled clinical trial. Arthritis Rheum 1999;42(6):1194–203.

[7] Denton CP, Merkel PA, Furst DE, et al. Recombinant human anti-transforming growth factor beta1 antibody therapy in systemic sclerosis: a multicenter, randomized, placebo-controlled phase I/II trial of CAT-192. Arthritis Rheum 2007;56(1):323–33.

[8] Shand L, Lunt M, Nihtyanova S, et al. Relationship between change in skin score and disease outcome in diffuse cutaneous systemic sclerosis: application of a latent linear trajectory model. Arthritis Rheum 2007;56(7):2422–31.

[9] Merkel PA, Silliman NP, Clements PJ, et al. Performance of the modified Rodnan skin score in clinical trials of scleroderma [abstract]. ACR Annual Meeting 2005 Presentation number 696.

[10] Steen VD, Medsger TA Jr. Improvement in skin thickening in systemic sclerosis associated with improved survival. Arthritis Rheum 2001;44(12):2828–35.

[11] Allison AC. Mechanisms of action of mycophenolate mofetil. Lupus 2005;14:s2–8.

[12] Stratton RJ, Wilson H, Black CM. Pilot study of anti-thymocyte globulin plus mycophenolate mofetil in recent-onset diffuse scleroderma. Rheumatology 2001;40(1):84–8.

[13] Tashkin DP, Elashoff R, Clements PJ, et al. Effects of 1-year treatment with cyclophosphamide on outcomes at 2 years in scleroderma lung disease. Am J Respir Crit Care Med 2007 [Epub ahead of print].

[14] Pakas I, Ioannidis JP, Malagari K, et al. Cyclophosphamide with low or high dose prednisolone for systemic sclerosis lung disease. J Rheumatol 2002;29(2):298–304.

[15] Griffiths B, Miles S, Moss H, et al. Systemic sclerosis and interstitial lung disease: a pilot study using pulse intravenous methylprednisolone and cyclophosphamide to assess the effect on high resolution computed tomography scan and lung function. J Rheumatol 2002;29(11): 2371–8.

[16] van den Hoogen FH, Boerbooms AM, Swaak AJ, et al. Comparison of methotrexate with placebo in the treatment of systemic sclerosis: a 24 week randomized double-blind trial, followed by a 24 week observational trial. Br J Rheumatol 1996;35(4):364–72.

[17] Pope JE, Bellamy N, Seibold JR, et al. A randomized, controlled trial of methotrexate versus placebo in early diffuse scleroderma. Arthritis Rheum 2001;44(6):1351–8.

[18] Clements P, Khanna D, Burger C, et al. Rapamycin (rapa) vs methotrexate (mtx) in early diffuse systemic sclerosis (ssc): a 48-week randomized, single-blind pilot safety study [abstract]. ACR Annual Meeting 2006 Presentation number 1257.

[19] Clements PJ, Lachenbruch PA, Sterz M, et al. Cyclosporine in systemic sclerosis. Results of a forty-eight-week open safety study in ten patients. Arthritis Rheum 1993;36(1):75–83.

[20] Furst DE, Clements PJ, Hillis S, et al. Immunosuppression with chlorambucil, versus placebo, for scleroderma. Results of a three-year, parallel, randomized, double-blind study. Arthritis Rheum 1989;32(5):584–93.

[21] Denton CP, Sweny P, Abdulla A, et al. Acute renal failure occurring in scleroderma treated with cyclosporin A: a report of three cases. Br J Rheumatol 1994;33(1):90–2.

[22] Siberil S, Elluru S, Negi VS, et al. Intravenous immunoglobulin in autoimmune and inflammatory diseases: more than mere transfer of antibodies. Transfus Apher Sci 2007;37(1): 103–7.

[23] Levy Y, Sherer Y, Langevitz P, et al. Skin score decrease in systemic sclerosis patients treated with intravenous immunoglobulin – a preliminary report. Clin Rheumatol 2000;19(3):207–11.

[24] Levy Y, Amital H, Langevitz P, et al. Intravenous immunoglobulin modulates cutaneous involvement and reduces skin fibrosis in systemic sclerosis: an open-label study. Arthritis Rheum 2004;50(3):1005–7.

[25] Nacci F, Righi A, Conforti ML, et al. Intravenous immunoglobulins improve the function and ameliorate joint involvement in systemic sclerosis: a pilot study. Ann Rheum Dis 2007;66(7):977–9.

[26] Tyndall A, Gratwohl A. Blood and marrow stem cell transplants in autoimmune disease. A consensus report written on behalf of the European League Against Rheumatism (EULAR) and the European Group for Blood and Marrow Transplantation (EBMT). Br J Rheumatol 1997;36(3):390–2 [review].

[27] Ermann J, Fathman CG. Autoimmune diseases: genes, bugs and failed regulation. Nat Immunol 2001;2(9):759–61.

[28] Burt RK, Slavin S, Burns WH, et al. Induction of tolerance in autoimmune diseases by hematopoietic stem cell transplantation: getting closer to a cure? Blood 2002;99(3):768–84 [review].

[29] Burt RK, Marmont A, Oyama Y, et al. Randomized controlled trials of autologous hematopoietic stem cell transplantation for autoimmune diseases: the evolution from myeloablative to lymphoablative transplant regimens. Arthritis Rheum 2006;54(12):3750–60 [review].

[30] Binks M, Passweg JR, Furst D, et al. Phase I/II trial of autologous stem cell transplantation in systemic sclerosis: procedure related mortality and impact on skin disease. Ann Rheum Dis 2001;60(6):577–84.

[31] Farge D, Passweg J, van Laar JM, et al. Autologous stem cell transplantation in the treatment of systemic sclerosis: report from the EBMT/EULAR registry. Ann Rheum Dis 2004;63(8):974–81.

[32] Vonk MC, Marjanovic Z, van den Hoogen FH, et al. Long-term follow-up results after autologous haematopoietic stem cell transplantation for severe systemic sclerosis. Ann Rheum Dis 2008;67(2):280.

[33] McSweeney PA, Nash RA, Sullivan KM, et al. High-dose immunosuppressive therapy for severe systemic sclerosis: initial outcomes. Blood 2002;100(5):1602–10.

[34] Nash RA, McSweeney PA, Crofford LJ, et al. High-dose immunosuppressive therapy and autologous hematopoietic cell transplantation for severe systemic sclerosis: long-term follow-up of the US multicenter pilot study. Blood 2007;110(4):1388–96.

[35] Tehlirian CV, Hummers LK, White B, et al. High dose cyclophosphamide without stem cell rescue in scleroderma. Ann Rheum Dis 2007 [Epub ahead of print].

[36] Mohty M. Mechanisms of action of antithymocyte globulin: T-cell depletion and beyond. Leukemia 2007;21(7):1387–94 [review].

[37] Balaban EP, Sheehan RG, Lipsky PE, et al. Treatment of cutaneous sclerosis and aplastic anemia with antithymocyte globulin. Ann Intern Med 1987;106(1):56–8.

[38] Matteson EL, Shbeeb MI, McCarthy TG, et al. Pilot study of antithymocyte globulin in systemic sclerosis. Arthritis Rheum 1996;39(7):1132–7.

[39] Hawrylko E, Spertus A, Mele CA, et al. Increased interleukin-2 production in response to human type I collagen stimulation in patients with systemic sclerosis. Arthritis Rheum 1991;34(5):580–7.

[40] Warrington KJ, Nair U, Carbone LD, et al. Characterisation of the immune response to type I collagen in scleroderma. Arthritis Res Ther 2006;8(4):R136.

[41] McKown KM, Carbone LD, Bustillo J, et al. Induction of immune tolerance to human type I collagen in patients with systemic sclerosis by oral administration of bovine type I collagen. Arthritis Rheum 2000;43(5):1054–61.

[42] Postlethwaite AE, Furst DE, Wong WK, et al. Oral tolerance (OT) induction to type I collagen (CI) significantly reduces the skin score in patients with diffuse systemic sclerosis (SSc) with late-phase disease. Results of a NIAMS/NIAID multicenter phase II placebo-controlled double blind clinical trial [abstract]. ACR Annual Meeting 2005 Presentation number L28.

[43] Denton CP, Engelhart M, Tvede N, et al. An open-label pilot study of infliximab therapy in diffuse cutaneous systemic sclerosis [abstract]. ACR Annual Meeting 2006 Presentation number 1256.

[44] Lam GK, Hummers LK, Woods A, et al. Efficacy and safety of etanercept in the treatment of scleroderma-associated joint disease. J Rheumatol 2007;34(7):1636–7.

[45] Lafyatis R, Kissin E, Viger K, et al. Rituximab treatment for patients with diffuse cutaneous systemic sclerosis – a phase I study [abstract]. ACR Annual Meeting 2006 Presentation number 1255.

[46] Krasagakis K, Dippel E, Ramaker J, et al. Management of severe scleroderma with long-term extracorporeal photopheresis. Dermatology 1998;196(3):309–15.

[47] Knobler RM, French LE, Kim Y, et al. A randomized, double-blind, placebo-controlled trial of photopheresis in systemic sclerosis. J Am Acad Dermatol 2006;54(5):793–9.

[48] Robertson LP, Marshall RW, Hickling P. Treatment of cutaneous calcinosis in limited systemic sclerosis with minocycline. Ann Rheum Dis 2003;62(3):267–9.

[49] Mayes MD, O'Donnell D, Rothfield NF, et al. Minocycline is not effective in systemic sclerosis: results of an open-label multicenter trial. Arthritis Rheum 2004;50(2):553–7.

[50] Grassegger A, Schuler G, Hessenberger G, et al. Interferon-gamma in the treatment of systemic sclerosis: a randomized controlled multicentre trial. Br J Dermatol 1998;139(4): 639–48.

[51] Black CM, Silman AJ, Herrick AI, et al. Interferon-alpha does not improve outcome at one year in patients with diffuse cutaneous scleroderma: results of a randomized, double-blind, placebo-controlled trial. Arthritis Rheum 1999;42(2):299–305.

[52] Samuel CS, Hewitson TD, Unemori EN, et al. Drugs of the future: the hormone relaxin [review]. Cell Mol Life Sci 2007;64(12):1539–57.

[53] Seibold JR, Korn JH, Simms R, et al. Recombinant human relaxin in the treatment of scleroderma. A randomized, double-blind, placebo-controlled trial. Ann Intern Med 2000;132(11): 871–9.

[54] Varga J, Abraham D. Systemic sclerosis: a prototypic multisystem fibrotic disorder [review]. J Clin Invest 2007;117(3):557–67.

[55] Pannu J, Gore-Hyer E, Yamanaka M, et al. An increased transforming growth factor beta receptor type I: type II ratio contributes to elevated collagen protein synthesis that is resistant to inhibition via a kinase-deficient transforming growth factor beta receptor type II in scleroderma. Arthritis Rheum 2004;50(5):1566–77.

[56] Hasegawa M, Sato S, Takehara K. Augmented production of transforming growth factor-beta by cultured peripheral blood mononuclear cells from patients with systemic sclerosis. Arch Dermatol Res 2004;296(2):89–93.

[57] Dziadzio M, Smith RE, Abraham DJ, et al. Circulating levels of active transforming growth factor beta1 are reduced in diffuse cutaneous systemic sclerosis and correlate inversely with the modified Rodnan skin score. Rheumatology (Oxford) 2005;44(12):1518–24.

[58] Dziadzio M, Usinger W, Leask A, et al. N-terminal connective tissue growth factor is a marker of the fibrotic phenotype in scleroderma. QJM 2005;98(7):485–92.

[59] Farina G, Widom RL, Benvenuto R, et al. COMP as a marker of active fibrosis in scleroderma: immunohistochemical analysis of skin, lung, and kidney tissue [abstract]. ACR Annual Meeting 2006 Presentation number 1836.

[60] McHugh NJ, Distler O, Giacomelli R, et al. Non organ based laboratory markers in systemic sclerosis. Clin Exp Rheumatol 2003;21(3 Suppl 29):S32–8 [review].

[61] Balbir-Gurman A, Denton CP, Nichols B, et al. Non-invasive measurement of biomechanical skin properties in systemic sclerosis. Ann Rheum Dis 2002;61(3):237–41.

[62] Falanga V, Bucalo B. Use of a durometer to assess skin hardness. J Am Acad Dermatol 1993; 29(1):47–51.

[63] Kissin EY, Merkel PA, Lafyatis R. Myofibroblasts and hyalinized collagen as markers of skin disease in systemic sclerosis [abstract]. ACR Annual Meeting 2006 Presentation number 1141.

[64] Akesson A, Hesselstrand R, Scheja A, et al. Longitudinal development of skin involvement and reliability of high frequency ultrasound in systemic sclerosis. Ann Rheum Dis 2004; 63(7):791–6.

[65] Moore TL, Lunt M, McManus B, et al. Seventeen-point dermal ultrasound scoring system— a reliable measure of skin thickness in patients with systemic sclerosis. Rheumatology (Oxford) 2003;42(12):1559–63.

[66] Hesselstrand R, Westergren-Thorsson G, Scheja A, et al. The association between changes in skin echogenicity and the fibroblast production of biglycan and versican in systemic sclerosis. Clin Exp Rheumatol 2002;20(3):301–8.

ELSEVIER
SAUNDERS

Rheum Dis Clin N Am
34 (2008) 181–190

RHEUMATIC
DISEASE CLINICS
OF NORTH AMERICA

The Heart in Scleroderma

Hunter C. Champion, MD, PhD

*Division of Cardiology, Department of Medicine, The Johns Hopkins Medical Institutions,
Johns Hopkins University School of Medicine, 720 Rutland Avenue, Ross 850, Baltimore,
MD 21205, USA*

Just as scleroderma can affect multiple organ systems, the cardiac manifestations of the disease are diverse. Although only relatively recently recognized, the heart is a major organ involved in scleroderma and the presence of cardiac involvement generally portends poorly for the patient. Cardiac involvement can generally be divided into direct myocardial effects and the indirect effect of other organ involvement (ie, pulmonary hypertension and renal crisis). Direct myocardial disease includes myositis, cardiac failure, cardiac fibrosis, coronary artery disease, conduction system abnormalities, and pericardial disease.

The involvement of the heart in scleroderma was first identified in 1926 by Heine [1], followed by Weiss and colleagues [2], who described nine cases of systemic sclerosis (SSc) with congestive heart failure; it was first postulated that cardiac fibrosis was the etiology. Historically, the cardiac manifestations of scleroderma have been confined to a progressive myocardial fibrosis that was observed on autopsy sectioning of the heart [1,2]. Since these initial observations, it has been established that SSc can involve the myocardium, coronary arteries, pericardium, and the conduction system.

Clinical presentation

Like any presentation of cardiac disease, the symptoms of patients with cardiac involvement in SSc are varied. In patients presenting with signs of

Dr. Champion is supported in part by the Bernard A. and Rebecca S. Bernard Foundation, a scientist development grant from the American Heart Association, the WW Smith Foundation, and National Institutes of Health grant P50 HL084946.

Dr. Champion is a Fellow of the American Heart Association and the Pulmonary Vascular Research Institute. He is a recipient of the Zipes Distinguished Young Investigator Award of the American College of Cardiology, the Shin Chun-Wang Young Investigator Award and the Giles F. Filley Memorial Award from the American Physiologic Society.

E-mail address: hcc@jhmi.edu

left heart failure, pulmonary congestion, and elevated left heart filling pressures, the most common complaints are dyspnea with exertion, paroxysms of nocturnal dyspnea or orthopnea and, if chronic in nature, possible presentation with ascites and pedal edema. Patients with pulmonary hypertension and subsequent right heart failure usually present with symptoms of indolent, progressive shortness of breath, pedal edema and ascites, and congestive hepatomegaly. When there is right heart failure in the absence of left heart involvement, patients generally do not experience orthopnea or paroxysms of nocturnal dyspnea. In patients with severe pulmonary hypertension, syncope and sudden cardiac death can occur, likely as a result of arrhythmias or acute right ventricular failure. Other signs and symptoms of cardiac involvement with SSc may be similar to myocardial ischemia, with dyspnea and chest pain. This chest pain may be atypical in nature, but the presence of coronary artery disease must always be considered in this patient population. Patients with arrhythmias may experience palpitations, caused either by bradycardia or tachycardia, or merely perceive a pounding of the heart beat in sinus rhythm, which is also common [3–5].

Prevalence and prognosis of cardiac involvement in systemic sclerosis

The presence of cardiac involvement in SSc is often underestimated because of the occult nature of the signs and symptoms, and reports of the prevalence of cardiac disease vary depending on the methods used. Moreover, symptoms of cardiac manifestations are often attributed to noncardiac causes, such as pulmonary, musculoskeletal, or esophageal involvement. More recent studies suggest that clinical evidence of myocardial disease may be seen in 20% to 25% of patients with SSc [4,6–8]. Autopsy studies have observed myocardial fibrosis and pericardial disease to be most prevalent, but like any autopsy study this likely represents patients with more advanced disease [4,9–12]. Other modalities of study in living patients have been used as well. With thallium scintigraphy, the estimated prevalence of clinical cardiac involvement in SSc is much higher [13–20].

Other modalities, such as single photon emission computed tomography thallium imaging have been noted in nearly all SSc patients tested [16–21], but the clinical implications of these defects remain uncertain. In addition to thallium and MRI studies, echocardiography has been used to screen SSc patients for asymptomatic cardiac abnormalities. In a study of 54 patients, 69% were found to have an abnormality by echocardiogram [22], the most common of which were elevated right ventricular (RV) systolic pressure, pericardial effusion, increased RV dimension, and left atrial enlargement. In addition to structural defects, 24-hour ambulatory monitoring has detected arrhythmias and conduction system abnormalities in SSc patients with or without symptoms [23,24].

The presence of clinical cardiac involvement in SSc is a harbinger of a poor prognosis. Medsger and Masi [25] showed that clinical cardiac disease in SSc was associated with a 70% mortality at 5 years. Certainly the presence of pulmonary arterial hypertension is a poor prognostic sign and is associated with a higher mortality rate in patients with SSc than idiopathic pulmonary arterial hypertension (PAH), as shown in the Johns Hopkins cohort from 2001 to 2005 [26,27]. In general, higher risk findings in patients with SSc include the presence of clinical heart failure, poor RV function [27], pulmonary arterial hypertension, low cardiac index, high right atrial pressure, and documented ventricular arrhythmia. Steen and colleagues [28] followed 48 patients who had undergone cardiac evaluation, and found that thallium perfusion defect scores were the single most powerful predictor of mortality and the subsequent development of clinical cardiac disease in patients with either limited or diffuse scleroderma [4].

Direct myocardial involvement: fibrosis and myositis

Studies of the cardiac manifestations of SSc have been limited for a number of reasons. Most histochemic studies involve autopsy specimens and likely do not reflect the cardiac involvement in patients with subclinical disease. Moreover, imaging studies have been limited because of the fact that there were no endomyocardial biopsies performed to correlated histopathologic fibrosis, hypertrophy, or myositis with imaging techniques. In general, myocardial fibrosis is considered to be the hallmark of cardiac involvement in SSc. The fibrosis tends to be patchy but distributed throughout the myocardium in both ventricles [4,6,9,29–31]. It has been noted that fibrosis in cardiac SSc can be distinguished from the fibrosis present in atherosclerotic coronary artery disease because in SSc the fibrosis may involve the immediate subendocardial layer (which is typically spared in atherosclerosis), while hemosiderin deposits (which are commonly observed in atherosclerotic disease) are not seen in SSc [4,6,8,9,29–31]. In general, the findings of fibrosis are often observed with cardiac hypertrophy. The presence of hypertrophy is nonspecific and may indirectly reflect elevated pulmonary or systemic pressures.

Some patients with SSc have features of polymyositis, and reports of SSc patients with coexisting myocardial disease and myositis suggest that there may be an association between myocarditis and peripheral myositis [2,32]. In another study, patients with an elevated creatine kinase (CK) at any time had an increased frequency of cardiac dysfunction, congestive heart failure, and cardiac death when compared with patients with no CK elevation [4,33]. However, the lack of an elevated CK does not rule out the presence of cardiac inflammation. In the author's experience, the presence of low grade inflammation (evidenced by the lack of elevated plasma troponin or CK-MB levels, but with cellular infiltrate on biopsy sample) is often found in many RV biopsies of SSc patients, suggesting that cardiac inflammation may be more common than originally appreciated. Moreover, the fibrotic process may be secondary to chronic inflammation of the heart (H.C. Champion, unpublished observation, 2008).

Left ventricular systolic and diastolic dysfuction

Left ventricular (LV) systolic dysfunction is not an uncommon finding in advanced scleroderma, but the time course and susceptibility for this is not well understood. Systolic and diastolic dysfunction can occur as a result of myocardial fibrosis, but the role of ongoing low-grade myocarditis in this process is less well characterized. Anecdotally, patients with reduced ejection fraction and normal coronary arteries may benefit from increasing the patient's immunosupression. It has been observed that patients with scleroderma with reduced ejection fraction and normal LV chamber size may improve their LV function with an increase in their immunosuppression regimen and a concomitant institution of appropriate drugs to treat heart failure (angiotensin-converting enzyme or angiotensin receptor blockers, beta blockade, aldosterone antagonist) (H.C. Champion, unpublished observation, 2008). Overt congestive heart failure occurs in more advanced disease, but systolic dysfunction is often clinically occult. In four studies using radionuclide ventriculography to evaluate left ventricular ejection fraction (LVEF), only 9 of 85 (11%) subjects had an abnormal LVEF under resting conditions [4,14,17,18,21]. As would be expected, there is a marked difference in symptoms and hemodynamics with exertion: in one study 46% of subjects had a reduced LVEF with exercise, while only 15% of this group had reduced function at rest [33].

More recently, there has been an increased awareness of nonsystolic heart failure (diastolic dysfunction) in scleroderma. Armstrong and colleagues [34] and Valentini and colleagues [35] showed echocardiographic findings in scleroderma patients consistent with diastolic dysfunction, and this correlated with disease duration, but the prognostic significance of these findings is unknown. Moreover, it was found that patients with scleroderma had impaired LV diastolic relaxation that was worsened with exercise. More recently, using gated myocardial perfusion single photon emission computed tomography scans, Nakajima and colleagues [36] found that diastolic dysfunction was found in more than half of patients with scleroderma, even in the absence of myocardial ischemia, and it correlated with the severity of cutaneous disease. This observation has subsequently been confirmed using tissue doppler imaging [37].

Comorbid conditions that predispose scleroderma patients to diastolic dysfunction are systemic hypertension, sleep disordered breathing, renal disease, and left ventricular hypertrophy or fibrosis. Echocardiographic signs of diastolic dysfunction are E wave/A wave reversal of the mitral inflow pattern and left atrial enlargement. Chronically, elevated LV diastolic pressures can lead to increased pulmonary artery pressures via increased pulmonary capillary wedge pressures [38]. Given the fact that diastolic dysfunction may not be clinically present at rest, it is recommended that patients undergo confrontational assessment of diastolic dysfunction by exercising right heart catheterization if clinically suspected.

Right heart failure

Right heart failure is most commonly the result of pulmonary hypertension. Pulmonary hypertension is a common manifestation of scleroderma and a poor prognostic sign. It is the ability of the right ventricle to function under this increased load that determines both the severity of symptoms and survival [39–42]. Signs and symptoms of right heart failure by history, echocardiogram, and catheterization are associated with a significantly increased risk of death. In studies addressing hemodynamic variables and survival with PAH, a low cardiac index and high mean right atrial pressure are consistently associated with poorer survival [40,43]. The mean pulmonary arterial pressure is also a determinant of survival, but only when the elevation is extremely severe. Several echocardiography-derived parameters have been reported to correlate with poor outcome, particularly with scleroderma [44–46]. Right atrial area index, the diastolic eccentricity index, and the presence of a pericardial effusion were all predictors of the combined endpoint of death or transplantation; right atrial area index and pericardial effusion were also independent predictors of mortality. However, although these indices usually reflect profound RV failure, they are crude at best. With this in mind, novel and practical ways to assess the presence and extent of subclinical RV failure are desperately needed before the stage of overt RV failure [47]. Recently, the use of TAPSE (Tricuspid Annular Plane Systolic Excursion) has been correlated to mortality in patients with SSc and idiopathic PAH [27]. Moreover, the role of pulmonary vascular stiffening and wave reflectance in increasing RV hydraulic load appears to be under-recognized, and may be particularly important in PAH-SSc patients in whom there is a significant degree of large artery stiffening in the pulmonary vascular tree [38].

Coronary vasculature and myocardial perfusion

The prevalence of atherosclerotic coronary artery disease is not increased in SSc [4,6], However, in patients with scleroderma and coronary disease, the likelihood of coronary vasospasm is significantly higher than in the general population. It is possible that coronary involvement in scleroderma is not in epicardial vessels, but rests in small arterial segments. Normal coronary angiograms have been demonstrated in patients with exercise-induced perfusion defects, suggesting that abnormal resistance to flow at the level of the microcirculation or myocardial interstitium may account for the observed abnormal perfusion [4,6,14,28,48].

Myocardial Raynaud's phenomenon (RP) has been postulated in scleroderma, but the available findings suggest that it is different from peripheral RP. Peripheral RP appears to involve significant anatomic narrowing of the vessels [49,50]. In contrast, SSc patients with myocardial ischemia demonstrate only infrequent luminal narrowing of the small arteries in the heart

[49,50]. A number of studies have examined the effect of cold pressor prov-
ocation on myocardial function and perfusion in SSc subjects to assess the
presence of possible cold-induced coronary vasospasm, but the results of
these studies have been mixed and the clinical and prognostic significance,
if any, require further investigation [4,50].

Pericardial disease

Pericardial abnormalities in scleroderma have noted fibrinous pericarditis,
fibrous pericarditis, pericardial adhesions, and pericardial effusions at the
time of autopsy [4]. However, clinically symptomatic pericardial disease
(5%–16%) is much less frequent than autopsy-demonstrated pericardial
involvement (33%–72%) [9,11,14,22,31,48,51–53]. Asymptomatic pericardial effusions commonly occur in scleroderma [54]. Moreover, there also
have been large effusions causing tamponade, which can even occur before
skin thickening and the diagnosis of scleroderma [55,56]. Pericardial effusions are also frequently associated with pulmonary hypertension and may
be the presenting feature of pulmonary hypertension in scleroderma [50].
Large pericardial effusions can lead to pericardial tamponade and are
a marker for poor outcome. If an inflammatory component is thought to
be the cause of the effusion, immunosuppression therapy can markedly reduce the volume of the effusion. Moreover, if clinical heart failure is present,
the effusion can be reduced with diuresis. However, if the pericardial effusion
is present in the setting of significant pulmonary hypertension, it has been the
experience at Johns Hopkins that attempts at percutaneous drainage should
be avoided, as this is associated with an increased risk of hemodynamic compromise and death (H.C. Champion, unpublished observation, 2008).

Conduction system disease

Conduction defects and arrhythmias are seen frequently in scleroderma
patients and are thought to be a result of fibrosis or ischemia of the conduction system [50]. Zakopoulos and colleagues [57] found that there was no
difference in the cumulative 24-hour heart rate and blood pressure when
comparing scleroderma patients with control subjects, while Wranicz and
colleagues [58] found that scleroderma patients had a higher mean heart
rate. Depending on the underlying cardiac involvement, increased numbers
and frequency of ventricular ectopic beats, as well as episodes of ventricular
tachycardia, can be seen in scleroderma [59,60]. Paradiso and colleagues
[61], using signal averaged electrocardiography, found that 46% of the
scleroderma subjects (versus 8% of control subjects) had late ventricular
potentials (LVPs), and Morelli and colleagues [62] also found an increase
in LVPs in scleroderma patients (20%) who frequently had a septal infarct
pattern on their electrocardiogram.

Cardiac involvement with a cardiomyopathy and ventricular arrhythmias is cause for great concern in scleroderma, given the increased likelihood for sudden death. Electrophysiologic studies are recommended in this patient population and automatic implantable cardioverter defibrillator implantation is recommended in patients with inducible ventricular tachycardia or reduced LVEF.

Valvular disease

Prior studies using echocardiography, as well as studies on autopsy samples, have suggested a relatively minor valvular involvement in SSc [4]. Nodular thickening of the mitral valve was shown in 38% of their autopsy subjects with SSc [11]. Shortening of the chordae tendinae of the mitral valve has been noted, as well as mitral and tricuspid valve vegetations in some autopsy samples [11,31,52,53]. Nodular thickening of the mitral and aortic valves with regurgitation and mitral valve prolapse have also been noted [22,54,63].

Summary

In summary, while the influence of scleroderma on cardiac function has been known for nearly a century, only recently have we begun to gain a new understanding of the prevalence and prognosis in this patient population. Through new and more refined imaging modalities, as well as more frequent use of invasive hemodynamics, we will be able to better assess patients for subclinical disease and gain new insight as to the long-term prognosis in patients with SSc. Moreover, early detection will allow us to improve quality of life and longevity in patients with cardiac involvement in scleroderma.

References

[1] Heine J. Uber ein eigenartiges Krankheitsbild von deiffuser Sklerosis der haut and innerer organe. Virchows Arch 1926;262:1.
[2] Weiss S, Stead E, Warren J. Scleroderma heart disease, with a consideration of certain other visceral manifestations of scleroderma. Arch Intern Med 1943;71:1.
[3] Clements P. Clinical aspects of localized and systemic sclerosis. Curr Opin Rheumatol 1992; 4:843–50.
[4] Deswal A, Follansbee WP. Cardiac involvement in scleroderma. Rheum Dis Clin North Am 1996;22:841–60.
[5] Ferri C, Bernini L, Bongiorni MG, et al. Noninvasive evaluation of cardiac dysrhythmias, and their relationship with multisystemic symptoms, in progressive systemic sclerosis patients. Arthritis Rheum 1985;28:1259–66.
[6] Follansbee WP. The cardiovascular manifestations of systemic sclerosis (scleroderma). Curr Probl Cardiol 1986;11:241–98.
[7] Follansbee WP, Curtiss EI, Rahko PS, et al. The electrocardiogram in systemic sclerosis (scleroderma). Study of 102 consecutive cases with functional correlations and review of the literature. Am J Med 1985;79:183–92.

[8] Follansbee WP, Miller TR, Curtiss EI, et al. A controlled clinicopathologic study of myocardial fibrosis in systemic sclerosis (scleroderma). J Rheumatol 1990;17:656–62.

[9] Bulkley BH, Ridolfi RL, Salyer WR, et al. Myocardial lesions of progressive systemic sclerosis. A cause of cardiac dysfunction. Circulation 1976;53:483–90.

[10] Bulkley BH, Klacsmann PG, Hutchins GM. Angina pectoris, myocardial infarction and sudden cardiac death with normal coronary arteries: a clinicopathologic study of 9 patients with progressive systemic sclerosis. Am Heart J 1978;95:563–9.

[11] D'Angelo W, Fries J, Masi A, et al. Pathologic observations in systemic sclerosis (scleroderma). A study of fifty-eight autopsy cases and fifty-eight matched controls. Am J Med 1969;46:428–40.

[12] McWhorter JE, LeRoy EC. Pericardial disease in scleroderma (systemic sclerosis). Am J Med 1974;57:566–75.

[13] Alexander EL, Firestein GS, Weiss JL, et al. Reversible cold-induced abnormalities in myocardial perfusion and function in systemic sclerosis. Ann Intern Med 1986;105:661–8.

[14] Follansbee W, Curtiss E, Medsger TJ, et al. Physiologic abnormalities of cardiac function in progressive systemic sclerosis with diffuse scleroderma. N Engl J Med 1984;310:142–8.

[15] Gustafsson R, Mannting F, Kazzam E, et al. Cold-induced reversible myocardial ischaemia in systemic sclerosis. Lancet 1989;2:475–9.

[16] Kahan A, Devaux J, Amor B, et al. Pharmacodynamic effect of dipyridamole on thallium-201 myocardial perfusion in progressive systemic sclerosis with diffuse scleroderma. Ann Rheum Dis 1986;45:718–25.

[17] Kahan A, Devaux J, Amor B, et al. Nicardipine improves myocardial perfusion in systemic sclerosis. J Rheumatol 1988;15:1395–400.

[18] Kahan A, Devaux J, Amor B, et al. Nifedipine and thallium-201 myocardial perfusion in progressive systemic sclerosis. N Engl J Med 1986;314:1397–402.

[19] Kahan A, Devaux J, Amor B, et al. The effect of captopril on thallium 201 myocardial perfusion in systemic sclerosis. Clin Pharmacol Ther 1990;47:483–9.

[20] Kahan A, Nitenberg A, Foult J, et al. Decreased coronary reserve in primary scleroderma myocardial disease. Arthritis Rheum 1985;28:637–46.

[21] Kahan A, Devaux J, Amor B, et al. Pharmacodynamic effect of nicardipine on left ventricular function in systemic sclerosis. J Cardiovasc Pharmacol 1990;15:249–53.

[22] Smith J, Clements P, Levisman J, et al. Echocardiographic features of progressive systemic sclerosis (PSS). Correlation with hemodynamic and postmortem studies. Am J Med 1979;66:28–33.

[23] Clements P. Systemic sclerosis (scleroderma) and related disorders: clinical aspects. Baillieres Best Pract Res Clin Rheumatol 2000;14:1–16.

[24] Clements P, Furst D. Heart involvement in systemic sclerosis. Clin Dermatol 1994;12:267–75.

[25] Medsger TJ, Masi A. Survival with scleroderma. II. A life-table analysis of clinical and demographic factors in 358 male U.S. veteran patients. J Chronic Dis 1973;26:647–60.

[26] Fisher M, Mathai S, Champion H, et al. Clinical differences between idiopathic and scleroderma-related pulmonary hypertension. Arthritis Rheum 2006;54:3043–50.

[27] Forfia PR, Fisher MR, Mathai SC, et al. Tricuspid annular displacement predicts survival in pulmonary hypertension. Am J Respir Crit Care Med 2006;174:1034–41.

[28] Steen VD, Follansbee WP, Conte CG, et al. Thallium perfusion defects predict subsequent cardiac dysfunction in patients with systemic sclerosis. Arthritis Rheum 1996;39:677–81.

[29] Leinwand I. Generalized scleroderma; report with autopsy findings. Ann Intern Med 1951;34:226–38.

[30] Leinwand I, Duryee A, Richter M. Scleroderma; based on a study of over 150 cases. Ann Intern Med 1954;41:1003–41.

[31] Sackner MA, Heinz ER, Steinberg AJ. The heart in scleroderma. Am J Cardiol 1966;17:542–59.

[32] Carette S, Turcotte J, Mathon G. Severe myositis and myocarditis in progressive systemic sclerosis. J Rheumatol 1985;12:997–9.

[33] Follansbee W, Zerbe T, Medsger TJ. Cardiac and skeletal muscle disease in systemic sclerosis (scleroderma): a high risk association. Am Heart J 1993;125:194–203.

[34] Armstrong GP, Whalley GA, Doughty RN, et al. Left ventricular function in scleroderma. Br J Rheumatol 1996;35:983–8.

[35] Valentini G, Vitale D, Giunta A, et al. Diastolic abnormalities in systemic sclerosis: evidence for associated defective cardiac functional reserve. Ann Rheum Dis 1996;55:455–60.

[36] Nakajima K, Taki J, Kawano M, et al. Diastolic dysfunction in patients with systemic sclerosis detected by gated myocardial perfusion SPECT: an early sign of cardiac involvement. J Nucl Med 2001;42:183–8.

[37] Plazak W, Zabinska-Plazak E, Wojas-Pelc A, et al. Heart structure and function in systemic sclerosis. Eur J Dermatol 2002;12:257–62.

[38] Mahmud M, Champion HC. Right ventricular failure complicating heart failure: pathophysiology, significance, and management strategies. Curr Cardiol Rep 2007;9:200–8.

[39] Gaine SP, Rubin LJ. Primary pulmonary hypertension. Lancet 1998;352:719–25.

[40] MacNee W. Right ventricular function in cor pulmonale. Cardiology 1988;75(Suppl 1):30.

[41] Nakamura Y, Nishikawa Y, Miyazaki T, et al. Behavior of the right ventricle against pressure loading: on its plasticity. Jpn Circ J 1985;49:255–60.

[42] Rubin LJ. Primary pulmonary hypertension. N Engl J Med 1997;336:111–7.

[43] Ramirez A, Varga J. Pulmonary arterial hypertension in systemic sclerosis: clinical manifestations, pathophysiology, evaluation, and management. Treat Respir Med 2004;3:339–52.

[44] Badui E, Robles E, Hernandez C, et al. Cardiovascular manifestations in progressive systemic sclerosis). Arch Inst Cardiol Mex 1985;55:263–8 [in Spanish].

[45] Wigley FM. Raynaud's phenomenon and other features of scleroderma, including pulmonary hypertension. Curr Opin Rheumatol 1996;8:561–8.

[46] Wigley FM, Lima JA, Mayes M, et al. The prevalence of undiagnosed pulmonary arterial hypertension in subjects with connective tissue disease at the secondary health care level of community-based rheumatologists (the UNCOVER study). Arthritis Rheum 2005;52:2125–32.

[47] Chin KM, Kim NH, Rubin LJ. The right ventricle in pulmonary hypertension. Coron Artery Dis 2005;16:13–8.

[48] Follansbee W, Curtiss E, Medsger TJ, et al. Myocardial function and perfusion in the CREST syndrome variant of progressive systemic sclerosis. Exercise radionuclide evaluation and comparison with diffuse scleroderma. Am J Med 1984;77:489–96.

[49] Steen V. Clinical manifestations of systemic sclerosis. Semin Cutan Med Surg 1998;17:48.

[50] Steen V. The heart in systemic sclerosis. Curr Rheumatol Rep 2004;6:137–40.

[51] Gaffney F, Anderson R, Nixon J, et al. Cardiovascular function in patients with progressive systemic sclerosis (scleroderma). Clin Cardiol 1982;5:569–76.

[52] Oram S, Stokes W. The heart in scleroderma. Br Heart J 1961;23:243–59.

[53] Sackner MA, Akgun N, Kimbel P, et al. The pathophysiology of scleroderma involving the heart and respiratory system. Ann Intern Med 1964;60:611–30.

[54] Gottdiener J, Moutsopoulos H, Decker J. Echocardiographic identification of cardiac abnormality in scleroderma and related disorders. Am J Med 1979;66:391–8.

[55] Gowda R, Khan I, Sacchi T, et al. Scleroderma pericardial disease presented with a large pericardial effusion—a case report. Angiology 2001;52:59–62.

[56] Langley R, Treadwell E. Cardiac tamponade and pericardial disorders in connective tissue diseases: case report and literature review. J Natl Med Assoc 1994;86:149–53.

[57] Zakopoulos N, Kotsis V, Gialafos E, et al. Systemic sclerosis is not associated with clinical or ambulatory blood pressure. Clin Exp Rheumatol 2003;21:199–204.

[58] Wranicz J, Strzondała M, Zielińska M, et al. Evaluation of early cardiovascular involvement in patients with systemic sclerosis). Przegl Lek 2000;57:389–92 [in Polish].

[59] Morelli S, Piccirillo G, Fimognari F, et al. Twenty-four hour heart period variability in systemic sclerosis. J Rheumatol 1996;23:643–5.

[60] Morelli S, Sgreccia A, Ferrante L, et al. Relationships between electrocardiographic and echocardiographic findings in systemic sclerosis (scleroderma). Int J Cardiol 1996;57:151–60.

[61] Paradiso M, Di Franco M, Musca A, et al. Ventricular late potentials in systemic sclerosis: relationship with skin involvement. J Rheumatol 2002;29:1388–92.

[62] Morelli S, Sgreccia A, De Marzio P, et al. Noninvasive assessment of myocardial involvement in patients with systemic sclerosis: role of signal averaged electrocardiography. J Rheumatol 1997;24:2358–63.

[63] Kinney E, Reeves W, Zellis R. The echocardiogram in scleroderma endocarditis of the mitral valve. Arch Intern Med 1979;139:1179–80.

ELSEVIER
SAUNDERS

Rheum Dis Clin N Am
34 (2008) 191–197

RHEUMATIC
DISEASE CLINICS
OF NORTH AMERICA

Treatment of Pulmonary Arterial Hypertension Due to Scleroderma: Challenges for the Future

Lewis J. Rubin, MD

University of California, San Diego School of Medicine, 9300 Campus Point Drive, La Jolla, CA 92032, USA

Remarkable advances have been achieved in elucidating the pathogenesis of pulmonary arterial hypertension (PAH) over the past two decades, leading to the development of disease-targeted therapies for this condition. Despite these achievements, the response to therapy is often incomplete in many patients who have PAH, particularly those who have connective tissue diseases, and survival remains poor. Accordingly, new treatment strategies must be developed for PAH that optimize the treatments currently available and capitalize on the identification of novel pathogenic pathways for PAH. This article provides an overview of the challenges faced in treatment of PAH caused by scleroderma and a glimpse into the future, based on recent developments in the field that hold promise for enhancing the treatment of this disease.

Early diagnosis

The prognosis of PAH in the setting of scleroderma is particularly poor, with estimates of survival generally measured in months to several years [1,2]. As with other forms of PAH, the signs and symptoms of pulmonary hypertension in scleroderma are nonspecific and subtle, leading to delays in diagnosis and initiation of treatment. Because the prevalence of PAH in scleroderma is high, likely approximately 20% to 30% [3], this population may be considered at risk and therefore worthy of screening methods to detect the presence of disease at an earlier stage, when therapeutic intervention may improve outcome [4]. Recent studies suggest that screening echocardiography may be useful in identifying scleroderma patients who have

---

E-mail address: ljrubin@ucsd.edu

0889-857X/08/$ - see front matter © 2008 Elsevier Inc. All rights reserved.
doi:10.1016/j.rdc.2007.11.003
rheumatic.theclinics.com

abnormalities suggestive of incipient PAH [5]. Long-term clinical trials in scleroderma PAH are needed, however, to determine whether earlier diagnosis and initiation of therapy alter the natural history of this condition.

Novel pathways in the pathogenesis of pulmonary arterial hypertension

Identification of mutations in the bone morphogenetic protein receptor-2 (BMPR2) in most cases of familial PAH (FPAH) has been a major advance in the elucidation of the pathogenic sequence in PAH [6]. Fewer than 20% of individuals who have a BMPR2 mutation develop FPAH, however, and most individuals who have PAH do not have an identifiable mutation [7,8]; genetic predispositions for scleroderma recently have been suggested that may provide insight into unique pathways for disease development and progression in this population [9,10].

It is likely that other factors, including genes and environmental stimuli (a second hit), are needed to initiate the pathological sequence that leads to vascular injury and the pulmonary hypertensive state. Both the role of these other factors in initiating the vascular injury and the mechanisms through which they interface with genetic abnormalities are unknown [11]. Various cellular pathway abnormalities have been described that may play important roles in the development and progression of PAH [12–17]. These include altered synthesis of nitric oxide, prostacyclin and endothelin, impaired potassium channel and growth factor receptor function, altered serotonin transporter regulation, increased oxidant stress, and enhanced matrix production. The relative importance of each of these processes is unknown, however, and the interactions between these various pathways need to be explored. Additionally, the intermediate steps involved in the transduction of signals related to BMPR2 are unknown; clarification of these pathways will lead to a more complete understanding of how impaired BMPR2 signaling, both inherited and acquired, leads to hypertensive pulmonary vascular disease.

Novel therapeutic targets in pulmonary arterial hypertension caused by scleroderma

Less than a decade ago, the treatment of PAH was based on a limited understanding of the disease pathogenesis and was largely empiric and usually ineffective. The treatment of PAH has advanced dramatically since then, with a number of well-designed clinical trials demonstrating efficacy of several therapies that target specific abnormalities present in various forms of PAH, including PAH associated with scleroderma [18–22]. Furthermore, the complexity of these treatments has devolved from continuous intravenous (IV) delivery to oral and inhaled modes of drug delivery. Future studies targeting newly identified alterations in endothelial and smooth muscle cell function may provide novel treatments. Several of the most promising targets are discussed.

Serotonin receptor and transporter function

Serotonin (5-Hydroxytryptamine, 5-HT) is a potent vasoconstrictor and mitogen that long has been suspected to play a pathogenic role in PAH [23]. Recent work suggests that the 5HT2 receptors may be up-regulated in PAH [24], providing a novel therapeutic target, because antagonists to these receptors have been developed. Others have shown that the serotonin transporter, a molecule that facilitates transmembrane transport of serotonin into the cell, is up-regulated in PAH [17]; additionally, the fenfluramine anorexigens, which are known to increase the risk of developing PAH, produce an up-regulation of the serotonin transporter in vitro, supporting a pathogenic mechanism for this system in PAH. Drugs that down-regulate the serotonin transporter, such as the selective serotonin reuptake inhibitors (SSRIs), may be worth exploring as treatment options in the future.

Vasoactive intestinal polypeptide

Vasoactive intestinal polypeptide (VIP) is a substance produced by various cells that exerts cellular antiproliferative effects. VIP is also a neuropeptide with potent vasodilating properties [25]. VIP deficiency has been described in lung tissues from patients who had IPAH [26]. In a preliminary case series, eight patients with IPAH who were treated with inhaled VIP at daily doses of 200 μg in four single inhalations showed marked clinical and hemodynamic improvement [26]. Further studies confirming these encouraging preliminary findings, particularly in other patient subsets, and clarifying optimal dosing and long-term safety, are being contemplated.

Rho kinase inhibitors

Rho kinase is part of a family of enzymes that is involved in the processes of cellular growth and, in particular, smooth muscle tone. Studies in animal models of pulmonary hypertension suggest that fasudil, an inhibitor of Rho kinase, may ameliorate the hemodynamic and pathologic severity of pulmonary vascular injury and provide rationale for clinical development of this agent in PAH [27,28].

Inhibitors of growth factor synthesis

PAH is characterized pathologically by uncontrolled angiogenesis, a process that is reminiscent of malignant transformation. In support of this concept, monoclonal expansion has been demonstrated in the plexiform lesion of IPAH [29]. Of the mediators of interest to target in PAH, perhaps none are more relevant to scleroderma PAH than chemokines and growth factors, which have been implicated in the pathogenesis of this disease. Recently published reports in which imatinib, a kinase inhibitor that is approved for the treatment of hematopoietic malignancies, produced improvement in an animal model of pulmonary hypertension [30] and a handful of PAH patients refractory of other available treatments [31] suggest that this novel approach may be of benefit in PAH. Imatinib warrants further study.

Adrenomedullin is a peptide that causes vasodilation and inhibits proliferation of pulmonary vascular smooth muscle cells [32,33]. Both intravenous and inhaled adrenomedullin lower pulmonary vascular resistance in patients who have IPAH [33,34]. Long-term data are not available, but the substance has the potential of a promising future treatment for PAH [24].

Cell-based therapy

Several recent publications have demonstrated that infusions of endothelial progenitor cells in animal models of pulmonary hypertension attenuate the injury, particularly when these cells are transfected with nitric oxide synthase, the enzyme responsible for the generation of nitric oxide from L-arginine precursor [35]. Thus, while cell-based therapies have yet to fulfill their promise in clinical studies, particularly in cardiovascular diseases, pilot safety and efficacy trials are underway with progenitor cell infusions in patients who have severe PAH refractory to medical therapy [36].

Drugs currently marketed to treat other conditions may have effects that are beneficial in PAH also. For example, the hydroxymethylglutaryl-coenzyme-A reductase inhibitors manifest pleiotropic effects that have been suggested to be responsible for a component of their benefit in arteriosclerotic disease [37], and these agents attenuate the pulmonary arteriopathy induced by the administration of monocrotaline to experimental animals [38,39]. Formal clinical studies with the statins, therefore, may be appropriate. Similarly, currently available platelet inhibitors (ie, aspirin) and newer antithrombotic agents may have a role for treating PAH, in light of the beneficial effects (and inherent risks) of anticoagulation with warfarin in idiopathic PAH.

As with other diseases with a complex pathogenesis, targeting a single pathway in PAH is unlikely to be uniformly successful. With the development of several pathway-specific therapies, the opportunity exists for evaluating multidrug therapy in PAH. Uncontrolled, small trials have suggested that the addition of bosentan to patients failing oral or inhaled prostanoid therapy, with beraprost or iloprost, respectively, resulted in improved exercise capacity. Similarly, the addition of sildenafil to inhaled iloprost therapy resulted in potentiation of the clinical effects. Recently, randomized clinical trials have demonstrated that the addition of inhaled iloprost to background therapy with bosentan [40], or oral sildenafil to background intravenous epoprostenol therapy, resulted in further improvement in hemodynamics, exercise capacity, and time to clinical worsening [41].

Unresolved questions exist regarding combination therapy for PAH:

- Which combinations are the most potent? Put another way, which pathways are the most relevant targets for treatment, and how many should be targeted?

- What is the optimal timing for combination therapy? Should combination therapy be initiated early in the course of the disease to maximize the response, or should it be considered only if monotherapy fails to achieve the desired clinical response? This question is of particular relevance to patients who have PAH caused by scleroderma, in whom responses to monotherapy appear to be less robust and in whom outcome remains poor.
- What are the appropriate criteria for assessing response to therapy?

Measuring outcomes and monitoring the course of therapy

The development of treatments for PAH has prompted the challenge of how to best assess and monitor the efficacy of long-term therapy. Because it is believed that randomized, placebo-controlled trials using survival as an end point would be unethical to perform in PAH, alternative strategies are required to measure and compare the relative effects of the available treatments. Similarly, noninvasive markers of disease severity, either biomarkers, imaging studies, or physiological tests, are needed that can be applied widely to reliably monitor clinical course. Studies that assess the value of these outcome measures, alone or in combination, will enable physicians to time and select therapy in a more structured fashion. Furthermore, more attention needs to be focused on the state of right ventricular function in PAH, because this is arguably the single most important determinant of outcome [42].

Summary

Although major advances in the understanding of the mechanism of disease development and in the treatment of PAH have been achieved over the past decade, substantial gaps in knowledge remain. Bringing together physicians and scientists representing multiple disciplines and expertise, all sharing an interest in PAH, affords the opportunity to explore areas of mutual interest and collaboration that will, it is hoped, narrow these gaps of knowledge in the future.

References

[1] Kawut SM, Taichman DB, Archer-Chicko CL, et al. Hemodynamics and survival in patients with pulmonary arterial hypertension related to systemic sclerosis. Chest 2003;123:344–50.
[2] MacGregor AJ, Canavan R, Knight C, et al. Pulmonary hypertension in systemic sclerosis: risk factors for progression and consequences for survival. Rheumatology 2001;40:453–9.
[3] Fagan KA, Badesch DB. Pulmonary hypertension associated with connective tissue disease. Prog Cardiovasc Dis 2002;45(3):225–34.
[4] McGoon M, Gutterman D, Steen V, et al. Screening, early detection, and diagnosis of pulmonary arterial hypertension: ACCP evidence-based clinical practice guidelines. Chest 2004;126(1 Suppl):14S–34S.

[5] de Groote P, Gressin V, Hachulla E, et al. Evaluation of cardiac abnormalities by Doppler echocardiography in a large nationwide multicentric cohort of patients with systemic sclerosis. Ann Rheum Dis 2008;67:31–6.

[6] Deng Z, Morse JH, Slager SL, et al. Familial primary pulmonary hypertension (gene PPH1) is caused by mutations in the bone morphogenetic protein receptor-II gene. Am J Hum Genet 2000;67:737–44.

[7] Lane KB, Machado RD, Pauciulo MW, et al. Heterozygous germline mutations in BMPR2, encoding a TGF-beta receptor, cause familial primary pulmonary hypertension. The International PPH Consortium. Nat Genet 2000;26:81–4.

[8] Thomson JR, Machado RD, Pauciulo MW, et al. Sporadic primary pulmonary hypertension is associated with germline mutations of the gene encoding BMPR2, a receptor member of the TGF-beta family. J Med Genet 2000;37:741–5.

[9] Nakerakanti SS, Kapanadze B, Yamasaki M, et al. Fli1 and Ets1 have distinct roles in connective tissue growth factor/CCN2 gene regulation and induction of the profibrotic gene program. J Biol Chem 2006;281:25259–69.

[10] Fonseca C, Renzoni E, Sestini P, et al. Endothelin axis polymorphisms in patients with scleroderma. Arthritis Rheum 2006;54:3034–42.

[11] Yuan JX, Rubin LJ. Pathogenesis of pulmonary artery hypertension: need for multiple hits. Circulation 2005;111:534–8.

[12] Christman BW, McPherson CD, Newman JH, et al. An imbalance between the excretion of thromboxane and prostacyclin metabolites in pulmonary hypertension. N Engl J Med 1992; 327:70–5.

[13] Tuder RM, Cool CD, Geraci MW, et al. Prostacyclin synthase expression is decreased in lungs from patients with severe pulmonary hypertension. Am J Respir Crit Care Med 1999;159:1925–32.

[14] Yuan JX, Aldinger AM, Juhaszova M, et al. Dysfunctional voltage gated K^+ channels in pulmonary artery smooth muscle cells of patients with primary pulmonary hypertension. Circulation 1998;98:400–6.

[15] Mandegar M, Remillard CV, Yuan JX. Ion channels in pulmonary arterial hypertension. Prog Cardiovasc Dis 2002;45:81–114.

[16] Denton C. Therapeutic targets in systemic sclerosis. Arthritis Res Ther 2007;(9 Suppl 2): S6.

[17] Eddhaibi S, Humbert M, Fadel E, et al. Serotonin transporter overexpression is responsible for pulmonary artery smooth muscle hyperplasia in primary pulmonary hypertension. J Clin Invest 2001;108:1141–50.

[18] Barst RJ, Rubin LJ, Long WA, et al. A comparison of continuous intravenous epoprostenol (prostacyclin) with conventional therapy for primary pulmonary hypertension. N Engl J Med 1996;334:296–301.

[19] Rubin LJ, Badesch DB, Barst RJ, et al. Bosentan therapy for pulmonary arterial hypertension. N Engl J Med 2002;346:896–903.

[20] Galie N, Humbert M, Vachiery JL, et al. Effects of beraprost sodium, an oral prostacyclin analogue, in patients with pulmonary arterial hypertension: a randomized, double-blind, placebo-controlled trial. J Am Coll Cardiol 2002;39:1496–502.

[21] Olschewski H, Simonneau G, Galie N, et al. Inhaled iloprost for severe pulmonary hypertension. N Engl J Med 2002;347:322–9.

[22] Galiè N, Ghofrani HN, Torbicki A, et al. Sildenafil citrate therapy for pulmonary arterial hypertension. N Engl J Med 2005;353:2148–57.

[23] Fanburg BL, Lee SL. A new role for an old molecule: serotonin as a mitogen. Am J Physiol 1997;272:L795–806.

[24] Long L, MacLean MR, Jeffery TK, et al. Serotonin increases susceptibility to pulmonary hypertension in BMPR2-deficient mice. Circ Res 2006;98:818–27.

[25] Said SI. Mediators and modulators of pulmonary arterial hypertension. Am J Physiol Lung Cell Mol Physiol 2006;291:547–58.

[26] Petkov V, Mosgeoller W, Ziesche, et al. Vasoactive intestinal polypeptide as a new drug for treatment of primary pulmonary hypertension. J Clin Invest 2003;111:1339–46.

[27] Oka M, Homma N, Taraseviciene-Stewart L, et al. Rho kinase-mediated vasoconstriction is important in severe occlusive pulmonary arterial hypertension in rats. Circ Res 2007;100: 923–9.

[28] Abe K, Shimokawa H, Morikawa K, et al. Long-term treatment with a Rho-kinase inhibitor improves monocrotaline-induced fatal pulmonary hypertension in rats. Circ Res 2004;94: 385–93.

[29] Yeager ME, Halley GR, Golpon HA, et al. Microsatellite instability of endothelial cell growth and apoptosis genes within plexiform lesions in primary pulmonary hypertension. Circ Res 2001;88:2–11.

[30] Schermuly RT, Dony E, Ghofrani HA, et al. Reversal of experimental pulmonary hypertension by PDGF inhibition. J Clin Invest 2005;115:2811–21.

[31] Ghofrani HA, Seeger W, Grimminger F. Imatinib for the treatment of pulmonary arterial hypertension. N Engl J Med 2005;353:1412–3.

[32] Nagaya N, Kangawa K. Adrenomedullin in the treatment of pulmonary hypertension. Peptides 2004;25:2013–8.

[33] von der Hardt K, Kandler MA, Chada M, et al. Brief adrenomedullin inhalation leads to sustained reduction of pulmonary artery pressure. Eur Respir J 2004;24:615–23.

[34] Nagayaa N, Nishikimib T, Uematsua M, et al. Haemodynamic and hormonal effects of adrenomedullin in patients with pulmonary hypertension. Heart 2000;84:653–8.

[35] Zhao YD, Courtman DW, Deng Y, et al. Rescue of monocrotaline-induced pulmonary arterial hypertension using bone marrow-derived endothelial-like progenitor cells: efficacy of combined cell and eNOS gene therapy in established disease. Circ Res 2005;96:442–50.

[36] Wang XX, Zhang FR, Shang YP, et al. Transplantation of autologous endothelial progenitor cells may be beneficial in patients with idiopathic pulmonary arterial hypertension: a pilot randomized controlled trial. J Am Coll Cardiol 2007;49:1566–71.

[37] Indolfi C, Cioppa A, Stabile E, et al. Effects of hydroxymethylglutaryl coenzyme-A reductase inhibitor simvastatin on smooth muscle cell proliferation in vitro and neointimal formation in vivo after vascular injury. J Am Coll Cardiol 2000;35:214–21.

[38] Nishimura T, Faul JL, Berry GJ, et al. Simvastatin attenuates smooth muscle neointimal proliferation and pulmonary hypertension in rats. Am J Respir Crit Care Med 2002;166: 1403–8.

[39] Nishimura T, Vaszar LT, Faul JL, et al. Simvastatin rescues rats from fatal pulmonary hypertension by inducing apoptosis in neointimal smooth muscle. Circulation 2003;108: 1640–5.

[40] McLaughlin VV, Oudiz RJ, Frost A, et al. A randomized, double-blind, placebo-controlled study of iloprost inhalation as add-on therapy to bosentan in pulmonary arterial hypertension. Am J Respir Crit Care Med 2006;174:1257–63.

[41] Simonneau G, Rubin LJ, Galie N, et al. Safety and efficacy of sildenafil–epoprostenol combination therapy in patients with pulmonary arterial hypertension [abstract]. Am J Respir Crit Care Med 2007;175:A300.

[42] Voelkel NF, Quaife RA, Leinwand LA, et al. Right ventricular function and failure: report of a National Heart, Lung, and Blood Institute working group on cellular and molecular mechanisms of right heart failure. Circulation 2006;114:1883–91.

ELSEVIER
SAUNDERS

Rheum Dis Clin N Am
34 (2008) 199–220

RHEUMATIC
DISEASE CLINICS
OF NORTH AMERICA

Scleroderma-like Fibrosing Disorders

Francesco Boin, MD[a],*, Laura K. Hummers, MD[b]

[a]*Division of Rheumatology, Johns Hopkins University School of Medicine,
5200 Eastern Avenue, Mason F. Lord Building, Center Tower, Suite 4100,
Room 405, Baltimore, MD 21224, USA*
[b]*Division of Rheumatology, Johns Hopkins University School of Medicine, 5501 Hopkins
Bayview Circle, Room 1B.7, Baltimore, MD 21224, USA*

Scleroderma (systemic sclerosis or SSc) is a relatively rare connective tissue disorder characterized by skin fibrosis, obliterative vasculopathy, and distinct autoimmune abnormalities. The word scleroderma derives from Greek (skleros = hard and derma = skin), highlighting the most apparent feature of this disease, which is excessive cutaneous collagen deposition and fibrosis. Many other clinical conditions present with substantial skin fibrosis and may be confused with SSc, sometimes leading to a wrong diagnosis. As summarized in Box 1, the list of SSc-like disorders is extensive, including other immune-mediated diseases (eosinophilic fasciitis, graft-versus-host disease), deposition disorders (scleromyxedema, scleredema, nephrogenic systemic fibrosis/nephrogenic fibrosing dermopathy, systemic amyloidosis), toxic exposures including occupational and iatrogenic (aniline-denatured rapeseed oil, L-tryptophan, polyvinyl chloride, bleomycin, carbidopa) and genetic syndromes (progeroid disorders, stiff skin syndrome). In most cases, even when the etiology is known or suspected, the precise pathogenetic mechanisms leading to skin and tissue fibrosis remain elusive. Importantly, an attentive and meticulous clinical assessment may allow one to distinguish these conditions from SSc and from each other. The distribution and the quality of skin involvement, the presence of Raynaud's or nailfold capillary microscopy, and the association with particular concurrent diseases or specific laboratory parameters can be of substantial help in refining the diagnosis. In most cases, a deep, full-thickness skin-to-muscle biopsy is necessary to confirm the clinical suspicion. Effective therapies are available for some of these conditions. For this reason, a prompt

This work was supported by the Scleroderma Research Foundation (Francesco Boin) and by the NIH 5K23AR52742-3 (Laura Hummers) awards.

* Corresponding author.
E-mail address: fboin1@jhmi.edu (F. Boin).

doi:10.1016/j.rdc.2007.11.001

Box 1. Spectrum of scleroderma-like fibrosing skin disorders

Immune-mediated/inflammatory
Eosinophilic fasciitis
Graft-versus-host disease
Lichen sclerosus et atrophicus
POEMS syndrome
Overlap (SLE, dermatomyositis)

Metabolic
Phenylketonuria
Porphyria cutanea tarda
Hypothyroidism (myxedema)

Deposition
Scleromyxedema
Systemic amyloidosis
Nephrogenic systemic fibrosis (or nephrogenic fibrosing
    dermopathy)
Scleredema adultorum
Lipodermatosclerosis

Occupational
Polyvinyl chloride
Organic solvents
Silica
Epoxy resins

Genetic
Progeroid disorders (progeria, acrogeria, Werner's syndrome)
Stiff skin syndrome (or congenital fascial dystrophy)

Toxic or iatrogenic
Bleomycin
Pentazocine
Carbidopa
Eosinophilia–myalgia syndrome (L-tryptophan)
Toxic oil syndrome (aniline denaturated rapeseed oil)
Postradiation fibrosis

Abbreviations: SLE, systemic lupus erythematosus; POEMS, polyneuropathy, organomegaly, endocrinopathy, monoclonal gammopathy, and skin changes.

---

diagnosis is important to spare patients from ineffective treatments and inadequate management.

Some SSc-like diseases are obsolete and mostly of historical interest (ie, toxic oil syndrome, L-tryptophan eosinophilia-myalgia syndrome); others are extremely rare (ie, genetic disorders). For this article, the authors reviewed the most common diseases mimicking SSc, such as nephrogenic fibrosing dermopathy/nephrogenic systemic fibrosis, eosinophilic fasciitis, scleromyxedema, and scleredema. General practitioners often detect the onset and initial progression of these conditions. A prompt referral to specialized centers is extremely important to refine or confirm the diagnosis and to initiate the appropriate treatment.

Nephrogenic systemic fibrosis (nephrogenic fibrosing dermopathy)

Nephrogenic fibrosing dermopathy (NFD) or nephrogenic systemic fibrosis (NSF) was unknown before 1997 when the first few cases were observed in California and subsequently reported in 2000 [1]. These patients were presenting with a rapid confluent fibrotic skin induration associated with lumpy–nodular plaques, pigmentary changes, and flexion contractures of the extremities. The lesions were characterized histologically by fibroblast proliferation, thickened collagen bundles, and mucin deposition, similar to those observed in scleromyxedema. The common denominator for these patients was a history of renal failure and hemodialysis treatment. Their renal disease was secondary to multiple etiologies, and in some cases previous (failing) renal transplantation was present. Despite the initial geographical clustering, patients with similar presentation have been reported worldwide without any ethnic background predilection. Both genders are affected equally (female to male ratio 1:1), with a broad age range (8 to 87 years), including several pediatric cases [2]. In the United States, a NSF registry has been established, with more then 200 cases collected to date [3]. It is likely, however, that the real incidence is much higher and that many existing cases have not been diagnosed or reported.

The disorder initially was called nephrogenic fibrosing dermopathy, indicating the association with renal disease and the apparent involvement of the skin [4]. Subsequent evidence, however, indicated that the fibrosing process was present within muscles, myocardium, lungs, kidneys, and testes [5]. Thus, the term nephrogenic systemic fibrosis now is preferred to recognize the potential systemic nature of this disorder.

Renal disease is invariably present in NSF, but neither the underlying cause nor its duration seems to be relevant. In general, at the time of diagnosis, 90% of patients have been already on hemo- or peritoneal dialysis for a variable period, following acute or chronic renal failure. No other specific clinical conditions have been temporally associated with NSF, with the exception, in different case series, of previous renal transplantation (often malfunctioning), hypercoagulable states, thromboembolic manifestations and vascular surgery or procedures [3]. Some authors have speculated about of the almost concurrent emergence of NSF with new dialysis components (eg, dialysate fluids or membranes) or treatments for patients who have renal failure (eg, erythropoietin and angiotensin-converting enzyme [ACE] inhibitors), without convincing correlation [6,7]. It also was also noted, however, that gadolinium-enhanced MRI or magnetic resonance angiography (MRA) started to be employed commonly in the clinical setting and in particular in renal patients during the early-mid 1990s right before NSF identification. Over the past 2 years, evidence for an association between use of gadolinium and subsequent development of NSF has been growing.

Etiopathogenesis

A strong association between exposure to gadolinium-containing contrast agents and the development of NSF in patients who have renal failure (hemodialysis or glomerular filtration rate [GFR] less than 15 mL/min) initially was reported by two retrospective European studies in 2006, and subsequently confirmed by other authors [8–10]. Recently, deposits of gadolinium and other metals have been shown within NSF skin lesions, strengthening the relevance of the epidemiological observations [11]. Gadolinium (Gd) normally is complexed into chelates (eg, Gadodiamide or Gd-DTPA-BMA or Omniscan), which are soluble and thus suitable for clinical use. In patients who have renal failure Gd half-life is increased substantially (from 1.3 hours up to 120 hours), and Gd-chelate complexes tend to be displaced by excess of certain metal ions such as iron, copper, or zinc (transmetallation) [12]. This dissociation may be enhanced further by a persistent underlying metabolic acidosis. Free Gd ions are less soluble and have a propensity to precipitate into different tissues through direct interaction with cation-binding sites on cellular membranes and extracellular matrix (ECM), or through microembolization in aggregate form [13]. This would explain the presence of Gd deposits in the skin and soft tissues of patients who have had prior exposure to this contrast material. A direct pathogenetic role of Gd in NSF has yet to be proven. Nevertheless, in December 2006, the US Food and Drug Administration issued a public health advisory recommending avoidance of Gd-based contrast agents in patients who have moderate to end-stage kidney disease [14].

The typical histology of NSF skin lesions is characterized by thickened disorganized collagen bundles separated by large clefts and surrounded by dominant fibroblast-like epitheliod or stellate cells (spindle cells), with positive staining for procollagen-I and CD34+ and abundant mucin deposition (Fig. 1A). Inflammatory infiltrates are usually absent, but dendritic and multinucleated giant cells are sometimes present. The infiltrative process usually extends into subcutaneous structures such as adipose interlobular septa, fascial planes (fasciitis), and even deeper into muscle layers, where fibrosis and atrophy can be detected (Fig. 1B). Interestingly, CD34 is a specific marker for adult hematopoietic stem cells, suggesting that these spindle fibroblast-like cells (called fibrocytes) may be circulating and derive from the bone marrow [15]. The mechanisms of fibrocyte recruitment into affected tissues are unknown and may result from active (chemotaxis) or passive

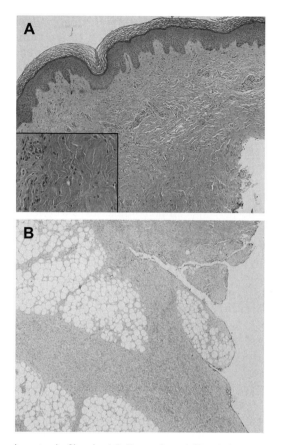

Fig. 1. Nephrogenic systemic fibrosis. (*A*) Dense dermal fibrosis is present under a normal epidermis. Disorganized collagen bundles are separated by large clefts and surrounded by numerous fibroblast-like (spindle) cells. Minimal perivascular inflammatory infiltrate is present. (*B*) The infiltrative process is deep, extending into subcutaneous adipose interlobular septa.

transmigration. The association with high doses of erythropoietin use in patients with NSF has been reported [7]. Despite the fact that this hormone has the ability to mobilize hematopoietic progenitors from the bone marrow, including mesenchymal precursors, and contribute to fibrin-induced wound healing, its role in the pathogenesis of NSF has yet to be elucidated [16].

Clinical features

The cutaneous lesions of NSF usually develop over a short period of time (days to weeks), and subsequently assume a chronic, unremitting course. The distribution often is symmetrical, commonly involving the lower extremities up to the knees and the upper extremities up to the elbows. More proximal spread and extension to the trunk is possible. The face usually is spared. The skin is characterized by a lumpy–nodular thickening with a tendency to form indurated irregular plaques. During early stages, these areas may appear slightly edematous with peau d'orange and erythematous surface features, and can be confounded easily with cellulitis, lymphangitis, or chronic (lymph) edema, not unusual in nephropathic patients. Over time, the skin tends to become bowed-down, with a cobblestone appearance and brawny hyperpigmentation. Objectively, the affected areas and subcutaneous tissues are extremely hard, woody, and can be slightly warm to the touch. The joints underlying NSF lesions usually are involved by a deep fibrotic process, causing severe flexion contractures (particularly hands, wrists, ankles and knees) with substantial loss of range of motion and significant disability. Even ambulation can become compromised severely, and patients can be confined to a wheelchair.

The symptoms in NSF are usually dramatic. The skin and the joints involved by the tight fibrotic process are extremely tender. Pruritus and a burning sensation are very common over affected areas. Nerve conduction studies seem to confirm the presence of a true peripheral neuropathy, further complicating the management of the underlying pain syndrome, which is usually very difficult to control.

Even if no specific diagnostic test is available, the detection in the right clinical context (renal failure) of the characteristic skin changes with unremarkable laboratory findings is adequate to prompt a reasonable suspicion for NSF. In most cases, the distinctive histopathology is confirmatory. Imaging, and in particular MRI (without contrast), can be very helpful to define the extension of the deep fibrosing process and the presence of calcifications. An increased T1 signal is often present within the muscles underlying affected surfaces suggesting presence atrophy and fat degeneration. In addition, fat suppression protocols (eg, fat-suppressed fast T2 weighted sequences) can reveal presence of fascial and muscular edema, particularly during early phases of the disease.

Different from SSc, in NSF serological markers for autoimmunity are absent, and nailfold capillary microscopy examination is normal (Table 1). The body distribution can be similar to SSc (ie, hands can be fully involved), but the face usually is spared. The cobblestone appearance and brawny hyperpigmentation tend to differ from typical SSc skin lesions. Raynaud's phenomenon is usually not present.

Treatment and prognosis

No effective treatment is available for patients who have NSF. In some cases, the normalization of kidney function has been associated with arrest of disease progression and partial reversal of skin lesions, but this is not the rule. Numerous publications have been suggesting favorable therapeutic strategies [17]. These were most exclusively anecdotal reports or very small patient series, however. The reported responses were invariably modest and

Table 1
Differentiating features between scleroderma and scleroderma-like fibrosing disorders

		Scleromyxedema	Scleredema	Eosinophilic fasciitis	Nephrogenic systemic fibrosis
Skin findings					
Quality	Indurated, thick	Papular, waxy	Indurated, doughy	Woody induration	Cobblestone, nodular, indurated plaques
Distribution	Fingers, hands, extremities, face, chest; back spared	Face, neck, extremities, fingers	Neck, back, face	Extremities, trunk; Hands and feet spared	Extremities, trunk, hand, feet; face spared
Systemic disease					
Raynaud's phenomenon	Almost universal	Not common	No	Unusual	Unusual
Nailfold capillaries	Universally abnormal	Normal	Normal	Normal	Normal
Antinuclear antibody	Positive 95% to 100%	Uncommon	Negative	Uncommon	Negative
Neurologic disease	Rare	Seizures, dementia, coma	None	Carpal tunnel syndrome	Peripheral neuropathy
Histological changes					
Mucin on biopsy	No	Yes	Yes	No	Yes
Fibrosis	Dermal, epidermal	Dermal	Dermal	Dermal, hypodermal	Dermal, epidermal
Fibrocytes	No (possible)	Yes	No	No	Yes
Inflammation	Perivascular	Perivascular	No	Yes, with/without eosinophils	No
Clinical associations		Monoclonal gammopathy	Infection, monoclonal gammopathy, diabetes	Morphea, immune-mediated cytopenias, hematologic and solid malignancies	Acute or chronic renal failure, renal transplant, exposure to gadolinium-based contrast agents

incomplete. Often, important details about concurrent changes of the underlying kidney function were missing. Most importantly, the results obtained have not been replicated consistently by different centers.

Immunosuppression (ie, cyclophosphamide, thalidomide, mycophenolate mofetil) does not seem to introduce any substantial advantage, even during early stages, when the lesions tend to evolve more rapidly. Interestingly, patients with renal transplantation experience development or progression of NSF despite being on potent antirejection immunosuppressive medications (ie, prednisone, cyclosporine, tacrolimus, or rapamycin). Topical preparations, including corticosteroids creams, are of limited help.

Extracorporeal photopheresis (ECP) has been reported as effective by different groups, but usually requires long periods (months) of administration and achieves mild results [18,19]. Plasmapheresis, intravenous immunoglobulins (IVIG) and ultraviolet (UV-A1) phototherapy also have been proposed [20–22]. In the authors' experience, these treatment strategies have been overall disappointing. A recent report indicates that intravenous sodium thiosulfate is beneficial [23]. This is of interest, because dystrophic dermal calcifications similar to those seen in calciphylaxis are observed in NSF patients.

Aggressive physical therapy remains the most important recommendation and plays a fundamental role in preventing progression of flexion contractures, muscular atrophy, and overall disability. Pain management is extremely challenging, often requiring a combination of agents targeting musculoskeletal and neuropathic pain. Narcotics are often used at high doses, but their efficacy is never satisfactory and decreases over time. Newer drugs with direct antifibrotic effects are being considered in NSF treatment. Substantial skin improvement has been reported with the use of imatinib mesylate [24].

Eosinophilic fasciitis

In 1974, Shulman reported two patients presenting with scleroderma-like skin changes and painful induration of subcutaneous tissues involving the extremities associated with hypergammaglobulinemia, striking peripheral eosinophilia, and histological evidence of diffuse fasciitis [25]. This syndrome was later named eosinophilic fasciitis (EF) by Rodnan and colleagues [26]. Other names used to designate this clinical entity are Shulman's syndrome or diffuse fasciitis with eosinophilia. Since the very first description, there have been more then 250 cases reported in literature; however the true incidence remains unknown. The only substantial case series (52 patients) was from the Mayo Clinic (Rochester, Minn.), published in 1988 [27]. EF tends to be more frequent in males (2:1 ratio), affecting adults in their second to sixth decade of life. More than 30 pediatric cases have been reported, with clinical characteristics similar to those of the adult occurrence, except with higher prevalence in females [28]. EF is largely more prevalent in Caucasians, but sporadically it has been observed in

Asian, African, and African American patients. Epidemics of two clinical entities similar to EF and resulting from the ingestion of toxic contaminants such as aniline-denaturated rapeseed oil and L-tryptophan have been identified in the past [29,30]. Specifically, the toxic oil syndrome (Spain, 1981) and the eosinophilia–myalgia syndrome (United States, 1989) were characterized by eosinophilia, skin fibrosis, and pathologic evidence of fasciitis. Different from EF, these cases presented a more acute course, with fever, severe multisystem involvement, and a high mortality rate. No new cases have been reported over the past decade, and these conditions are now mostly of historical significance.

Etiopathogenesis

The fibrotic changes of EF develop rapidly in the context of an exaggerated immune response and proinflammatory environment. Peripheral blood and tissue eosinophilia, hypergammaglobulinemia, and elevated inflammatory markers are dominant features and correlate with disease activity and response to treatment [27].

The classic histopathologic changes in EF are dermal–hypodermic sclerosis associated with fibrotic thickening of the subcutaneous adipose lobular septa, superficial fascia, and perimysium. The epidermis usually is spared. The adjacent muscles can present mild inflammation without evidence of necrosis. The fibroblastic proliferation is associated with an inflammatory infiltrate, characterized predominantly by macrophages and CD8+ T cells exhibiting an activated cytotoxic phenotype [31]. Eosinophils can be enriched within affected tissues, but they may not be present when biopsies are obtained after institution of corticosteroid therapy. Elevated serum levels of type 2 cytokines such as interleukin (IL)-5 and other profibrotic molecules (transforming growth factor beta [TGF-β]) have been reported in patients who have active disease [32,33]. IL-5 plays an important role in the chemotaxis, activation, and regulation of eosinophil effector function [34]. Tissue-infiltrating eosinophils can generate important local fibrogenic stimuli by increasing their expression of TGF-β and by releasing toxic cationic proteins upon degranulation. In vitro studies have shown the ability of eosinophils to stimulate matrix production in dermal fibroblasts [35]. An activated phenotype, along with increased collagen expression, has been shown in fascial fibroblasts isolated from EF lesions [36].

Different potential triggers have been considered for EF. An antecedent history of vigorous exercise or trauma is present in about 50% of the cases [27]. A positive serology for *Borrelia burgdorferi* has been reported, and spirochetal organisms have been identified in some EF lesions [37,38]. These findings, however, have not been reproduced consistently [39]. Toxic exposures other than aniline-denaturated rapeseed oil and L-tryptophan have not been proven. The association between EF and other autoimmune manifestations such as immune-mediated cytopenias and localized scleroderma has been observed. Morphea in particular often is reported in conjunction with EF [40,41]. Commonly, it presents in the generalized form or with discrete areas of deeper fibrosis sparing the superficial skin layers (morphea profunda). EF and morphea can have an asynchronous clinical course. In up to 10% to 15% of patients who have EF, underlying hematological disorders or malignancies have been found [27]. A causal relationship between EF and these potential triggers or associated conditions remains unclear and, to date, unproven.

Clinical features

The classic onset of EF is usually acute with rapid and symmetric spreading of skin changes over the extremities within a short period of time (days to weeks), in particular over forearms and calves. Less frequently, the disease process can be confined exclusively to the legs or the arms, or affect an individual limb. The trunk and the neck also can be involved. The hands and face generally are spared, except for some isolated reports [27]. During the early inflammatory phase, the skin is edematous, with dimpling and a peau d'orange appearance. This is followed by a progressive induration of subcutaneous tissues, which can acquire a marble-like consistency. Tethering of the dermis to the fascial and muscular layers causes skin puckering and venous furrowing (Fig. 2A). These are very typical in EF and particularly visible over the medial aspect of arms and thighs. Importantly, the more superficial layers of the skin are not affected by the fibrotic process, and wrinkling of the epidermis still can be elicited by gentle pinching. Hair loss is common in affected areas.

Deeper involvement and fibrosis of periarticular structures can prompt severe flexion contractures and disturbances secondary to peripheral nerve compression, such as carpal tunnel syndrome. Raynaud's phenomenon can be present, but the nailfold capillary microscopy examination is normal. True joint inflammation has been reported, presenting as a symmetric polyarthritis of the small joints (hands) or as oligo-monoarthritis (knees) [27]. Constitutional symptoms such as profound fatigue and weight loss can be observed in patients who have aggressive disease presentation. EF usually does not manifest with visceral involvement. Extensive trunk fibrosis or neck/laryngeal scarring, however, can be associated with significant breathing or swallowing difficulties.

Peripheral eosinophilia is commonly present in up to 80% of cases but is not a prerequisite for diagnosis. Other relevant laboratory findings include polyclonal hypergammaglobulinemia, increased inflammatory markers (ie, erythrocyte sedimentation rate and C-reactive protein), and, occasionally, elevated muscular enzymes (aldolase and creatine phosphokinase), suggesting the presence of underlying muscular involvement. Antinuclear antibodies are rarely positive, and SSc-specific autoantibodies are usually absent. Presence of cytopenias, isolated or in combination, always warrants

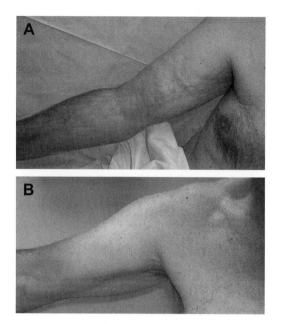

Fig. 2. Eosinophilic fasciitis. (*A*) Patient presenting bilateral involvement of upper extremities with typical woody induration of the skin and puckering. (*B*) The same patient after 12 months of corticosteroid treatment.

further investigation, because they may be secondary to underlying hematological disorders, including immune-mediated anemia or thrombocytopenia, pure red cell aplasia, aplastic anemia, myelodysplastic syndromes, and lymphoproliferative processes (T or B cell lymphoma, multiple myeloma) [42–46]. To obtain a definitive diagnosis, an incisional full-thickness biopsy should be pursued. MRI can be very useful to confirm the diagnosis of EF, to monitor the response to therapy or to evaluate patients when disease relapse is suspected [47]. Appropriate MRI image sequences (ie, fluid-sensitive) can show in great detail the presence of fascial thickening and edema, and the involvement of muscular structures.

Compared with SSc, the epidermis in EF is spared by the fibrotic process. Raynaud's phenomenon and visceral involvement are uncommon (see Table 1). Nailfold capillary microscopy is normal. Autoimmune serology is negative. Corticosteroids are rapidly effective.

Treatment and prognosis

There is substantial agreement among published cases or case series that corticosteroids are the first-line treatment for EF and usually effective in more then 70% of patients (Fig. 2B) [27,48]. Other therapies, including nonsteroidal anti-inflammatory drugs, antihistamines (cimetidine), D-penicillamine or antimalarials (hydroxychloroquine) have been reported, but their efficacy has not been confirmed [27]. Spontaneous resolution also has been observed in some cases.

The ultimate goal in treating EF patients is a complete resolution of the fibrotic manifestations, and this is predicated on an early initiation of the treatment followed by slow tapering. Prednisone (or equivalent corticosteroid) is usually initiated at doses ranging from 0.5 to 1 mg/kg daily. This is maintained until the clinical response is evident, in general within few weeks. Subsequent tapering is slow, particularly with doses below 20 mg daily, and it may take up to 12 to 18 months to achieve a satisfactory or full response. In patients who have aggressive presentation such as extensive body surface involvement, significant weight loss, or when trunk or neck are affected, the authors usually start corticosteroids at the highest doses, often in combination with a second immunosuppressive drug such as methotrexate or mycophenolate mofetil. This strategy allows faster control of the disease and, in the long run, avoidance of excessive cumulative steroid load. A second agent is also useful to achieve further benefit in refractory (unusual) or relapsing cases. In a recent review of 88 published EF cases, clinical variables associated with poor outcome (defined as refractory disease or residual skin fibrosis despite prolonged treatment) were young (pediatric) age of onset, presence of morphea lesions, and trunk involvement [40]. Importantly, the absence of a response should prompt further investigation to rule out presence of an underlying malignancy. Physical therapy plays an important role throughout the disease course to limit the long-term consequences of flexion contractures and disability. Overall, the prognosis of EF is good. Even if prolonged treatment is necessary, most patients usually achieve full disease remission and cure.

Scleromyxedema

Scleromyxedema (papular mucinosis) is a condition of mucinous deposition in the skin associated with a presence of a monoclonal gammopathy characterized by a flesh-colored, papular skin eruption. The exact prevalence of scleromyxedema is unknown, as no formal epidemiologic studies have been performed. It is thought to be quite rare, however, with approximately 150 cases described in the English medical literature. Even this number is difficult to interpret, given that the terminology for this condition has varied with time, and many cases may have been misclassified. For example, early cases of nephrogenic systemic fibrosis may have been misdiagnosed as scleromyxedema before the condition was defined. New terminology proposed by Rongioletti and Rebora [49] in 2001 defined lichen myxedematosus as a broader term under which both scleromyxedema (diffuse, systemic form) and papular mucinosis (focal form) fall. The largest series of scleromyxedema cases to date was published from the Mayo clinic in 1995, where 26 patients evaluated at their institution from 1966 to 1990 were reviewed [50]. This series found that the average age of onset was 55 years, and there was a roughly equal distribution by gender. In the author's center, where 12 patients have been evaluated, the authors found that the average age of onset is 51 plus or minus 12 years (range 35 to 74 years) and the female-to-male ratio is 3:1. This illness has not been reported in children.

Etiopathogenesis

Histological findings reveal three key features: extensive interstitial mucin deposition throughout the dermis with thickened collagen bundles and wide intercollagenous spaces, an increased number of fibroblast-like cells (fibrocytes), and an enhanced inflammatory infiltrate [51]. The etiology of scleromyxedema is unknown. In almost every reported case, there has been demonstration of a monoclonal protein in the peripheral blood. In one scleromyxedema patient who had absent circulating paraprotein, evidence of a monoclonal protein was found in the affected skin lesions [52]. Not surprisingly, given the striking association with circulating paraproteins, several groups have investigated the possible direct pathogenic role these proteins may play. Ferrarini and colleagues [53] demonstrated stimulation of fibroblast cells by serum from one scleromyxedema patient. Another study found that serum from scleromyxedema patients can stimulate in vitro fibroblast proliferation [54]. These results, however, could not be replicated using purified immunoglobulin from the patient's sera. These conflicting data would perhaps suggest that the measurable paraprotein does not have a direct role in the pathogenesis of scleromyxedema through direct tissue fibroblast stimulation. A study of five patients who underwent peripheral blood stem cell transplant (PBSCT) showed that only two patients had an eradication of their monoclonal protein and that there was no relationship between clinical improvement and monoclonal band disappearance [55]. Additionally, as the authors and others have observed, the level of paraprotein does not decrease even after effective treatment, and there seems to be no dose-dependant relationship between paraprotein quantity and clinical effects. Ferrarini [53] suggested an intrinsic abnormality of the scleromyxedema fibroblasts, because they were exhibiting an increased glycosaminoglycan (GAG) synthesis at baseline compared with controls, but this was not increased with addition of serum. Taken together, these data suggest that in scleromyxedema there may be an intrinsic fibroblast defect or possibly other (unknown) circulating factors that can activate fibroblasts in the pathogenesis of this disease.

Clinical features

The cutaneous findings in scleromyxedema are fairly uniform in appearance and location among different patients. The skin is indurated and papular in quality with a cobblestone feel, and its involvement occurs in a characteristic distribution, with the glabellum, posterior auricular area, and neck being affected most commonly (Fig. 3). Other areas include the

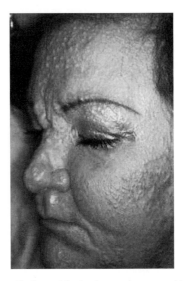

Fig. 3. Scleromyxedema. Patient with classic papular-waxy skin eruption of the face.

back and extremities, and distribution may be similar to scleroderma. One important difference, however, is that the middle portion of the back, commonly affected in scleromyxedema, almost never is involved in scleroderma patients. Sclerodactyly can be present, although papular in quality. In addition to skin findings, patients may have organ involvement that seems to mimic the pattern of scleroderma. Raynaud's phenomenon, esophageal dysmotility, and myopathy have been reported [50]. Less common but potentially life- threatening complications may involve the neurological system in the form of encephalopathy, seizures, coma, and psychosis [56–60]. Additionally, pulmonary hypertension also has been described in patients who have scleromyxedema. The texture of the skin and the histological findings (deep incisional biopsy) remain the most important features distinguishing these two conditions (see Table 1).

Treatment and prognosis

The natural history of this disease has not been defined well, but fatal cases have been reported, most commonly because of neurologic complications [50,59,61]. Various therapies have been employed to treat the symptoms of scleromyxedema with variable success. Historically, melphalan therapy has been the treatment of choice for this condition with multiple reports of benefit, but significant toxicity appears frequent [62–65]. Case reports cite variable improvement with other immunosuppressants including cyclophosphamide and cyclosporine [66–69]. There are multiple cases describing some benefit using thalidomide, although there remains a legitimate concern for the development of disabling peripheral neuropathy

[69–73]. More recent data note benefit of autologous stem cell transplantation in recalcitrant cases [55,74–76].

Multiple groups have reported clinical improvement in scleromyxedema patients following therapy with IVIG [56,61,77–80]. The first case report by Lister and colleagues [77] summarized two patients who were treated with 2 g/kg of IVIG monthly, with responses noted within two to three treatments and maintained by repeated infusions spaced at 10-week intervals. IVIG also has shown benefit in those patients who have complicated neurologic manifestations such as dementia [56]. None of the case reports document any significant long-lasting adverse effects following IVIG therapy. Although long-term follow-up (greater than 3 years) is lacking, these published cases suggest that IVIG is not only an effective treatment for scleromyxedema but safe also. In the authors' center, nine patients have been treated with IVIG, and success has been universal, although the authors also noted that maintenance therapy is necessary.

Scleredema

Scleredema also is associated with deposition of collagen and mucin in the dermis and seems to occur in the setting of three conditions: poorly controlled diabetes, monoclonal gammopathies, and after certain infections, particularly streptococcal pharyngitis. This condition causes scleroderma-like skin changes but in a distribution that is quite different than scleroderma.

Scleredema is a rare condition. Although the exact prevalence is unknown, there are approximately 175 cases in the English medical literature from 1966 to present. The nomenclature is variable, with scleredema adultorum and scleredema of Buschke often being used interchangeably to reflect presence of scleredema of any cause. Scleredema diabeticorum refers to scleredema related to diabetes only. The initial description by Buschke was a postinfectious case, and some authors limit the eponym to this subset. There are also some references subtyping scleredema into three categories according to the three clearly defined disease associations: type 1 in those patients where a preceding febrile illness is identified type 2 including those patients who have an identified circulating paraprotein, and type 3 in patients who have diabetes. There is no clear gender difference, and the disease has been reported in the United States, Europe, Asia, Africa, and Australia. Despite the name adultorum, there are many cases of postinfectious scleredema described in children [81].

It has been estimated that as many as 2.5% to 14% of diabetics have scleredema in some cross-sectional studies, so it is thought that this subset may be under-reported [82–84]. Diabetic patients can be either type 1 or type 2, but commonly tend to be poorly controlled, insulin-requiring and have evidence of diabetic complications such as microangiopathy and retinopathy. In one review of seven cases of diabetes-associated scleredema, the ratio of males to females was 4:3. The mean age at onset was 54 years;

the mean duration of diabetes was 13 years, and there was a high frequency of diabetic complications [85].

Etiopathogenesis

Most literature reports find this disease to be associated with febrile illness, monoclonal gammopathies, or diabetes. Some cases, however, do not fit into one of these three diagnostic categories, and other atypical causal relationships have been considered such as mechanical stress and use of certain medications (infliximab) [86,87]. In patients with type 2 disease, multiple types of monoclonal gammopathies have been described, including multiple myeloma (IgG and IgA), monoclonal gammopathy of undetermined significance, Waldenstrom's macroglobulinemia, and generalized hypergammaglobulinemia [88–90]. Poor diabetic control and presence of microvascular complications (retinopathy, neuropathy) seem to be key risk factors among diabetic patients.

The pathology of scleredema is notable for marked thickening of the upper and lower dermis and mucin deposition between thickened collagen bundles. There are no clear histopathological differences between the different subtypes of scleredema. In diabetes, it is thought that the abnormal metabolic state in the tissues leads to fibroblast activation and increased collagen synthesis. Like in scleromyxedema, the monoclonal proteins found in some patients who have type 2 scleredema do not have a clear pathogenic role. Multiple infectious agents have been associated with type 1 disease, including *Streptococcus,* influenza, varicella, measles, and mumps. Other series only describe preceding febrile illness by history. No one has determined any clear direct relationship between these pathogens and the development of scleredema, but no thorough investigation has been conducted.

Clinical features

Scleredema causes a non-pitting, doughy or woody induration of the skin that typically involves the neck, back, interscapular region, face, and chest (Fig. 4). In one case series from China of 12 patients, 75% had neck involvement; 42% had back involvement, and 17% had shoulder involvement [91]. In this series, 83% of patients were diabetic; none had previous infection, and none had an identified paraprotein. Typically, the extremities, and in particular the distal portion are spared, but some cases of widespread involvement have been reported. In contrast with scleroderma, the mid-back commonly is involved, while the hands and fingers are not (see Table 1). Some cases have demonstrated marked involvement of the face causing ocular muscle palsy, diminished oral aperture, and periorbital edema [92,93]. Systemic involvement has been reported only infrequently, but some case reports highlight involvement of the tongue, pharynx, and upper esophagus [93,94]. Others have reported cardiac dysfunction with myocarditis [95,96].

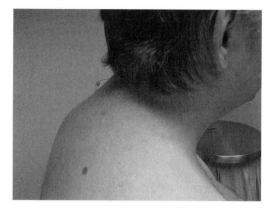

Fig. 4. Scleredema. Patient with diabetes mellitus type 2 and skin induration of the neck and upper back.

Treatment and prognosis

The natural progression of scleredema depends on the underlying associated condition. Patients with infection-related disease are noted to have a rapid onset of symptoms days to months after the infection, with a course that typically resolves in several months to 2 years. Patients who have type 2 disease tend to have a very insidious onset with gradual progression of symptoms over many years. Also in diabetes-associated scleredema, the onset is typically slow, but some improvement may occur as control of diabetes is established [97].

Because most cases of type 1, infection-associated scleredema resolve spontaneously, there is little information regarding treatment. Some recommend the use of penicillin in cases where recent streptococcal infection is demonstrated. In diabetic patients, there are data suggesting that improvement of glycemic control can impact the course of scleredema and reverse skin changes, but this is not a universal phenomenon [98]. Various immunosuppressants such as corticosteroids and methotrexate have been tried without clear benefit [98,99]. Ultraviolet light therapy, in several forms, has been reported to be beneficial, including UVA-1 treatment, PUVA therapy (bath, cream, oral) and photophoresis [100–105]. Several authors also reported some benefit with various types of radiation therapy [106–108].

Summary

There are many conditions that can mimic the appearance of scleroderma. This article highlighted four scleroderma-like conditions that are often detected in the primary care setting and referred to rheumatologists for further evaluation. Rheumatologists must be able to promptly recognize these distinct entities to provide valuable prognostic information and treatment options for affected patients.

References

[1] Cowper SE, Robin HS, Steinberg SM, et al. Scleromyxoedema-like cutaneous diseases in renal–dialysis patients. Lancet 2000;356(9234):1000–1.

[2] Jan F, Segal JM, Dyer J, et al. Nephrogenic fibrosing dermopathy: two pediatric cases. J Pediatr 2003;143(5):678–81.

[3] Cowper SE. Nephrogenic fibrosing dermopathy [NFD/NSF Website]. 2001–2007. Available at: http://www.icnfdr.org. Accessed May 11, 2007.

[4] Cowper SE, Su LD, Bhawan J, et al. Nephrogenic fibrosing dermopathy. Am J Dermatopathol 2001;23(5):383–93.

[5] Ting WW, Stone MS, Madison KC, et al. Nephrogenic fibrosing dermopathy with systemic involvement. Arch Dermatol 2003;139(7):903–6.

[6] Fazeli A, Lio PA, Liu V. Nephrogenic fibrosing dermopathy: are ACE inhibitors the missing link? Arch Dermatol 2004;140(11):1401.

[7] Swaminathan S, Ahmed I, McCarthy JT, et al. Nephrogenic fibrosing dermopathy and high-dose erythropoietin therapy. Ann Intern Med 2006;145(3):234–5.

[8] Marckmann P, Skov L, Rossen K, et al. Nephrogenic systemic fibrosis: suspected causative role of gadodiamide used for contrast-enhanced magnetic resonance imaging. J Am Soc Nephrol 2006;17(9):2359–62.

[9] Grobner T. Gadolinium—a specific trigger for the development of nephrogenic fibrosing dermopathy and nephrogenic systemic fibrosis? Nephrol Dial Transplant 2006;21(4):1104–8.

[10] Khurana A, Runge VM, Narayanan M, et al. Nephrogenic systemic fibrosis: a review of 6 cases temporally related to gadodiamide injection (omniscan). Invest Radiol 2007;42(2):139–45.

[11] High WA, Ayers RA, Chandler J, et al. Gadolinium is detectable within the tissue of patients with nephrogenic systemic fibrosis. J Am Acad Dermatol 2007;56(1):21–6.

[12] Grobner T, Prischl FC. Gadolinium and nephrogenic systemic fibrosis. Kidney Int 2007;72(3):260–4.

[13] Barnhart JL, Kuhnert N, Bakan DA, et al. Biodistribution of GdCl3 and Gd-DTPA and their influence on proton magnetic relaxation in rat tissues. Magn Reson Imaging 1987;5(3):221–31.

[14] Food and Drug Administration. Public health advisory: gadolinium-containing contrast agents for magnetic resonance imaging (MRI). 2006. Available at: http://www.fda.gov/cder/drug/infopage/gcca/default.htm. Accessed December 28, 2007.

[15] Quan TE, Cowper S, Wu SP, et al. Circulating fibrocytes: collagen-secreting cells of the peripheral blood. Int J Biochem Cell Biol 2004;36(4):598–606.

[16] Haroon ZA, Amin K, Jiang X, et al. A novel role for erythropoietin during fibrin-induced wound-healing response. Am J Pathol 2003;163(3):993–1000.

[17] Galan A, Cowper SE, Bucala R. Nephrogenic systemic fibrosis (nephrogenic fibrosing dermopathy). Curr Opin Rheumatol 2006;18(6):614–7.

[18] Richmond H, Zwerner J, Kim Y, et al. Nephrogenic systemic fibrosis: relationship to gadolinium and response to photopheresis. Arch Dermatol 2007;143(8):1025–30.

[19] Gilliet M, Cozzio A, Burg G, et al. Successful treatment of three cases of nephrogenic fibrosing dermopathy with extracorporeal photopheresis. Br J Dermatol 2005;152(3):531–6.

[20] Baron PW, Cantos K, Hillebrand DJ, et al. Nephrogenic fibrosing dermopathy after liver transplantation successfully treated with plasmapheresis. Am J Dermatopathol 2003;25(3):204–9.

[21] Chung HJ, Chung KY. Nephrogenic fibrosing dermopathy: response to high-dose intravenous immunoglobulin. Br J Dermatol 2004;150(3):596–7.

[22] Kafi R, Fisher GJ, Quan T, et al. UV-A1 phototherapy improves nephrogenic fibrosing dermopathy. Arch Dermatol 2004;140(11):1322–4.

[23] Yerram P, Saab G, Karuparthi PR, et al. Nephrogenic systemic fibrosis: a mysterious disease in patients with renal failure—role of gadolinium-based contrast media in causation and the beneficial effect of intravenous sodium thiosulfate. Clin J Am Soc Nephrol 2007; 2(2):258–63.

[24] Kay J. Imatinib mesylate treatment improves skin changes of nephrogenic systemic fibrosis. Arthritis Rheum 2007;56(9):S64.

[25] Shulman LE. Diffuse fasciitis with hypergamaglobulinemia and eosinophilia: a new syndrome? J Rheumatol 1974;1(Suppl 1):46.

[26] Rodnan GP, DiBartolomeo AG, Medsger TA, et al. Eosinophilic fasciitis: report of seven cases of a newly recognized scleroderma-like syndrome. Arthritis Rheum 1975;18(4):422.

[27] Lakhanpal S, Ginsburg WW, Michet CJ, et al. Eosinophilic fasciitis: clinical spectrum and therapeutic response in 52 cases. Semin Arthritis Rheum 1988;17(4):221–31.

[28] Grisanti MW, Moore TL, Osborn TG, et al. Eosinophilic fasciitis in children. Semin Arthritis Rheum 1989;19(3):151–7.

[29] Tabuenca JM. Toxic–allergic syndrome caused by ingestion of rapeseed oil denatured with aniline. Lancet 1981;2(8246):567–8.

[30] Slutsker L, Hoesly FC, Miller L, et al. Eosinophilia–myalgia syndrome associated with exposure to tryptophan from a single manufacturer. JAMA 1990;264(2):213–7.

[31] Toquet C, Hamidou MA, Renaudin K, et al. In situ immunophenotype of the inflammatory infiltrate in eosinophilic fasciitis. J Rheumatol 2003;30(8):1811–5.

[32] Viallard JF, Taupin JL, Ranchin V, et al. Analysis of leukemia inhibitory factor, type 1, and type 2 cytokine production in patients with eosinophilic fasciitis. J Rheumatol 2001;28(1): 75–80.

[33] Dziadzio L, Kelly EA, Panzer SE, et al. Cytokine abnormalities in a patient with eosinophilic fasciitis. Ann Allergy Asthma Immunol 2003;90(4):452–5.

[34] Kariyawasam HH, Robinson DS. The eosinophil: the cell and its weapons, the cytokines, its locations. Semin Respir Crit Care Med 2006;27(2):117–27.

[35] Birkland TP, Cheavens MD, Pincus SH. Human eosinophils stimulate DNA synthesis and matrix production in dermal fibroblasts. Arch Dermatol Res 1994;286(6):312–8.

[36] Kahari VM, Heino J, Niskanen L, et al. Eosinophilic fasciitis. Increased collagen production and type I procollagen messenger RNA levels in fibroblasts cultured from involved skin. Arch Dermatol 1990;126(5):613–7.

[37] Granter SR, Barnhill RL, Hewins ME, et al. Identification of *Borrelia burgdorferi* in diffuse fasciitis with peripheral eosinophilia: borrelial fasciitis. JAMA 1994;272(16):1283–5.

[38] Hashimoto Y, Takahashi H, Matsuo S, et al. Polymerase chain reaction of *Borrelia burgdorferi* flagellin gene in Shulman syndrome. Dermatology 1996;192(2):136–9.

[39] Anton E. Failure to demonstrate *Borrelia burgdorferi*-specific DNA in lesions of eosinophilic fasciitis. Histopathology 2006;49(1):88–90.

[40] Endo Y, Tamura A, Matsushima Y, et al. Eosinophilic fasciitis: report of two cases and a systematic review of the literature dealing with clinical variables that predict outcome. Clin Rheumatol 2007;26(9):1445–51.

[41] Bielsa I, Ariza A. Deep morphea. Semin Cutan Med Surg 2007;26(2):90–5.

[42] Garcia VP, de Quiros JF, Caminal L. Autoimmune hemolytic anemia associated with eosinophilic fasciitis. J Rheumatol 1998;25(9):1864–5.

[43] Bachmeyer C, Monge M, Dhote R, et al. Eosinophilic fasciitis following idiopathic thrombocytopenic purpura, autoimmune hemolytic anemia and Hashimoto's disease. Dermatology 1999;199(3):282.

[44] Junca J, Cuxart A, Tural C, et al. Eosinophilic fasciitis and non-Hodgkin lymphoma. Eur J Haematol 1994;52(5):304–6.

[45] Eklund KK, Anttila P, Leirisalo-Repo M. Eosinophilic fasciitis, myositis, and arthritis as early manifestations of peripheral T-cell lymphoma. Scand J Rheumatol 2003;32(6):376–7.

[46] Khanna D, Verity A, Grossman JM. Eosinophilic fasciitis with multiple myeloma: a new haematological association. Ann Rheum Dis 2002;61(12):1111–2.

[47] Moulton SJ, Kransdorf MJ, Ginsburg WW, et al. Eosinophilic fasciitis: spectrum of MRI findings. AJR Am J Roentgenol 2005;184(3):975–8.

[48] Antic M, Lautenschlager S, Itin PH. Eosinophilic fasciitis 30 years after—what do we really know? Report of 11 patients and review of the literature. Dermatology 2006;213(2): 93–101.

[49] Rongioletti F, Rebora A. Updated classification of papular mucinosis, lichen myxedematosus, and scleromyxedema. J Am Acad Dermatol 2001;44(2):273–81.

[50] Dinneen AM, Dicken CH. Scleromyxedema. J Am Acad Dermatol 1995;33(1):37–43.

[51] Pomann JJ, Rudner EJ. Scleromyxedema revisited. Int J Dermatol 2003;42(1):31–5.

[52] Clark BJ, Mowat A, Fallowfield ME, et al. Papular mucinosis: is the inflammatory cell infiltrate neoplastic? The presence of a monotypic plasma cell population demonstrated by in situ hybridization. Br J Dermatol 1996;135(3):467–70.

[53] Ferrarini M, Helfrich DJ, Walker ER, et al. Scleromyxedema serum increases proliferation but not the glycosaminoglycan synthesis of dermal fibroblasts. J Rheumatol 1989;16(6): 837–41.

[54] Harper RA, Rispler J. Lichen myxedematosus serum stimulates human skin fibroblast proliferation. Science 1978;199(4328):545–7.

[55] Lacy MQ, Hogan WJ, Gertz MA, et al. Successful treatment of scleromyxedema with autologous peripheral blood stem cell transplantation. Arch Dermatol 2005;141(10): 1277–82.

[56] Shergill B, Orteu CH, McBride SR, et al. Dementia associated with scleromyxoedema reversed by high-dose intravenous immunoglobulin. Br J Dermatol 2005;153(3):650–2.

[57] Berger JR, Dobbs MR, Terhune MH, et al. The neurologic complications of scleromyxedema. Medicine (Baltimore) 2001;80(5):313–9.

[58] Nieves DS, Bondi EE, Wallmark J, et al. Scleromyxedema: successful treatment of cutaneous and neurologic symptoms. Cutis 2000;65(2):89–92.

[59] Godby A, Bergstresser PR, Chaker B, et al. Fatal scleromyxedema: report of a case and review of the literature. J Am Acad Dermatol 1998;38(2):289–94.

[60] Webster GF, Matsuoka LY, Burchmore D. The association of potentially lethal neurologic syndromes with scleromyxedema (papular mucinosis). J Am Acad Dermatol 1993;28(1): 105–8.

[61] Majeski C, Taher M, Grewal P, et al. Combination oral prednisone and intravenous immunoglobulin in the treatment of scleromyxedema. J Cutan Med Surg 2005;9(3):99–104.

[62] Feldman P, Shapiro L, Pick AI, et al. Scleromyxedema. A dramatic response to melphalan. Arch Dermatol 1969;99(1):51–6.

[63] Harris RB, Perry HO, Kyle RA, et al. Treatment of scleromyxedema with melphalan. Arch Dermatol 1979;115(3):295–9.

[64] Helm F, Helm TN. Iatrogenic myelomonocytic leukemia following melphalan treatment of scleromyxedema. Cutis 1987;39(3):219–23.

[65] Gabriel SE, Perry HO, Oleson GB, et al. Scleromyxedema: a scleroderma-like disorder with systemic manifestations. Medicine (Baltimore) 1988;67(1):58–65.

[66] Kuldeep CM, Mittal AK, Gupta LK, et al. Successful treatment of scleromyxedema with dexamethasone cyclophosphamide pulse therapy. Indian J Dermatol Venereol Leprol 2005;71(1):44–5.

[67] Rongioletti F, Hazini A, Rebora A. Coma associated with scleromyxoedema and interferon alfa therapy. Full recovery after steroids and cyclophosphamide combined with plasmapheresis. Br J Dermatol 2001;144(6):1283–4.

[68] Saigoh S, Tashiro A, Fujita S, et al. Successful treatment of intractable scleromyxedema with cyclosporin A. Dermatology 2003;207(4):410–1.

[69] Sansbury JC, Cocuroccia B, Jorizzo JL, et al. Treatment of recalcitrant scleromyxedema with thalidomide in 3 patients. J Am Acad Dermatol 2004;51(1):126–31.

[70] Caradonna S, Jacobe H. Thalidomide as a potential treatment for scleromyxedema. Arch Dermatol 2004;140(3):277–80.

[71] Thyssen JP, Zachariae C, Menne T. Successful treatment of scleromyxedema using thalidomide. J Eur Acad Dermatol Venereol 2006;20(10):1396–7.

[72] Jacob SE, Fien S, Kerdel FA. Scleromyxedema, a positive effect with thalidomide. Dermatology 2006;213(2):150–2.

[73] Amini-Adle M, Thieulent N, Dalle S, Blade J, et al. Scleromyxedema: successful treatment with thalidomide in two patients. Dermatology 2007;214(1):58–60.

[74] Iranzo P, Lopez-Lerma I, Blade J, et al. Scleromyxoedema treated with autologous stem cell transplantation. J Eur Acad Dermatol Venereol 2007;21(1):129–30.

[75] Donato ML, Feasel AM, Weber DM, et al. Scleromyxedema: role of high-dose melphalan with autologous stem cell transplantation. Blood 2006;107(2):463–6.

[76] Illa I, de la Torre C, Rojas-Garcia R, et al. Steady remission of scleromyxedema 3 years after autologous stem cell transplantation: an in vivo and in vitro study. Blood 2006; 108(2):773–4.

[77] Lister RK, Jolles S, Whittaker S, et al. Scleromyxedema: response to high-dose intravenous immunoglobulin (hdIVIg). J Am Acad Dermatol 2000;43(2):403–8.

[78] Righi A, Schiavon F, Jablonska S, et al. Intravenous immunoglobulins control scleromyxoedema. Ann Rheum Dis 2002;61(1):59–61.

[79] Kulczycki A, Nelson M, Eisen A, et al. Scleromyxoedema: treatment of cutaneous and systemic manifestations with high-dose intravenous immunoglobulin. Br J Dermatol 2003;149(6):1276–81.

[80] Wojas-Pelc A, Blaszczyk M, Glinska M, et al. Tumorous variant of scleromyxedema. Successful therapy with intravenous immunoglobulins. J Eur Acad Dermatol Venereol 2005;19(4):462–5.

[81] Greenberg LM, Geppert C, Worthen HG, et al. Scleredema adultorum in children. Report of three cases with histochemical study and review of world literature. Pediatrics 1963;32: 1044–54.

[82] Sattar MA, Diab S, Sugathan TN, et al. Scleroedema diabeticorum: a minor but often unrecognized complication of diabetes mellitus. Diabet Med 1988;5(5):465–8.

[83] Vijayasingam SM, Thai AC, Chan HL. Noninfective skin associations of diabetes mellitus. Ann Acad Med Singapore 1988;17(4):526–35.

[84] Cole GW, Headley J, Skowsky R. Scleredema diabeticorum: a common and distinct cutaneous manifestation of diabetes mellitus. Diabetes Care 1983;6(2):189–92.

[85] Tate BJ, Kelly JW, Rotstein H. Scleredema of Buschke: a report of seven cases. Australas J Dermatol 1996;37(3):139–42.

[86] Tsunemi Y, Ihn H, Fujita H, et al. Square-shaped scleredema in the back: probably induced by mechanical stress. Int J Dermatol 2005;44(9):769–70.

[87] Ranganathan P. Infliximab-induced scleredema in a patient with rheumatoid arthritis. J Clin Rheumatol 2005;11(6):319–22.

[88] Beers WH, Ince A, Moore TL. Scleredema adultorum of Buschke: a case report and review of the literature. Semin Arthritis Rheum 2006;35(6):355–9.

[89] Kovary PM, Vakilzadeh F, Macher E, et al. Monoclonal gammopathy in scleredema. Observations in three cases. Arch Dermatol 1981;117(9):536–9.

[90] Ratip S, Akin H, Ozdemirli M, et al. Scleredema of Buschke associated with Waldenstrom's macroglobulinaemia. Br J Dermatol 2000;143(2):450–2.

[91] Leung CS, Chong LY. Scleredema in Chinese patients: a local retrospective study and general review. Hong Kong Med J 1998;4(1):31–5.

[92] Ioannidou DI, Krasagakis K, Stefanidou MP, et al. Scleredema adultorum of Buschke presenting as periorbital edema: a diagnostic challenge. J Am Acad Dermatol 2005; 52(2 Suppl 1):41–4.

[93] Ulmer A, Schaumburg-Lever G, Bauer J, et al. Scleredema adultorum Buschke. Case report and review of the literature. Hautarzt 1998;49(1):48–54.

[94] Wright RA, Bernie H. Scleredema adultorum of Buschke with upper esophageal involvement. Am J Gastroenterol 1982;77(1):9–11.

[95] Paz RA, Badra RE, Marti HM, et al. Systemic Buschke's scleredema with cardiomyopathy, monoclonal IgG kappa gammopathy and amyloidosis. Case report with autopsy. Medicina (B Aires) 1998;58(5 Pt 1):501–3.

[96] Livieri C, Monafo V, Bozzola M, et al. Buschke's scleredema and carditis: a clinical case. Pediatr Med Chir 1982;4(6):695–7.

[97] Rho YW, Suhr KB, Lee JH, et al. A clinical observation of scleredema adultorum and its relationship to diabetes. J Dermatol 1998;25(2):103–7.

[98] Venencie PY, Powell FC, Su WP, et al. Scleredema: a review of thirty-three cases. J Am Acad Dermatol 1984;11(1):128–34.

[99] Breuckmann F, Appelhans C, Harati A, et al. Failure of low-dose methotrexate in the treatment of scleredema diabeticorum in seven cases. Dermatology 2005;211(3):299–301.

[100] Nakajima K, Iwagaki M, Ikeda M, et al. Two cases of diabetic scleredema that responded to PUVA therapy. J Dermatol 2006;33(11):820–2.

[101] Tuchinda C, Kerr HA, Taylor CR, et al. UVA1 phototherapy for cutaneous diseases: an experience of 92 cases in the United States. Photodermatol Photoimmunol Photomed 2006;22(5):247–53.

[102] Eberlein-Konig B, Vogel M, Katzer K, et al. Successful UVA1 phototherapy in a patient with scleredema adultorum. J Eur Acad Dermatol Venereol 2005;19(2):203–4.

[103] Grundmann-Kollmann M, Ochsendorf F, Zollner TM, et al. Cream PUVA therapy for scleredema adultorum. Br J Dermatol 2000;142(5):1058–9.

[104] Hager CM, Sobhi HA, Hunzelmann N, et al. Bath-PUVA therapy in three patients with scleredema adultorum. J Am Acad Dermatol 1998;38(2 Pt 1):240–2.

[105] Stables GI, Taylor PC, Highet AS. Scleredema associated with paraproteinaemia treated by extracorporeal photopheresis. Br J Dermatol 2000;142(4):781–3.

[106] Konemann S, Hesselmann S, Bolling T, et al. Radiotherapy of benign diseases—scleredema adultorum Buschke. Strahlenther Onkol 2004;180(12):811–4.

[107] Bowen AR, Smith L, Zone JJ. Scleredema adultorum of Buschke treated with radiation. Arch Dermatol 2003;139(6):780–4.

[108] Tobler M, Leavitt DD, Gibbs FA Jr. Dosimetric evaluation of a specialized radiotherapy treatment technique for scleredema. Med Dosim 2000;25(4):215–8.

ELSEVIER
SAUNDERS

Rheum Dis Clin N Am
34 (2008) 221–238

RHEUMATIC
DISEASE CLINICS
OF NORTH AMERICA

Often Forgotten Manifestations of Systemic Sclerosis

Ami A. Shah, MD[a],*, Fredrick M. Wigley, MD[a,b]

[a]Division of Rheumatology, Johns Hopkins University, 5200 Eastern Avenue, Mason F. Lord
Building, Center Tower, Suite 4100, Baltimore, MD 21224, USA
[b]Johns Hopkins Scleroderma Center, Johns Hopkins University, 5200 Eastern Avenue,
Mason F. Lord Building, Center Tower, Suite 4100, Baltimore, MD 21224, USA

Given the multisystem nature of systemic sclerosis (scleroderma), there are several clinical manifestations that often go unrecognized; yet they can cause significant morbidity and are challenging to manage. The topics covered in this article include osteolysis, avascular necrosis of the wrist, oral manifestations, erectile dysfunction, pharyngeal weakness, fecal incontinence, nonscleroderma renal disease, liver disease, thyroid disease, and neurological disease in the scleroderma patient.

Osteolysis

Osteolysis, or bony resorption, may be seen in scleroderma in the terminal digital tufts of fingers [1,2] and occasionally toes [3], middle phalanges [1], the distal radius and ulna [1], the distal clavicle [1,4], ribs [2], mandibular angles resulting in decreased oral aperture and pathologic fracture [1,2], cervical spine [2], and even the shaft of tubular bones [5].

Acro-osteolysis, in particular, is a fairly common, undetected complication. It may create a phenotype of digital pseudoclubbing caused by bone resorption beginning in the terminal digital tuft, resulting in a sharpened phalanx and tapered fingers [1], and one even may observe by radiograph a pencil-in-cup deformity [6]. Patients usually present with asymptomatic gradual shortening of the involved digit (Fig. 1). Occasionally pain is a presenting complaint, or in the case of mandible involvement, deformity of facial features or difficulty with mastication is experienced. Deformity of a long bone can be mistaken for a bone malignant lesion (Fig. 2).

---

* Corresponding author.
E-mail address: ashah32@jhmi.edu (A.A. Shah).

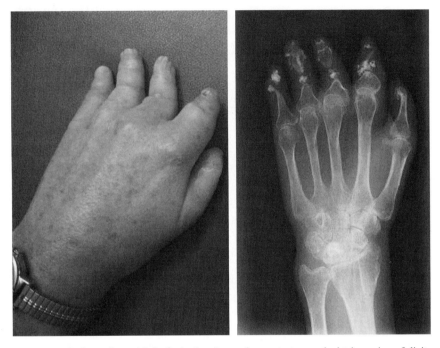

Fig. 1. Hand of a patient with limited scleroderma demonstrates marked telescoping of digits (*left*). Radiographic evidence of profound osteolysis, resorption of terminal digital tufts, and shortening of involved digits (*right*).

In a study evaluating hand radiographs of 120 consecutive patients who had scleroderma, acro-osteolysis was noted in 22% of subjects [1]. Acro-osteolysis was associated significantly with extra-articular calcification, digital ulcers, and pulmonary arterial hypertension [1]. In another study evaluating differences between 105 patients who had limited and diffuse scleroderma, there was no significant difference in the frequency of fingertip osteolysis by hand radiography [7].

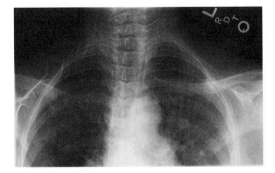

Fig. 2. Prominent right-sided clavicular resorption mimicking bony metastasis.

Although the pathogenic mechanism of osteolysis in scleroderma is unknown, theories include microvasculopathy and vascular insufficiency from recurrent vasospasm, and pressure ischemia due to skin tightening and muscular atrophy [2]. No treatment is shown to alter the course of osteolysis, but vasodilator therapy, bisphosphonates and anti-inflammatory medications are tried. Physical and occupational therapies are helpful, and dental consultation is necessary when the mandible is involved.

Avascular necrosis of the wrist

Avascular necrosis (AVN) can mimic commonly seen problems in scleroderma including arthropathy, fibrosis of tendons, and inflammatory polyarthritis [8]. Avascular necrosis is caused by death of the bone, likely caused by interrupted circulation to the marrow and trabeculae [9]. It rarely can occur in scleroderma, probably secondary to both macro- and microvascular abnormalities that are part of the underlying disease process [10].

Initial case reports of bilateral hip [8,11–14] and bilateral ankle [11] ischemic necrosis in scleroderma were notable in the absence of significant corticosteroid therapy, arthropathy, vasculitis, or anticardiolipin antibodies. Fewer reports describe osteonecrosis of the wrist in scleroderma. One report of AVN of the carpal scaphoid was in a patient treated with 25 g of prednisone over 8 years [15]. Another subject who suffered bilateral lunate osteonecrosis had severe Raynaud's phenomenon and vasculitis [16]. In the authors' center, three patients, two of whom had no corticosteroid exposure, developed osteonecrosis of the lunate [17]. These patients presented with a painful wrist with minimal inflammatory signs. Diagnosis was made by radiographs of the symptomatic area. All had sclerosis of the lunate on radiographs, and loss of signal intensity of the lunate was demonstrated by MRI in two patients. Treatment included a vascularized bone graft into the lunate in one patient and a proximal row carpalectomy in another. Since this report, the authors have seen three other cases of AVN of the wrist in patients who have had either limited and diffuse scleroderma.

Other risk factors for AVN were not identified in these patients, and the unusual involvement of the lunate suggests that circulatory impairment caused by scleroderma vascular disease may have caused bone injury. The authors believe this may be an under-recognized complication of scleroderma presenting as joint pain that is attributed to arthritis or tendonitis. It is important to recognize AVN early, because revascularization of the involved bone may prevent bone death. Surgical removal of damaged bone and stabilization may be needed to treat pain and improve function.

Oral manifestations

Oral complications are experienced commonly by the patient who has scleroderma but often are not managed well. Facial changes are uniform in diffuse scleroderma, with decreased oral aperture, thinning and retraction of the lips, vertical wrinkling around the mouth, and sclerosis of the skin that can make the face have a thin puckered to grimaced appearance. These changes can be cosmetically unpleasant, and they can affect eating by reducing the capacity to incise large parcels of solid food and causing a fatigue sensation with chewing. The decreased oral aperture also makes daily oral hygiene and dental treatment more challenging. Dilated capillaries very frequently are noted on the mucous membranes of patients who have either limited or diffuse scleroderma; these lesions are a manifestation of the microvascular disease but usually are clinically silent with very rare episodes of rupture and bleeding.

In one study, 31 female patients who had scleroderma and 30 age- and sex-matched control subjects underwent clinical and radiographic oral examinations [18]. The intercommissural distance, the interincisal distance, and the maximum oral aperture were reduced in patients who had scleroderma compared with controls. Xerostomia was present in 70% of the patients and was associated with an increased frequency of dental caries. Mobile teeth and periodontal disease were more prevalent in patients who had scleroderma than in control subjects. Loosening of teeth because of loss of normal periodontal attachment to alveolar bone may cause early tooth loss (Fig. 3). Periodontal membrane width was increased in patients who had scleroderma and involved all groups of teeth [18]. Periodontal disease often becomes a problem because of the combination of these membrane abnormalities along with decreased saliva content and the antimicrobial properties of such. Mandibular erosions or thinning of normal contours were seen in 9 of 31 patients and involved the mandibular angle, the condylar head, the coronoid process, the posterior ramus, and the digastric region [18]. Another study of 21 patients demonstrated a prevalence of periodontal ligament space widening of 33%, bone resorption of 9.5%, and tooth root resorption in 4 (33%) of the 12 dentate patients [19].

Nineteen patients who had scleroderma were surveyed, and over 50% complained of xerostomia and limited oral opening [20]. Several were

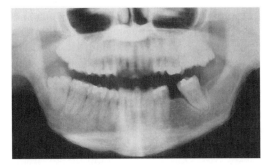

Fig. 3. Loosened tooth caused by loss of normal periodontal attachment to alveolar bone.

refused dental care because of limited accessibility to the oral cavity. Prominent lingual and buccal mucosal crenations and loss of tongue mobility with fibrotic induration were noted in a quarter of the patients. Three of the patients who had advanced disease exhibited foci of severe gingival recession because of fibrous strictures and stripping of the attached gingiva [20].

Several surveys have investigated the prevalence of sicca symptoms in patients with scleroderma [21–23]. Features of Sjögren's syndrome (SS) were sought in 26 patients who had systemic sclerosis and in age- and sex-matched control subjects. Numerous patients and control subjects showed various individual symptoms and signs of lacrimal and salivary disorders, but these features alone were not felt to be sufficient for the diagnosis of SS [21].

Forty-four sequential, unselected patients who had scleroderma were evaluated prospectively for evidence of coexistent SS using lip biopsy findings for diagnosis [22]. Ten patients had a high score of focal lymphocytic infiltration consistent with SS; three had a low score. Seventeen had mild to moderate fibrosis only, and 14 had normal tissue. Pure fibrosis in the biopsy was felt to be secondary to the scleroderma process of tissue fibrosis [22]. Of note, anti-Ro (SSA) antibodies were detected in 33.3% of the patients felt to have secondary SS and only 11.8% of those who had fibrosis only.

In a survey of 133 scleroderma patients, 91 (68%) had sicca symptoms; 50 of these 91 had histological findings of labial tissue fibrosis. Fourteen percent (19 of 133) met criteria for SS, and 18 of these 19 had limited scleroderma and anticentromere antibodies [23].

All oral tissues can be affected by scleroderma; therefore, treatment of the oral manifestations requires early referral to an experienced dentist or dental specialist for preventive and regular dental and periodontal care. Dental prophylaxis with fluoride treatment every 3 months is recommended. Tooth stabilization procedures are available to stabilize loosening teeth. Adjustment of the diet to softer foods, smaller portions, and adequate fluids often are needed. Avoiding aggravating medications such as anticholinergic medications that can dry membranes, controlling severe gastrointestinal (GI) reflux, and recognizing that the chronic use of calcium channel blockers can cause gingival hypertrophy can be helpful. Pilocarpine and cevimeline are stimulators of muscarinic cholinergic receptors that can increase saliva and improve the symptoms of xerostomia.

Erectile dysfunction

Erectile dysfunction (ED), a common problem in scleroderma, has an estimated prevalence as high as 81%, with mean disease onset 3 years after scleroderma diagnosis [24]. Lally and Jimenez initially reported ED as an early manifestation of scleroderma in five patients in 1981; some of these patients had simultaneous onset of Raynaud's phenomenon, and the authors hypothesized a vascular or autonomic neuropathic etiology [25].

Since then, numerous case reports, pathologic and epidemiologic studies, and vascular diagnostic tests have hinted at possible etiologic mechanisms of ED in scleroderma subjects without psychogenic or medication-induced causes. Rossman described three patients in whom the dominant pathological feature was collagenization of the corporal smooth muscle and arterial insufficiency, the latter demonstrated by atresia of the internal pudendal artery and nonvisualization of the cavernous artery on arteriogram in one subject. Two of these patients did not respond to intracorporeal papaverine, arguing against a purely neurologic etiology [26]. In another patient who had scleroderma, Nehra and colleagues [27] demonstrated extensive corporeal fibrosis, luminal stenosis of medium sized arteries, and myointimal proliferation pathologically. In addition, computer-assisted color histomorphometry showed a significant decrease in the ratio of trabecular smooth muscle area to total erectile tissue area as compared with normal individuals [27]. Abnormal penile blood pressures have been demonstrated in subjects who have scleroderma [28]. Although atherosclerosis could contribute to these deviations, a recent study evaluating 15 subjects who had scleroderma showed abnormal blood flow velocities in the cavernous artery after pharmacostimulation in subjects with no early evidence of atherosclerosis as assessed by intima media thickness of the common carotid artery [29]. Penile thermal testing in scleroderma subjects has been notable for lower baseline penile temperatures and a slower recovery from cooling compared with healthy controls, suggesting abnormal thermoregulation [30]. Other hypotheses regarding the etiology of erectile dysfunction in scleroderma have included higher levels of endothelin in scleroderma, autonomic dysfunction, hypogonadism caused by testicular fibrosis or gonadal vascular disease, penile fibrosis altering penile compliance, and lower cavernosal arterial perfusion pressure caused by scleroderma vascular disease [31–33].

Initial evaluation of erectile dysfunction in scleroderma should include a hormonal profile, diagnostic intracavernosal injection of vasoactive agents to rule out neuropathic etiologies, penile brachial index and Doppler ultrasound assessment of vascular insufficiency, and potentially pharmacocavernosometry to evaluate for corporal veno-occlusive dysfunction [31,33]. Psychogenic and medication-induced causes also should be considered. Rarely, corpus cavernosum biopsy may be indicated.

ED treatments in scleroderma have included intracavernous vasoactive therapy, vacuum erection devices, penile prostheses with variable success and risk of perforation because of underlying fibrotic tissue, and attempts at surgical revascularization that often do not succeed because of microcirculatory defects and smooth muscle noncompliance [26,27,31,33,34]. One case report also has documented success with nitroglycerin patch application on the penis [35]. Currently, there is insufficient literature on the use of phosphodiesterase inhibitors to treat ED in scleroderma, with lack of success documented in one report [36]. The authors' experience with the use of phosphodiesterase inhibitors in the treatment of ED has been generally disappointing, but some cases have benefited.

Sexual dysfunction in females with scleroderma is not well-studied and often not discussed openly. Decreased sexual desire, painful and inflexible joints, general fatigue, dry vaginal membranes, and depression are common complaints that the authors have encountered. The authors' approach is to give supportive care while treating pain and any mood disorder. Gynecological consultation, discussion with the patient's spouse, and physical therapy are often helpful.

Pharyngeal weakness

Esophageal dysphagia, a common occurrence in scleroderma, may reflect primary oropharyngeal pathology, as an abnormality in one location may alter another site functionally [37]. Oropharyngeal dysphagia is known as transfer dysphagia caused by abnormal bolus transfer. Hila stated that it could be secondary to poor oral preparation or pharyngeal contraction, inadequate upper esophageal sphincter (UES) opening, or incoordination between pharyngeal contraction and UES relaxation [38]. This may manifest symptomatically as an immediate sensation of bolus holdup in the neck, postnasal regurgitation, a need to swallow repetitively, cough while eating, or dysphonia [38].

Montesi and colleagues studied 51 patients who had scleroderma using videofluoroscopy during barium swallow. Twenty six percent of patients demonstrated oropharyngeal swallowing abnormalities, which included oral leakage, retention, penetration, aspiration, and mild, transient aberrant UES behavior. An increased frequency of hiatal hernia, gastroesophageal reflux, esophagitis, and stricture was noted in subjects with oropharyngeal deglutition deficits compared with those without. As all 13 subjects with oropharyngeal pathology also had evidence of esophageal dysmotility, it was unclear whether these functional abnormalities were secondary to esophageal defects or perhaps a neurogenic cause. Unsurprisingly, these subjects also had more lung disease, presumably secondary to aspiration [39].

Other case reports exist of oropharyngeal swallowing defects in scleroderma. In one case, a woman could not relax her UES in response to pharyngeal contraction because of markedly thickened upper esophageal and pharyngeal constrictors, which pathologically revealed muscle fibers separated by an edematous collagenous matrix [40]. In another report of seven patients who had cricopharyngeal muscle abnormalities, the one patient with scleroderma had a myotomy with pathology notable for degeneration and regeneration of muscle fibers with interstitial fibrosis; however, these findings were not unique to the one patient who had scleroderma [41]. Additionally, one patient had swallowing deficits caused by D-penicillamine induced polymyositis, an idiosyncratic reaction [42]. Another scleroderma patient had severe oropharyngeal dysphagia requiring a feeding gastrostomy [43].

Initial evaluation of oropharyngeal dysphagia should include a spot radiograph to evaluate anatomy [37], plus videotaping a series of swallows using thickened barium and a solid bolus with anteroposterior and lateral radiographs to evaluate motility [38]. If the barium study suggests an obstructing lesion, endoscopy is necessary, but if the study suggests a motility disorder or is normal, manometry is indicated [38].

Fecal incontinence

Diarrhea, constipation, and abdominal discomfort associated with defecation are commonly recognized lower GI symptoms associated with scleroderma. Fecal incontinence, however, often is unrecognized. In a study by Trezza and colleagues [44], 38% of patients who had systemic sclerosis had fecal incontinence, and 19% felt this impacted their quality of life. Fecal incontinence was significantly associated with diarrhea at least once monthly in patients who had diffuse scleroderma.

The etiology of fecal incontinence in scleroderma is understood incompletely. In an autopsy study comparing 58 scleroderma cases with 58 controls matched for age, race, gender, hospital, and date of death, large intestinal muscle atrophy, dilation, or fibrosis was observed in 39% of scleroderma subjects and no controls [45]. Of note, 21% of scleroderma subjects in this study had manifestations of an overlap syndrome. Another pathologic study evaluating rectal histology in a patient who had scleroderma and passive fecal incontinence demonstrated collagenous replacement of the rectal muscularis propria [46]. An ultrastructural study of deep rectal biopsies in three scleroderma patients who had GI symptoms, one of whom had fecal incontinence, revealed signs of axonal degeneration, cytoskeletal abnormalities in bundles of unmyelinated fibers, degeneration of smooth muscle cells, partially degranulated mast cells, and vascular abnormalities but no collagenous replacement [47]. Abnormal plasma neurotransmitter levels also have been noted in scleroderma subjects [48].

In addition to histologic studies of the large bowel, many groups have investigated anorectal dysfunction by means of manometry in scleroderma patients with and without fecal incontinence [46,49–54]. Control groups in these studies have varied and included fecally incontinent and normal subjects. One of the most common outcome measures includes the rectoanal inhibitory reflex (RAIR), which is controlled by intrinsic innervation mediated by means of the enteric nervous system [51]. The RAIR represents the degree of relaxation of the internal anal sphincter in response to rectal distension [51], and an abnormal RAIR suggests neural impairment. Salient findings among scleroderma subjects include a higher voluntary external anal squeeze pressure [49], a significantly lower threshold for rectal sensation [49], and abnormal, often absent, RAIRs [46,49–53]. Investigators also have evaluated the internal anal sphincter, which is composed largely of smooth muscle that may be affected by scleroderma and which is an important barrier against leakage [49].

In a study evaluating colonic motility in 10 scleroderma subjects compared with 18 asymptomatic controls, subjects who had scleroderma demonstrated a lower tolerance for balloon distension of the colon and greater contractile activity after balloon distension than controls [55]. Poor tolerance for distension may be secondary to muscle atrophy and fibrosis of the colon resulting in decreased compliance, whereas the increased contractility may be mediated by the enteric plexus [55].

Initial evaluation of fecal incontinence should include a detailed history, plus perineal examination to assess sensation and perianal examination to identify hemorrhoids, other anal deformities, and possible rectal prolapse [56]. Digital rectal examination is important to identify fecal impaction and test anal sphincter tone and strength [56]. Functional testing with anorectal manometry and anatomic assessment with anal sonography or pelvic MRI are additional diagnostic tests to consider [56].

Rectal prolapse has been identified as a potential contributor to fecal incontinence in scleroderma, and surgical correction may result in improvement [49,52]. Successful treatment measures have included improving stool consistency [49,56], surface anal electromyographic biofeedback [49], sacral nerve stimulation [56,57], and posterior anal repair [50] in small numbers of subjects.

Nonscleroderma renal disease

Mild proteinuria without loss of renal function is the most common manifestation of scleroderma renal disease. It is recognized that patients who have scleroderma are at an increased risk to develop an acute scleroderma renal crisis secondary to microvascular disease, vasospasm of renal vessels, and associated tissue ischemia [58]. It is estimated that approximately 10% to 15% of patients, usually within the first 2 to 3 years of disease onset, will have a renal crisis that presents as malignant hypertension and rapidly progressive renal failure. Patients who have diffuse scleroderma, early active skin disease, the use of corticosteroids, and the presence of anti-RNA polymerase III [59] are at increased risk of having a scleroderma renal crisis.

A survey of 675 patients with diffuse scleroderma seen between 1972 and 1993 found that renal crisis occurred in 129 (19.5%) patients. Kidney function abnormalities or proteinuria were present in 173 patients (26%); 48% had no abnormalities. Most of the patients had a nonscleroderma-related cause for proteinuria including drug toxicity. Only 28 (4%) of these 675 patients had an unknown cause for their kidney dysfunction or proteinuria [60]. It was recommended that patients who have scleroderma without evidence of a renal crisis who have abnormal urinalysis, increased creatinine, or proteinuria should be evaluated carefully for nonscleroderma causes of kidney disease.

A recent case report emphasized that a subset of patients who have scleroderma can present normotensive with rapidly progressive renal failure secondary to antineutrophil cytoplasmic antibody-positive crescentic glomerulonephritis [61]. A patient who had diffuse scleroderma presented with acute renal failure secondary to antimyeloperoxidase (MPO) antibody-associated crescentic glomerulonephritis [61]. Renal biopsy revealed typical features of pauci-immune glomerulonephritis with crescent formation and fibrinoid necrosis. Several similar cases from Germany, Japan, Spain, and Australia suggest an association between normotensive MPO–ANCA-positive crescentic glomerulonephritis and progressive renal failure in scleroderma [62–65]. Three patients who had diffuse scleroderma presented in a manner identical to a scleroderma renal crisis with hypertension but were found to have antibodies to myeloperoxidase (anti-MPO) and crescentic glomerulonephritis [66]. These cases point out the need to carefully evaluate every patient with scleroderma for nonscleroderma causes of renal disease.

Although the absence of hypertension is a clue to nonscleroderma disease, the presence of malignant hypertension does not exclude other causes. Certainly, all causes of renal disease, including drug toxicity, need to be considered. Patients with scleroderma and lupus overlap with related immune complex–mediated glomerulonephritis also are reported [67]. The authors recommend special attention to abnormalities on urinalysis, particularly if there are findings beyond mild proteinuria; comprehensive serologies including anti-MPO should be ordered, and renal biopsy should be done in cases of unexplained changing renal function.

Liver

The liver is thought to be spared as a primary target organ in scleroderma, although it is reported that primary biliary cirrhosis associates with the limited subtype of scleroderma (CREST syndrome) [68,69]. Several recent reports suggest that autoimmune hepatitis also is associated with limited scleroderma [70–73]. The authors have seen three cases of autoimmune hepatitis at their center (F. Wigley, personal data); all have limited scleroderma and have responded to immunosuppressive therapy.

It is recommended that all patients who have scleroderma, particularly those who have limited skin disease, be screened for autoimmune-mediated liver disease. An elevated serum alkaline phosphatase suggests that cholestasis may be caused by the progressive destruction of small interlobular ducts secondary to the autoimmune process of primary biliary cirrhosis. Antimitochondrial antibodies are positive early in the disease, even before chemical evidence of liver disease. Ursodeoxycholic acid therapy is used, but its therapeutic benefit is still controversial [74]. Patients who have unexplained serum liver enzyme elevation may require liver biopsy. The presence of autoimmune hepatitis cannot be overlooked in that it usually responds to immunosuppressive therapy.

Thyroid

Thyroid gland fibrosis and hypothyroidism thought secondary to autoimmune thyroiditis are frequent and often unsuspected findings in scleroderma. A series of 77 ambulatory, clinically euthyroid patients who had systemic sclerosis was evaluated for clinical, chemical, and serologic evidence of thyroid disease [75]. Eight patients (10%) were chemically hypothyroid, but only four had antithyroid antibodies. A study of 56 patients with late-stage scleroderma found histologic evidence of severe fibrosis of the thyroid gland in 14% of cases compared with 2% of an age- and sex-matched control autopsy series from the same institution [76]. In this series, patients who had hypothyroidism, subcutaneous calcinosis, Raynaud's phenomenon, esophageal hypomotility, sclerodactyly, and multiple telangiectasias (the CREST syndrome) occurred more frequently than other variants of scleroderma. The combination of the CREST syndrome, primary biliary cirrhosis, autoimmune thyroiditis and SS is reported, emphasizing the likely association of these autoimmune disorders [69,77]. A large survey of patients who had systemic autoimmune diseases reported that 6% of patients who had scleroderma had Hashimoto's thyroiditis, and 3% had Grave's disease, a prevalence greater than found in a survey of the local general population [78].

It is clear that patients who have scleroderma may develop hypothyroidism [79–82] and that the presence of thyroid autoantibodies support an autoimmune process as the mechanism of gland disease [83,84]. A recent case–control study included 202 scleroderma patients documenting thyroid-stimulating hormone (TSH), free triiodothyronine, free thyroxine, antithyroglobulin and antithyroid-peroxidase (anti-TPO) autoantibodies, thyroid ultrasonography and blood flow, and fine needle aspiration [85]. They found that the odds ratio (OR) for female scleroderma patients versus controls was:

For subclinical hypothyroidism, 3.2 (95% CI = 1.8–5.7);
For clinical hypothyroidism, 14.5 (95% CI = 2.3–90.9);
For anti-TPO positivity, 2.7 (95% CI = 1.8–4.1);
For hypoechoic pattern, 3.2 (95% CI = 2.2–4.7);
For thyroid autoimmunity, 3.7 (95% CI = 2.6–5.4);
For thyroid volume <6 mL, 1.8 (95% CI = 1.2–2.7)

The OR for thyroid autoimmunity in male patients who had scleroderma versus controls was 10.8 (95% CI = 2.2–52.4). These investigators recommended that thyroid function, anti-TPO, and ultrasonography should be tested as part of the clinical evaluation of patients who have scleroderma.

Studies indicate that there is an increased frequency of sometimes previously unsuspected clinical and subclinical hypothyroidism in otherwise apparently stable scleroderma patients. Thyroid disease becomes more prevalent with increased disease duration and particularly in the subtype of limited skin disease. Therefore, careful examination and regular monitoring of the thyroid function in patients who have scleroderma is advisable in that appropriate management of thyroid disease is highly successful.

Neurological

Neurological involvement is thought to occur in a significant proportion of patients who have scleroderma [86]. Most of the reported cases concern trigeminal neuropathy [87,88] or peripheral nerve entrapment. One study surveyed 125 scleroderma patients for neurological involvement prospectively and found four cases of carpal tunnel syndrome and one each of peripheral neuropathy, trigeminal neuralgia, and mononeuritis multiplex [89]. A selected sample of 17 patients who had scleroderma without clinical symptoms or signs of peripheral neuropathy found that the mean distal sensory and motor conduction of the median, ulnar, sural, and tibial nerves were significantly lower than those of a control group, while no significant differences were found in the more proximal tracts of the same nerves [90]. A comprehensive neurologic examination in 14 patients revealed that quantitative sensory testing of the upper and lower extremity revealed increased cold or vibration detection thresholds in 8 of 14 patients [91]. Four of 32 (12.4%) patients who had scleroderma had sensory–motor nerve conduction studies of the upper and lower limbs that demonstrated a distal neuropathy of the upper limbs (one with unilateral and two with bilateral involvement of the median nerve and one bilateral involvement of the ulnar nerve) [92]. From a case–control study involving 536 patients who had the CREST syndrome, seven cases were identified as having peripheral neuropathy not attributable to another cause [93]. Sural nerve biopsy specimens demonstrated multifocal fiber loss and perivascular inflammation; one was diagnostic for necrotizing vasculitis, and two others were highly suggestive for necrotizing vasculitis. Peripheral neuropathy without histological evidence of vasculitis [93] but with the vasculopathy of small vessels [94,95] also is reported in scleroderma. These findings suggest that peripheral neuropathy occurs in patients who have scleroderma at a higher frequency than previously appreciated and that multiple causes need to be considered including entrapment and nerve injury from microvascular disease.

Central nervous system involvement is rare and usually secondary to complications of cardiopulmonary or renal disease. Using a standard electromyographic (EMG) technique in 35 scleroderma patients with no history or signs of cranial nerve impairment and 20 control subjects, six cases (18%) had delayed blink reflex responses suggesting occult central nervous system dysfunction [96].

Autonomic dysfunction has been implicated in scleroderma [97], particularly in the pathology of the GI tract dysmotility [98,99], cardiac disease

[100], skin [101], and abnormal vascular reactivity in various sites including Raynaud's phenomenon [102,103]. Studies into the pathogenesis of Raynaud's phenomenon suggest changes in the peripheral nervous system with loss of normal sensory nerve transmitters or increased alpha 2 receptor activity at the level of the vascular smooth muscle. These changes likely are linked to the profound abnormalities of vascular endothelial function.

Muscle weakness is a common cause of morbidity among patients who have scleroderma. The cause is usually a direct disease of the muscle without central nervous system disease. Multiple factors, including inflammatory polymyositis, disuse myopathy, malnutrition, medications, and in diffuse scleroderma a fibrosing myopathy are known to cause muscle dysfunction [104].

Summary

Scleroderma is a complex human disease that has the unique biological response of tissue fibrosis likely triggered by an inflammatory autoimmune process. Although Raynaud's phenomenon; skin fibrosis; and GI, cardiopulmonary, and musculoskeletal dysfunctions are recognized clinical problems, there are several important manifestations of this multisystem disease that often are overlooked. The topics covered in this article included some of these issues including osteolysis, avascular necrosis of the wrist, oral manifestations, ED, pharyngeal weakness, fecal incontinence, nonscleroderma renal disease, liver disease, thyroid disease, and neurological disease. Awareness of these often forgotten manifestations will help to design appropriate management strategies and hopefully improve clinical outcomes.

Acknowledgments

The authors thank Dr. James Scuibba for his expert review and advice, and Pamela Hill for help in preparing the manuscript.

References

[1] Avouac J, Guerini H, Wipff J, et al. Radiological hand involvement in systemic sclerosis. Ann Rheum Dis 2006;65(8):1088–92.
[2] Benitha R, Modi M, Tikly M. Osteolysis of the cervical spine and mandible in systemic sclerosis: a case report with computed tomography and magnetic resonance imaging findings. Rheumatology (Oxford) 2002;41(10):1198–200.
[3] Bassett LW, Blocka KL, Furst DE, et al. Skeletal findings in progressive systemic sclerosis (scleroderma). AJR Am J Roentgenol 1981;136(6):1121–6.
[4] Bertouch JV, Gordon TP, Henderson D, et al. Asymptomatic osteolysis of ribs and clavicles in progressive systemic sclerosis. Aust N Z J Med 1982;12(6):627–9.
[5] Olutola PS, Adelowo F. Osteolysis of the shaft of tubular bones in systemic scleroderma. Diagn Imaging Clin Med 1985;54(6):322–5.
[6] Wild W, Beetham WP Jr. Erosive arthropathy in systemic scleroderma. JAMA 1975;232(5): 511–2.

[7] Ostojic P, Damjanov N. Different clinical features in patients with limited and diffuse cutaneous systemic sclerosis. Clin Rheumatol 2006;25(4):453–7.

[8] Rodnan GP, Medsger TA. The rheumatic manifestations of progressive systemic sclerosis (scleroderma). Clin Orthop Relat Res 1968;57:81–93.

[9] Glimcher MJ, Kenzora JE. The biology of osteonecrosis of the human femoral head and its clinical implications: II. The pathological changes in the femoral head as an organ and in the hip joint. Clin Orthop Relat Res 1979;139:283–312.

[10] Campbell PM, LeRoy EC. Pathogenesis of systemic sclerosis: a vascular hypothesis. Semin Arthritis Rheum 1975;4(4):351–68.

[11] Fossaluzza V, Peressini A, De Vita S. Multifocal ischemic necrosis of bone in scleroderma. Clin Rheumatol 1991;10(1):95–7.

[12] Martinez-Cordero E. Avascular necrosis of bone in systemic sclerosis. Clin Rheumatol 1992;11(3):443–4.

[13] Taccari E, Spadaro A, Riccieri V, et al. Avascular necrosis of the femoral head in long-term follow-up of systemic sclerosis: report of two cases. Clin Rheumatol 1989;8(3):386–92.

[14] Wilde AH, Mankin HJ, Rodman GP. Avascular necrosis of the femoral head in scleroderma. Arthritis Rheum 1970;13(4):445–7.

[15] Kawai H, Tsuyuguchi Y, Yonenobu K, et al. Avascular necrosis of the carpal scaphoid associated with progressive systemic sclerosis. Hand 1983;15(3):270–3.

[16] Agus B. Bilateral aseptic necrosis of the lunate in systemic sclerosis. Clin Exp Rheumatol 1987;5(2):155–7.

[17] Matsumoto AK, Moore R, Alli P, et al. Three cases of osteonecrosis of the lunate bone of the wrist in scleroderma. Clin Exp Rheumatol 1999;17(6):730–2.

[18] Wood RE, Lee P. Analysis of the oral manifestations of systemic sclerosis (scleroderma). Oral Surg Oral Med Oral Pathol 1988;65(2):172–8.

[19] Rout PG, Hamburger J, Potts AJ. Orofacial radiological manifestations of systemic sclerosis. Dentomaxillofac Radiol 1996;25(4):193–6.

[20] Eversole LR, Jacobsen PL, Stone CE. Oral and gingival changes in systemic sclerosis (scleroderma). J Periodontol 1984;55(3):175–8.

[21] Rasker JJ, Jayson MI, Jones DE, et al. Sjögren's syndrome in systemic sclerosis. A clinical study of 26 patients. Scand J Rheumatol 1990;19(1):57–65.

[22] Drosos AA, Andonopoulos AP, Costopoulos JS, et al. Sjögren's syndrome in progressive systemic sclerosis. J Rheumatol 1988;15(6):965–8.

[23] Avouac J, Sordet C, Depinay C, et al. Systemic sclerosis-associated Sjögren's syndrome and relationship to the limited cutaneous subtype: results of a prospective study of sicca syndrome in 133 consecutive patients. Arthritis Rheum 2006;54(7):2243–9.

[24] Hong P, Pope JE, Ouimet JM, et al. Erectile dysfunction associated with scleroderma: a case–control study of men with scleroderma and rheumatoid arthritis. J Rheumatol 2004;31(3):508–13.

[25] Lally EV, Jimenez SA. Impotence in progressively systemic sclerosis. Ann Intern Med 1981; 95(2):150–3.

[26] Rossman B, Zorgniotti AW. Progressive systemic sclerosis (scleroderma) and impotence. Urology 1989;33(3):189–92.

[27] Nehra A, Hall SJ, Basile G, et al. Systemic sclerosis and impotence: a clinicopathological correlation. J Urol 1995;153(4):1140–6.

[28] Nowlin NS, Brick JE, Weaver DJ, et al. Impotence in scleroderma. Ann Intern Med 1986; 104(6):794–8.

[29] Aversa A, Proietti M, Bruzziches R, et al. The penile vasculature in systemic sclerosis: a duplex ultrasound study. J Sex Med 2006;3(3):554–8.

[30] Merla A, Romani GL, Tangherlini A, et al. Penile cutaneous temperature in systemic sclerosis: a thermal imaging study. Int J Immunopathol Pharmacol 2007;20(1):139–44.

[31] Lotfi MA, Varga J, Hirsch IH. Erectile dysfunction in systemic sclerosis. Urology 1995; 45(5):879–81.

[32] Nowlin NS, Zwillich SH, Brick JE, et al. Male hypogonadism and scleroderma. J Rheumatol 1985;12(3):605–6.

[33] Lally EV, Jimenez SA. Erectile failure in systemic sclerosis. N Engl J Med 1990;322(19): 1398–9.

[34] Klein LE, Posner MS. Progressive systemic sclerosis and impotence. Ann Intern Med 1981; 95(5):658–9.

[35] Ahmad S. Scleroderma and impotence: response to nitroglycerin applied to the fingers and penis. Southampt Med J 1990;83(12):1495.

[36] Ostojic P, Damjanov N. The impact of depression, microvasculopathy, and fibrosis on development of erectile dysfunction in men with systemic sclerosis. Clin Rheumatol 2007;26(10):1671–4.

[37] Rubesin SE. Oral and pharyngeal dysphagia. Gastroenterol Clin North Am 1995;24(2): 331–52.

[38] Hila A, Castell JA, Castell DO. Pharyngeal and upper esophageal sphincter manometry in the evaluation of dysphagia. J Clin Gastroenterol 2001;33(5):355–61.

[39] Montesi A, Pesaresi A, Cavalli ML, et al. Oropharyngeal and esophageal function in scleroderma. Dysphagia 1991;6(4):219–23.

[40] Rajapakse CN, Bancewicz J, Jones CJ, et al. Pharyngo-oesophageal dysphagia in systemic sclerosis. Ann Rheum Dis 1981;40(6):612–4.

[41] Cruse JP, Edwards DA, Smith JF, et al. The pathology of a cricopharyngeal dysphagia. Histopathology 1979;3(3):223–32.

[42] Barrera P, den Broeder AA, van den Hoogen FH, et al. Postural changes, dysphagia, and systemic sclerosis. Ann Rheum Dis 1998;57(6):331–8.

[43] Stainforth J, Goodfield MD. Severe oropharyngeal deglutition abnormalities in a patient with systemic sclerosis, managed with a gastrostomy. Br J Dermatol 1994;130(5):682–3.

[44] Trezza M, Krogh K, Egekvist H, et al. Bowel problems in patients with systemic sclerosis. Scand J Gastroenterol 1999;34(4):409–13.

[45] D'Angelo WA, Fries JF, Masi AT, et al. Pathologic observations in systemic sclerosis (scleroderma). A study of fifty-eight autopsy cases and fifty-eight matched controls. Am J Med 1969;46(3):428–40.

[46] Engel AF, Kamm MA, Talbot IC. Progressive systemic sclerosis of the internal anal sphincter leading to passive faecal incontinence. Gut 1994;35(6):857–9.

[47] Malandrini A, Selvi E, Villanova M, et al. Autonomic nervous system and smooth muscle cell involvement in systemic sclerosis: ultrastructural study of 3 cases. J Rheumatol 2000; 27(5):1203–6.

[48] Akesson A, Ekman R. Gastrointestinal regulatory peptides in systemic sclerosis. Arthritis Rheum 1993;36(5):698–703.

[49] Jaffin BW, Chang P, Spiera H. Fecal incontinence in scleroderma. Clinical features, anorectal manometric findings, and their therapeutic implications. J Clin Gastroenterol 1997; 25(3):513–7.

[50] Chiou AW, Lin JK, Wang FM. Anorectal abnormalities in progressive systemic sclerosis. Dis Colon Rectum 1989;32(5):417–21.

[51] Heyt GJ, Oh MK, Alemzadeh N, et al. Impaired rectoanal inhibitory response in scleroderma (systemic sclerosis): an association with fecal incontinence. Dig Dis Sci 2004;49(6): 1040–5.

[52] Leighton JA, Valdovinos MA, Pemberton JH, et al. Anorectal dysfunction and rectal prolapse in progressive systemic sclerosis. Dis Colon Rectum 1993;36(2):182–5.

[53] Hamel-Roy J, Devroede G, Arhan P, et al. Comparative esophageal and anorectal motility in scleroderma. Gastroenterology 1985;88(1 Pt 1):1–7.

[54] Lock G, Zeuner M, Lang B, et al. Anorectal function in systemic sclerosis: correlation with esophageal dysfunction? Dis Colon Rectum 1997;40(11):1328–35.

[55] Whitehead WE, Taitelbaum G, Wigley FM, et al. Rectosigmoid motility and myoelectric activity in progressive systemic sclerosis. Gastroenterology 1989;96(2 Pt 1):428–32.

[56] Wald A. Clinical practice. Fecal incontinence in adults. N Engl J Med 2007;356(16): 1648–55.

[57] Kenefick NJ, Vaizey CJ, Nicholls RJ, et al. Sacral nerve stimulation for faecal incontinence due to systemic sclerosis. Gut 2002;51(6):881–3.

[58] Steen VD. Scleroderma renal crisis. Rheum Dis Clin North Am 2003;29(2):315–33.

[59] Steen VD. Autoantibodies in systemic sclerosis. Semin Arthritis Rheum 2005;35(1):35–42.

[60] Steen VD, Syzd A, Johnson JP, et al. Kidney disease other than renal crisis in patients with diffuse scleroderma. J Rheumatol 2005;32(4):649–55.

[61] Arnaud L, Huart A, Plaisier E, et al. ANCA-related crescentic glomerulonephritis in systemic sclerosis: revisiting the normotensive scleroderma renal crisis. Clin Nephrol 2007; 68(3):165–70.

[62] Anders HJ, Wiebecke B, Haedecke C, et al. MPO-ANCA-positive crescentic glomerulonephritis: a distinct entity of scleroderma renal disease? Am J Kidney Dis 1999;33(4):E3.

[63] Kobayashi M, Saito M, Minoshima S, et al. A case of progressive systemic sclerosis with crescentic glomerulonephritis associated with myeloperoxidase-antineutrophil cytoplasmic antibody (MPO-ANCA) and antiglomerular basement membrane antibody (anti-GBM Ab). Nippon Jinzo Gakkai Shi 1995;37(3):207–11.

[64] Martinez Ara J, Picazo ML, Torre A, et al. Progressive systemic sclerosis associated with antimyeloperoxidase ANCA vasculitis with renal and cutaneous involvement. Nefrologia 2000;20(4):383–6.

[65] Katrib A, Sturgess A, Bertouch JV. Systemic sclerosis and antineutrophil cytoplasmic autoantibody-associated renal failure. Rheumatol Int 1999;19(1–2):61–3.

[66] Kamen DL, Wigley FM, Brown AN. Antineutrophil cytoplasmic antibody-positive crescentic glomerulonephritis in scleroderma—a different kind of renal crisis. J Rheumatol 2006;33(9):1886–8.

[67] Kameda H, Kuwana M, Hama N, et al. Coexistence of serum anti-DNA topoisomerase I and anti-Sm antibodies: report of 3 cases. J Rheumatol 1997;24(2):400–3.

[68] Hirakata M, Akizuki M, Miyachi K, et al. Coexistence of CREST syndrome and primary biliary cirrhosis. Serological studies of two cases. J Rheumatol 1988;15(7):1166–70.

[69] Nakamura T, Higashi S, Tomoda K, et al. Primary biliary cirrhosis (PBC)-CREST overlap syndrome with coexistence of Sjögren's syndrome and thyroid dysfunction. Clin Rheumatol 2007;26(4):596–600.

[70] Marie I, Levesque H, Tranvouez JL, et al. Autoimmune hepatitis and systemic sclerosis: a new overlap syndrome? Rheumatology (Oxford) 2001;40(1):102–6.

[71] Yabe H, Noma K, Tada N, et al. A case of CREST syndrome with rapidly progressive liver damage. Intern Med 1992;31(1):69–73.

[72] Ishikawa M, Okada J, Shibuya A, et al. CRST syndrome (calcinosis cutis, Raynaud's phenomenon, sclerodactyly, and telangiectasia) associated with autoimmune hepatitis. Intern Med 1995;34(1):6–9.

[73] West M, Jasin HE, Medhekar S. The development of connective tissue diseases in patients with autoimmune hepatitis: a case series. Semin Arthritis Rheum 2006;35(6):344–8.

[74] Goulis J, Leandro G, Burroughs AK. Randomised controlled trials of ursodeoxycholic-acid therapy for primary biliary cirrhosis: a meta-analysis. Lancet 1999;354(9184):1053–60.

[75] Kahl LE, Medsger TA Jr, Klein I. Prospective evaluation of thyroid function in patients with systemic sclerosis (scleroderma). J Rheumatol 1986;13(1):103–7.

[76] Gordon MB, Klein I, Dekker A, et al. Thyroid disease in progressive systemic sclerosis: increased frequency of glandular fibrosis and hypothyroidism. Ann Intern Med 1981; 95(4):431–5.

[77] Horita M, Takahashi N, Seike M, et al. A case of primary biliary cirrhosis associated with Hashimoto's thyroiditis, scleroderma and Sjögren's syndrome. Intern Med 1992;31(3): 418–21.

[78] Biro E, Szekanecz Z, Czirjak L, et al. Association of systemic and thyroid autoimmune diseases. Clin Rheumatol 2006;25(2):240–5.

[79] Kucharz EJ. Thyroid disorders in patients with progressive systemic sclerosis: a review. Clin Rheumatol 1993;12(2):159–61.

[80] De Keyser L, Narhi DC, Furst DE, et al. Thyroid dysfunction in a prospectively followed series of patients with progressive systemic sclerosis. J Endocrinol Invest 1990;13(2):161–9.

[81] Ghayad E, Tohme A, Haddad F, et al. Scleroderma with anomalies of the thyroid function. 7 cases. Ann Med Interne (Paris) 1997;148(4):307–10.

[82] Shahin AA, Abdoh S, Abdelrazik M. Prolactin and thyroid hormones in patients with systemic sclerosis: correlations with disease manifestations and activity. Z Rheumatol 2002; 61(6):703–9.

[83] Molteni M, Barili M, Eisera N, et al. Antithyroid antibodies in Italian scleroderma patients: association of antithyroid peroxidase (anti-TPO) antibodies with HLA-DR15. Clin Exp Rheumatol 1997;15(5):529–34.

[84] Innocencio RM, Romaldini JH, Ward LS. High prevalence of thyroid autoantibodies in systemic sclerosis and rheumatoid arthritis but not in the antiphospholipid syndrome. Clin Rheumatol 2003;22(6):494.

[85] Antonelli A, Ferri C, Fallahi P, et al. Clinical and subclinical autoimmune thyroid disorders in systemic sclerosis. Eur J Endocrinol 2007;156(4):431–7.

[86] Herrick AL. Neurological involvement in systemic sclerosis. Br J Rheumatol 1995;34(11): 1007–8.

[87] Teasdall RD, Frayha RA, Shulman LE. Cranial nerve involvement in systemic sclerosis (scleroderma): a report of 10 cases. Medicine (Baltimore) 1980;59(2):149–59.

[88] Farrell DA, Medsger TA Jr. Trigeminal neuropathy in progressive systemic sclerosis. Am J Med 1982;73(1):57–62.

[89] Lee P, Bruni J, Sukenik S. Neurological manifestations in systemic sclerosis (scleroderma). J Rheumatol 1984;11(4):480–3.

[90] Mondelli M, Romano C, Della Porta PD, et al. Electrophysiological evidence of "nerve entrapment syndromes" and subclinical peripheral neuropathy in progressive systemic sclerosis (scleroderma). J Neurol 1995;242(4):185–94.

[91] Poncelet AN, Connolly MK. Peripheral neuropathy in scleroderma. Muscle Nerve 2003; 28(3):330–5.

[92] Lori S, Matucci-Cerinic M, Casale R, et al. Peripheral nervous system involvement in systemic sclerosis: the median nerve as target structure. Clin Exp Rheumatol 1996;14(6):601–5.

[93] Badakov S. Ultrastructural changes of cutaneous nerves in scleroderma. Folia Med (Plovdiv) 1992;34(3–4):57–64.

[94] Dyck PJ, Hunder GG, Dyck PJ. A case–control and nerve biopsy study of CREST multiple mononeuropathy. Neurology 1997;49(6):1641–5.

[95] Di Trapani G, Tulli A, La Cara A, et al. Peripheral neuropathy in course of progressive systemic sclerosis. Light and ultrastructural study. Acta Neuropathol (Berl) 1986;72(2): 103–10.

[96] Casale R, Frazzitta G, Fundaro C, et al. Blink reflex discloses CNS dysfunction in neurologically asymptomatic patients with systemic sclerosis. Clin Neurophysiol 2004;115(8): 1917–20.

[97] Klimiuk PS, Taylor L, Baker RD, et al. Autonomic neuropathy in systemic sclerosis. Ann Rheum Dis 1988;47(7):542–5.

[98] Cohen S, Fisher R, Lipshutz W, et al. The pathogenesis of esophageal dysfunction in scleroderma and Raynaud's disease. J Clin Invest 1972;51(10):2663–8.

[99] Iovino P, Valentini G, Ciacci C, et al. Proximal stomach function in systemic sclerosis: relationship with autonomic nerve function. Dig Dis Sci 2001;46(4):723–30.

[100] Ferri C, Emdin M, Giuggioli D, et al. Autonomic dysfunction in systemic sclerosis: time and frequency domain 24-hour heart rate variability analysis. Br J Rheumatol 1997; 36(6):669–76.

[101] Raszewa M, Hausmanowa-Petrusewicz I, Blaszczyk M, et al. Sympathetic skin response in scleroderma. Electromyogr Clin Neurophysiol 1991;31(8):467–72.

[102] Terenghi G, Bunker CB, Liu YF, et al. Image analysis quantification of peptide–immuno-reactive nerves in the skin of patients with Raynaud's phenomenon and systemic sclerosis. J Pathol 1991;164(3):245–52.
[103] Wallengren J, Akesson A, Scheja A, et al. Occurrence and distribution of peptidergic nerve fibers in skin biopsies from patients with systemic sclerosis. Acta Derm Venereol 1996;76(2): 126–8.
[104] Clements PJ, Furst DE, Campion DS, et al. Muscle disease in progressive systemic sclerosis: diagnostic and therapeutic considerations. Arthritis Rheum 1978;21(1):62–71.

ELSEVIER
SAUNDERS

Rheum Dis Clin N Am
34 (2008) 239–255

RHEUMATIC
DISEASE CLINICS
OF NORTH AMERICA

Systemic Sclerosis and Localized Scleroderma in Childhood

Francesco Zulian, MD

Department of Pediatrics, Pediatric Rheumatology Unit, University of Padova,
Via Giustiniani 3, 35128 Padova, Italy

Juvenile systemic sclerosis

Juvenile systemic sclerosis (JSSc) is a chronic multisystemic connective tissue disease characterized by symmetrical thickening and hardening of the skin, associated with fibrous changes in internal organs. Although rare in children, it represents one of the most severe rheumatic conditions in pediatric rheumatology practice.

Classification

Very recently, a Committee on Classification Criteria for JSSc, including members of the Pediatric Rheumatology European Society (PRES), the American College of Rheumatology (ACR), and the European League Against Rheumatism (EULAR), developed new classification criteria to help standardize the conduct of clinical, epidemiological, and outcome research for this rare pediatric disease [1].

These criteria, which will supplant the adult criteria [2] that have been used until now, will help ensure an accurate diagnosis of JSSc.

The criteria were developed by using well-recognized consensus formation methodologies specifically designed to combine clinical and laboratory features of real patients with judgments from a group of experts. On the basis of the results obtained, a patient, aged less than 16 years, shall be classified as having JSSc if the one major, presence of proximal skin sclerosis/induration, and at least two of 20 minor criteria, grouped in nine main categories, are present. These classification criteria have a sensitivity of 90%, a specificity of 96% and kappa statistic value of 0.86 (Box 1). Although validated with actual patient data, the new classification criteria will need further validation using external prospective trials.

E-mail address: zulian@pediatria.unipd.it

0889-857X/08/$ - see front matter © 2008 Elsevier Inc. All rights reserved.
doi:10.1016/j.rdc.2007.11.004
rheumatic.theclinics.com

Box 1. Preliminary classification criteria for juvenile systemic sclerosis

Major criterion—proximal sclerosis/induration of the skin
Minor criteria
Skin
    sclerodactyly
Vascular
    Raynaud's phenomenon
    Nailfold capillary abnormalities
    Digital tip ulcers
Gastrointestinal
    Dysphagia
    Gastro–esophageal reflux
Renal
    Renal crisis
    New-onset arterial hypertension
Cardiac
    Arrhythmias
    Heart failure
Respiratory
    Pulmonary fibrosis (high resolution computed tomography/
        radiograph)
    Diffusing lung capacity for carbon monoxide
    Pulmonary hypertension
Musculoskeletal
    Tendon friction rubs
    Arthritis
    Myositis
Neurological
    Neuropathy
    Carpal tunnel syndrome
Serology
    Antinuclear antibodies.
    SSc-selective autoantibodies (anticentromere,
        antitopoisomerase I, antifibrillarin, anti-PM-Scl, ant-fibrillin
        or anti-RNA polymerase I or III)

A patient, aged less than 16 years, shall be classified as having juvenile systemic sclerosis if the one major and at least two of the 20 minor criteria are present. This set of classification criteria has a sensitivity of 90%, a specificity of 96%, and kappa statistic value of 0.86.

Clinical presentation

The onset of JSSc in childhood is very uncommon; children under 16 years of age account for less than 5% of all cases [3]. The onset occurs at a mean age of 8.1 years, and the peak age is between 10 and 16 years [3,4]. The disease is almost fourfold more frequent in girls, and there is no clear evidence for a racial predilection [4].

The onset is often insidious. The mean time between the first sign of the disease and the diagnosis of JSSc is between 1.9 to 2.8 years, with a range between 0 and 12.2 years [3,4]. Overlap syndromes, most frequently with polymyositis or dermatomyositis features, in one large study, accounted for 29% of all cases [3].

Raynaud's phenomenon (RP) is the first sign of the disease in 70% of the patients, and in 10% it is complicated by digital infarcts. Proximal skin induration is the second most frequent symptom, being present in 40% of cases. As expected, the association of RP and skin changes, eventually with some signs of internal organ involvement, are the key diagnostic features.

During the overall course of the disease, RP and skin induration are far the most frequent symptoms (84%), followed by involvement of the respiratory (42%) and gastrointestinal (GI) systems (30%), arthritis (27%), and cardiac involvement (15%). Rarely reported are scleroderma renal crisis (0.7%), renal failure (5%), and central nervous system involvement (3%).

Abnormalities on nailfold capillaroscopy are reported in approximately half of patients, but it is expected that these changes probably would be more frequent if the examination were preformed in a standardized way.

Distinctive features from the adult form

In general, a comparison with adult series is difficult, because in children the limited cutaneous form, which is the far most frequent in adults, is rare. It has now been shown, however, that a substantial number of patients who have childhood-onset JSSc have their diagnosis made either during adolescence or as young adults [3]. It is so possible that the limited cutaneous subset might be underdiagnosed in younger children because of the lack of a full expression of the clinical features.

Children, at the time of diagnosis, show a significantly less frequent visceral involvement compared with adults. The exception is for the prevalence of arthritis seen early in JSSc. Differences with adults become less evident during the follow-up, with the exception of interstitial lung involvement, gastroesophageal dysmotility, renal involvement, arterial hypertension, which are significantly much more common in adults. Other differences during the course of the disease include the prevalence of arthritis and myositis, which are slightly more common in children than adults, while Raynaud's phenomenon and skin sclerosis are fairly less frequent in the pediatric age [3–5].

Similar to adults, children who have JSSc commonly are found to have antinuclear antibodies (ANA) with a frequency of 81% to 97% [3,4]. Antitopoisomerase I autoantibodies are present in 28% to 34% of patients, while the prevalence of anticentromere antibodies is lower in children (7% to 8%) as compared with adults (21% to 23%) [3–5]. Interestingly, around one third of ANA-positive children have none of the SSc specific autoantibody reactivities [3,4]. The frequency of occurrence of rheumatoid factor (RF) and antiphospholipid antibodies (APL) is similar in adults and children who have SSc [4,5].

Treatment options

The pharmacologic management of patients who have JSSc is challenging, because no drug has been shown to be of unequivocal benefit in either children or adults who have systemic sclerosis. For this reason an EULAR task force of 18 SSc international experts, including two pediatric rheumatologists and two representatives of patients who had SSc very recently tried to establish some recommendations to provide guidelines for the management of SSc.

This task was done according to the EULAR guidelines and recommendations including the definition of research questions, and a systematic literature research with subsequent classification and establishment of a level of evidence for each article. A final consensus conference among international experts was held, and a final set of 14 recommendations for the treatment of SSc was established [6].

These recommendations subsequently were evaluated by a panel of 18 pediatric JSSc experts to test their agreement on the appropriateness for children. Through a Dephi survey, they were asked to approve, disapprove, or state the lack of experience for each of the 14 recommendations. For nine recommendations, a consensus greater than 85% among experts was reached [7].

Calcium channel blockers (CCB), usually oral nifedipine or nicardipine, should be considered as first-line therapy for RP, and iloprost, or other available intravenously delivered prostanoids, would be used for severe SSc-related RP and digital ulcers [8,9]. In fact, a recent study in children who had JSSc and other connective tissue diseases reported that intermittent infusions of iloprost were safe and effective in treatment of refractory RP and ischemic digits [10].

Despite the controversial results of recently published studies [11–13], and despite its known toxicity, the pediatric experts suggest that cyclophosphamide (CYC) should be considered for the treatment of SSc-related interstitial lung disease in children. According to the experience in juvenile SLE, CYC should be administered as intravenous pulse therapy at a dosage of 0.5 to 1 g/m^2 every 4 weeks for at least 6 months. To prevent cystitis, adequate hydration and frequent voiding must be emphasized. Indeed, prophylactic

MESNA should be considered to minimize contact of acrolein with the bladder mucosa.

Glucocorticoids, preferably prednisone at a dosage of 0.3 to 0.5 mg/kg/d, have very few indications in JSSc; indications do include the treatment of myositis, arthritis, and tenosynovitis. Because several studies suggest that steroids are associated with a higher risk of scleroderma renal crisis [14,15], patients on steroids should be monitored carefully for blood pressure and renal function.

Methotrexate, which is used widely for the treatment of many rheumatic conditions in children, has been shown to improve skin score in early diffuse SSc in adults [16]. According to the pediatric experts' opinion, methotrexate could be the treatment of choice for the skin manifestations also for children who have JSSc, especially in the early phase. Angiotensin-converting enzyme (ACE) inhibitors (eg, captopril, losartan) are unanimously considered effective for the long-term control of blood pressure and stabilization of renal function of scleroderma renal crisis [17]. Whether they should be used for preventing scleroderma renal crisis is not entirely clear.

Some recommendations for symptomatic treatments essentially are based on the principle of good clinical practice. They include the use of:

Proton pump inhibitors (PPIs), such as omeprazole and lansoprazole, for preventing gastroesophageal reflux disease (GERD) and esophageal ulcers

Prokinetic drugs, such as domperidone, for managing symptomatic motility disturbances

Rotating antibiotics, such as metronidazole, ciprofloxacin, and doxycycline, to treat malabsorption caused by bacterial overgrowth

As far as new experimental drugs (ie, bosentan for PAH and digital ulcers, sitaxsentan, and sildenafil), the pediatric experts expressed interest for future applications in pediatric clinical trials, although there is not enough experience, at present, to recommend their use [7].

In conclusion, most of the recommendations for the management of SSc in adults can be extended to the pediatric-onset SSc. An international cooperation, following standardized operative procedure, is needed to validate the strength of these and future recommendations.

Outcome

The prognosis of SSc in children appears better than in adults. The survival of childhood-onset SSc at 5, 10, 15 years after diagnosis is 89%, 80% to 87.4% and 74% to 87.4%, respectively, and is significantly higher than adult-onset disease [3,18]. The most common causes of death in children are related to the involvement of cardiac, renal, and pulmonary systems. In a series of 153 patients from the Padua PRES database, SSc in children may have two possible evolutions. Few patients have a rapid development of internal organ failure, leading to severe disability and eventually to death, while other patients experience a slow insidious course of the disease with lower mortality but higher morbidity [19]. Compared with studies in adults, the presence of antitopoisomerase I, anti-RNA polymerase III antibodies, and the male gender is not associated with poorer survival in children [18,19].

Conclusions

Compared with adult-onset disease, JSSc appears to be less severe with less internal organ involvement and to have less specific autoantibody profile and better long-term outcome. A multicenter and multispecialty collaboration is needed to better define the disease activity and damage outcome measures to standardize the clinical approach and treatment to this threatening disease.

Juvenile localized scleroderma

JLS, also know as morphea, comprises a group of conditions that involve essentially the skin and subcutaneous tissues. They have various features and range from very small plaques to extensive fibrotic lesions that may cause significant functional and cosmetic deformity.

Although JLS is relatively uncommon, it is far more common than systemic sclerosis in childhood, by a ratio of at least 10:1 [20]. There is a mild female predilection (female to male ratio 2.4: 1) [21]. The mean age at disease onset is 7.3 years, and a few cases with onset at birth, so-called congenital localized scleroderma (LS), have been described [22].

Clinical manifestations

The most widely used classification divides JLS into five general types: plaque morphea, generalized morphea, bullous morphea, linear sclero-derma, and deep morphea [23]. Some conditions, such as atrophoderma of Pasini Pierini, eosinophilic fasciitis, and lichen sclerosus et atrophicus, sometimes are classified among the subtypes of JLS, but this aspect is still controversial. This classification does not include the mixed forms of JLS where different type of lesions occur in the same individual. This subtype is more common than previously recognized, accounting for 15% of the whole group, as recently reported by a multicenter study in children [21].

A proposal for a new classification includes five subtypes: circumscribed morphea (CM), linear scleroderma, generalized morphea (GM), panscler-otic morphea, and the new mixed subtype where a combination of two or more of the previous subtypes is present [24].

CM is characterized by oval or round circumscribed areas of induration surrounded by a violaceous halo (Fig. 1). It is confined to the dermis, with

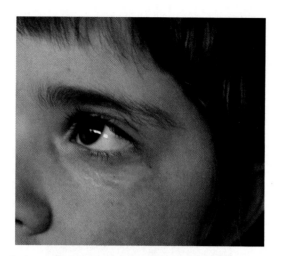

Fig. 1. Circumscribed morphea of the lower left eyelid, characterized by an area of induration with waxy consistence and ivory color, surrounded by an inflammatory edge.

only occasional involvement of the superficial panniculus. Sometimes, as in deep morphea, the entire skin feels thickened, taut, and bound down.

GM exists when there are four or more plaques with individual plaques that are larger than 3 cm and they become confluent involving at least two out of seven anatomic sites (head-neck, right upper extremity, left upper extremity, right lower extremity, left lower extremity, anterior trunk, posterior trunk) (Fig. 2). Unilateral GM has been proposed as an uncommon variant, usually beginning in childhood [4].

Linear scleroderma, the most common subtype in children and adolescents, is characterized by one or more linear streaks that can extend through the dermis, subcutaneous tissue, and muscle to the underlying bone, causing significant deformities (Fig. 3). The upper or lower extremities can be affected but also the face or scalp, as in the *en coup de sabre* variety (ECDS). The Parry Romberg syndrome (PRS), characterized by hemifacial atrophy of the skin and tissue below the forehead, with mild or absent involvement of the superficial skin, is considered the severe end of the spectrum of ECDS, and for this reason, it is included in subtype of linear scleroderma [25]. Evidence for this close relationship is the presence of associated disorders, including seizures, CNS abnormalities, dental and ocular abnormalities, reported with similar prevalence in both conditions [26–28].

Pansclerotic morphea, an extremely rare but severe subtype, is characterized by generalized full-thickness involvement of the skin of the trunk, extremities, face, and scalp with sparing of the fingertips and toes. It is more common in children than adults. Recent reports raised the attention on the possible evolution of chronic ulcers, frequently complicating pansclerotic morphea, to squamous cell carcinoma, a threatening complication already reported in SSc [29–31].

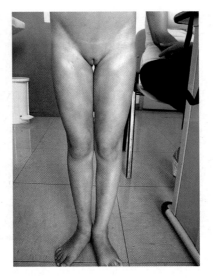

Fig. 2. Generalized morphea involving, symmetrically, the lower limbs in an 8-year-old girl.

Conversely to what has been reported for many years, JLS is not confined exclusively to the skin but can present many extracutaneous features. A recent multinational study, including 750 JLS patients, reported that 168 (22.4%) presented a total of 193 extracutaneous manifestations [32]. The overall distribution of extracutaneous manifestations was as follows: arthritis 19%, neurological findings 4%, other autoimmune conditions (eg, thyroiditis) 3%, vascular changes (eg, Raynaud's phenomenon, deep vein

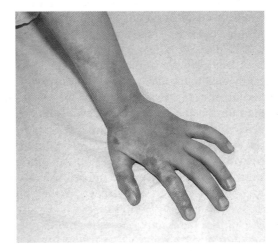

Fig. 3. Linear scleroderma of the right upper limb involving the forearm and the first and second fingers.

thrombosis) 2%, ocular and GI abnormalities 2%, and respiratory findings (restrictive lung disease) 1%. Systemic sclerosis developed in only one patient.

Articular involvement is the most frequent finding, especially in linear scleroderma. Children with JLS who develop arthritis often have a positive RF, and sometimes an elevated erythrocyte sedimentation rate (ESR) and circulating autoantibodies [32]. These children tend to have asymmetric joint involvement with no erosions, an accelerated course with predominant musculoskeletal disease and rapid development of contractures.

The most frequent neurological conditions are seizures and headaches, although behavioral changes and learning disabilities also have been described [32,33]. Abnormalities on MRI, such as calcifications, white matter changes, vascular malformations, and vasculitis, also have been reported [34,35]. Although most of the imaging abnormalities have little clinical relevance, biopsy findings have shown sclerosis, fibrosis, gliosis, and vasculitis [36]. Gastroesophageal reflux (GER) is the only GI complication reported so far [21,37,38].

JLS patients who have extracutaneous manifestations represent a new subset of JLS. The organ impairment is milder and not life-threatening as usually seen in SSc but, probably, indicates that JLS and JSS likely represent two ends of a continuous spectrum of the disease.

Autoantibodies

In a large cohort of patients, ANAs were found in 42.3% of patients who had JLS [21]. This frequency was lower than in adults who had LS [40] but higher than in normal population. In children there is no correlation between the presence of ANA and a particular subtype or the disease course [21].

Of interest, antitopoisomerase I antibodies (anti-Scl 70), a marker of SSc in adults, were found to be positive in 2% to 3% of children who had LS but not in adults who had LS [2,39]. Conversely, anticentromere antibodies (ACA) were found in 12% of adults who had LS but only in 1.7% of children [21,40]. Whether these antibodies are markers that reflect the immunological component of the disease process or can have a prognostic significance is unclear. It should be noted that none of SCL-70- or ACA-positive patients in the series of 750 JLS patients presented signs or symptoms of internal organ involvement after a mean follow-up of 3.4 years [21].

RF has been detected, at low titre, in 16% of the patients who had JLS, and significantly correlated with the presence of arthritis [21]. In adults, IgM RF is present in 30% of patients who have LS, particularly in those who have GM, and seems to be correlated with the disease severity [41].

One of the major autoantigens for ANA in LS is nuclear histone. Antihistone antibodies (AHA) have been detected in 47% of patients who have LS with a different prevalence in the various subtypes, higher in GM, lower in CM [39].

A recent study underlined the role of anti-DNA topoisomerase IIα (anti-topo IIα) autoantibodies in LS [42]. These autoantibodies were detected in 76% of patients who had LS and in 85% of those who had GM. Immuno-blotting showed no cross-reactivity of antitopo IIα with antitopo I autoan-tibodies, that are almost exclusively detected in SSc. Antitopo IIα, however, is not completely specific for LS being present also in 14% of the patients who have SSc, in 8% of those who have SLE and even in dermatomyositis (10%). Although it remains unknown why LS is associated with antitopo IIα but not antitopo I antibodies and vice-versa in SSc, these antibodies seem to play an important role in the fibrotic disorders as confirmed by their presence also in idiopathic pulmonary fibrosis [43].

Recently, Sato and colleagues [44] reported that 46% of the patients who had LS exhibited anticardiolipin antibodies (aCL), and exhibited 24% lupus anticoagulant (LAC), while beta2-glycoproteinI (β2GPI) antibodies were absent. Pulmonary embolism was seen in only one patient who had GM. In children, aCLs were found in 12.6% of the patients, but none had coag-ulation-related symptoms [21]. Although this frequency is lower than in adult patients, it is higher than in normal subjects, where it ranges from 1.5% to 9.4% [45].

Disease monitoring

The management of JLS is challenging, and the detection of disease activity and progression remains a fundamental problem. Clinical examination is subjective, and classical skin scoring methods, such as the modified Rodnan skin score widely used in the assessment of systemic sclerosis, cannot be ap-plied. A few, quite new tools have been developed but need proper validation.

Infrared thermography (IRT) has been shown to be of value in the detec-tion of active LS lesions in children [46]. This technique has shown to have a very high reproducibility, but it was found to yield false-positive results in the assessment of older lesions characterized by marked atrophy of the skin and subcutaneous tissues. In these cases, laser Doppler flowmetry (LDF) can help to discriminate real active lesions from false-positive changes [47]. LDF is a noninvasive method for measuring cutaneous microcircula-tion, and it is useful especially in a condition like scleroderma en coup de sabre. where no evident clinical signs of inflammation are present, even though the disease remains active and continues to progress.

A computerized skin score (CSS) method for measuring circumscribed lesions in LS recently has been proposed [48]. This technique consists in the demarcation of hyperemic and indurated borders of the lesions on an adhesive transparent film with different colors. The film, transferred over a cardboard, is scanned and recorded in a computer. Calculation of the affected area is performed by computer software. CSS has been shown to be a reliable method to assess the skin lesions in patients who have LS with very low intra- and interobserver variability.

MRI also is an important tool in the clinical management of JLS. MRI is clearly most useful when CNS or eye involvement is suspected but is also able to demonstrate the true depth of soft tissue lesions and the degree to which different tissue are involved in other sites [49].

Treatment

Over the years, many treatments have tried for LS. These have included topical, intralesional and systemic corticosteroids, topical and systemic calcipotriol, topical tacrolimus, hydroxychloroquine, sulfasalazine, penicillamine, gamma-interferon and methotrexate, and phototherapy with UVA light, with and without psoralens. Unfortunately, the rarity of this disease and the difficulty in assessing outcomes in an objective way have limited the interpretation of most of these studies.

CM generally is of cosmetic concern only, and therefore treatments with potentially significant toxicity are not justified. In general, these lesions will remit spontaneously with residual pigmentation as the only abnormality. Therefore, treatment should be directed mainly at topical therapies such as moisturizing agents, topical glucocorticoids, or calcipotriene [50]. Good results have been reported recently with topical Imiquimod, a novel immunomodulator that up-regulates interferon α and γ, inhibiting, in this way, the collagen production by fibroblasts, likely by down-regulating TGFβ [51].

The use of vitamin D or its analogs (topically and systemically) has been reported in several case series with encouraging results [52]; however, in the only randomized controlled trial, results indicated it was no more effective than placebo [53].

Phototherapy with ultraviolet (UV) represents another possible therapeutic choice for LS [54–59]. Treatment with UVA1 at low, medium, and high doses, with or without psoralens (PUVA) all seem to be effective clinically, although high doses seem somewhat better. There are various mechanisms of action by which UV phototherapy may work, and these include causing an increase in MMP1-collagenase activity, an increase expression of INFγ, and a decrease in TGFβ [58]. This approach seems to be much more effective for localized or superficial lesions than for the subtypes with deeper involvement such as linear or generalized scleroderma (Table 1) [54–59].

Because the rate of relapse after UV phototherapy discontinuation is not known, the need for prolonged maintenance therapy, leading to a high cumulative dosage of irradiation, and the increased risk for potential long-term effects such as skin aging and carcinogenesis [60,61] are clear limitations for its use in the pediatric age group.

When there is a significant risk for disability, such as in linear and deep subtypes, systemic treatment methotrexate (MTX) in combination with corticosteroids should be considered [62–66].

The treatment protocol usually consists in a combination of oral prednisone or intravenous methylprednisolone (IVMP 20 to 30 mg/kg/d for

Table 1
Treatment with phototherapy and methotrexate in localized scleroderma

Author (reference)	Study design	Treatment	Regimen	Number of patients (children)	Follow-up	Result	Assessment
Kersher et al [54]	Prospective, nonrandomized pilot	UVA1	UVA1 20 J/cm² for 12 weeks (total number of treatments: 30; cumulative UVA1 dose: 600 J/cm²	20 (0)	12 wks	Effective (90%)	Clinical judgment, 20 MHz US, histopathology
Kreuter et al [55]	Prospective, nonrandomized pilot	LdUVA1 + Vit D	UVA1 40 sessions in 10 wks; cumulative dose 800 J(cm²) + calcipotriol ointment 0.005% twice daily for 10 wks	19 (19)	10 wks	Effective (100%)	Clinical judgment, 20 MHz US
Gruss et al [56]	Prospective, nonrandomized pilot	UVA1	UVA1 20 J/cm², 4 times/wk for 6 wks, then once/wk for 6 wks	3 (0)	12 wks	Effective (100%)	Clinical judgment, photos
De Rie et al [57]	Prospective, nonrandomized pilot	UVA1	UVA1 = 48 J/cm², 4 times/wk for 5 weeks	8 (0)	12 wks	Effective (100%)	mRodnan skin score, cutometer, histopathology
El-Mofty et al [58]	Prospective, open, randomized controlled two arms	UVA	BB-UVA = 20 J/cm² or BB-UVA = 10 J/cm², 3 times/wk	21 (10)	7 kws	Effective (86%)	Clinical judgment

Study	Design	Treatment	Regimen	N (na)	Duration	Outcome	Measures
Kreuter et al [59]	Prospective, open, randomized controlled three arms	UVA1, UVB	LdUVA1 = 20 J/cm², MdUVA1 = 50 J/cm², NB-UVB 0,1-0,2 J/cm² 5 times/wk	64 (na)	8 wks	Effective (97%)	MSS, VAS, histopathology, 20 MHz US
Seyger et al [62]	Prospective, nonrandomized pilot	MTX	MTX 15 mg/wk orally	9 (0)	24 wks	Effective (67%)	MSS, durometer, patient's judgment VAS
Uziel et al [63]	Prospective, nonrandomized pilot	MTX + pulse steroids	MTX 0,3-0,6 mg/kg/wk os or sc + MPDN 30 mg/kg/day pulse for 3 days/mo for 3 mo	10 (10)	8-30 wks	Effective (90%)	Clinical judgment
Kreuter et al [64]	Prospective, nonrandomized pilot	MTX + pulse steroids	MTX 15 mg/wk orally + MPDN 1000 mg/day pulse for 3 days/mo for 6 mo	15 (0)	6-25 mo	Effective (93%)	MSS, patient's judgment VAS, 20 MHz US, histopathology
Fitch et al [65]	Retrospective	MTX ± steroids	MTX 0,4-1,0 mg/kg/wk os or sc ± PDN 1 mg/kg/day or every other day for 3-6 mo	17 (17)	6-60 mo	Effective (94%)	Clinical judgment, family telephone questionnaire
Wiebel et al [66]	Retrospective	MTX + steroids	MTX 10 mg/m²/wk ± PDN 1 mg/kg/d or every other day for 3-6 mo	34 (34)	24 mo	Effective (74%)	Clinical judgment, thermography

Abbreviations: BB-UVA, broad band UVA; LdUVA, low-dose UVA; MTX, methotrexate; US, ultrasonography; UVA, ultraviolet A.

3 days) and MTX (10 to 15 mg/m^2/week). Most patients show a response within 2 to 4 months, and the adverse effects are usually mild and associated more with corticosteroid use rather than with the MTX treatment. Unfortunately these studies were not controlled trials, and the series of treated patients very small (see Table 1).

Summary

JLS is a challenging but uncommon disorder among children. A new classification is now available that recognizes that many children have more than one type of LS (morphea and linear) and that a small subset of patients have evidence of internal organ disease. New techniques are available to assess and follow lesions. Therapy is based on open-labeled experiences, and controlled trials using new guidelines are needed to determine the best approach to disease modification.

References

[1] Zulian F, Woo P, Athreya BH, et al. The PRES/ACR/EULAR provisional classification criteria for juvenile systemic sclerosis. Arthritis Rheum 2007;57:203–12.

[2] Subcommittee for scleroderma criteria of the American Rheumatism Association Diagnostic and Therapeutic Criteria Committee. Preliminary criteria for the classification of systemic sclerosis (scleroderma). Arthritis Rheum 1980;23:581–90.

[3] Scalapino K, Arkachaisri T, Lucas M, et al. Childhood-onset systemic sclerosis: classification, clinical and serologic features, and survival in comparison with adult-onset disease. J Rheumatol 2006;33:1004–13.

[4] Martini G, Foeldvari I, Russo R, et al. Systemic sclerosis in childhood: clinical and immunological features of 153 patients in an international database. Arthritis Rheum 2006;54:3971–8.

[5] Della Rossa A, Valentini G, Bombardieri S, et al. European multicentre study to define disease activity criteria for systemic sclerosis. I. Clinical and epidemiological features of 290 patients from 19 centres. Ann Rheum Dis 2001;60:585–91.

[6] Kowal-Bielecka O, Landewe R, Avouac J, et al. EULAR/EUSTAR recommendations for the treatment of systemic sclerosis (SSc) [abstract]. Ann Rheum Dis 2007;66(SII): 213.

[7] Zulian F, Kowal-Bielecka O, Miniati I, et al. Preliminary agreement of the Pediatric Rheumatology European Society (PRES) on the EUSTAR/EULAR recommendations for the management of systemic sclerosis in children [abstract]. Proceedings of the 14th Pediatric Rheumatology Congress. Istanbul (Turkey), September 5–9, 2007.

[8] Thompson AE, Shea B, Welch V. Calcium channel blockers for Raynaud's phenomenon in systemic sclerosis. Arthritis Rheum 2001;44:1841–7.

[9] Pope J, Fenlon D, Thompson A, et al. Iloprost and cisaprost for Raynaud's phenomenon in progressive systemic sclerosis. Cochrane Database Syst Rev 2007;(2):[CD000953].

[10] Zulian F, Corona F, Gerloni V, et al. Safety and efficacy of iloprost for the treatment of ischaemic digits in paediatric connective tissue diseases. Rheumatology (Oxford) 2004; 43(2):229–33.

[11] Tashkin DP, Elashoff R, Clements PJ, et al. Cyclophosphamide versus placebo in scleroderma lung disease. N Engl J Med 2006;354:2655–66.

[12] Hoyles RK, Ellis RW, Wellsbury J, et al. A multicenter, prospective, randomized, double-blind, placebo-controlled trial of corticosteroids and intravenous cyclophosphamide followed by oral azathioprine for the treatment of pulmonary fibrosis in scleroderma. Arthritis Rheum 2006;54:3962–70.

[13] Nadashkevich O, Davis P, Fritzler M, et al. Randomized unblinded trial of cyclophosphamide (CYC) versus azathioprine (AZ) in the treatment of systemic sclerosis. Clin Rheumatol 2006;25:205–12.

[14] Steen VD, Medsger TA Jr. Case–control study of corticosteroids and other drugs that either precipitate or protect from the development of scleroderma renal crisis. Arthritis Rheum 1998;41:1613–9.

[15] DeMarco PJ, Weisman MH, Seibold JR, et al. Predictors and outcomes of scleroderma renal crisis: the high-dose versus low-dose D-penicillamine in early diffuse systemic sclerosis trial. Arthritis Rheum 2002;46:2983–9.

[16] Pope JE, Bellamy N, Seibold JR, et al. A randomized, controlled trial of methotrexate versus placebo in early diffuse scleroderma. Arthritis Rheum 2001;44:1351–8.

[17] Steen VD, Costantino JP, Shapiro AP, et al. Outcome of renal crisis in systemic sclerosis: relation to availability of angiotensin converting enzyme (ACE) inhibitors. Ann Intern Med 1990;113:352–7.

[18] Martini G, Zulian F. Clinical features and outcome in juvenile systemic sclerosis (JSSc): data from the international Padua database of 153 patients [abstract]. Clin Exp Rheumatol 2006; 24(1 Suppl 40):S57.

[19] Scussel-Lonzetti L, Joyal F, Raynauld JP, et al. Predicting mortality in systemic sclerosis. Analysis of a cohort of 309 French Canadian patients with emphasis on features at diagnosis as predictive factors for survival. Medicine 2002;81:154–67.

[20] Peterson LS, Nelson AM, Su WP, et al. The epidemiology of morphea (localized scleroderma) in Olmsted County 1960–1993. J Rheumatol 1997;24:73–80.

[21] Zulian F, Athreya BH, Laxer RM, et al. Juvenile localized scleroderma: clinical and epidemiological features in 750 children. An international study. Rheumatology (Oxford) 2006;45:614–20.

[22] Zulian F, Vallongo C, de Oliveira SKF, et al. Congenital localized scleroderma. J Pediatr 2006;149(2):248–51.

[23] Peterson LS, Nelson AM, Su WP. Subspecialty clinics: rheumatology and dermatology. Classification of morphea (localized scleroderma). Mayo Clin Proc 1995;70:1068–76.

[24] Zulian F, Ruperto N. Proceedings of the II Workshop on Juvenile Scleroderma Syndrome. Padua (Italy), June 3–6, 2004.

[25] Jablonska S, Blaszczyk M. Long-lasting follow-up favours a close relationship between progressive facial hemiatrophy and scleroderma en coup de sabre. J Eur Acad Dermatol Venereol 2005;19:403–4.

[26] Menni S, Marzano AV, Passoni E. Neurologic abnormalities in two patients with facial hemiathrophy and sclerosis coexisting with morphea. Pediatr Dermatol 1997;14:113–6.

[27] Blaszczyk M, Jablonska S. Linear scleroderma en coup de sabre: relationship with progressive facial hemiatrophy. Adv Exp Med Biol 1999;455:101–4.

[28] Sommer A, Gambichler T, Bacharach-Buhles M, et al. Clinical and serological characteristics of progressive facial hemiatrophy: a case series of 12 patients. J Am Acad Dermatol 2006; 54:227–33.

[29] Wollina U, Buslau M, Weyers W. Squamous cell carcinoma in pansclerotic morphea of childhood. Pediatr Dermatol 2002;19:151–4.

[30] Parodi PG, Roberti G, Draganic Stinco D, et al. Squamous cell carcinoma arising in a patient with long-standing pansclerotic morphea. Br J Dermatol 2001;144:417–9.

[31] Maragh SH, Davis MD, Bruce AJ, et al. Disabling pansclerotic morphea: clinical presentation in two adults. J Am Acad Dermatol 2005;53:S115–9.

[32] Zulian F, Vallongo C, Woo P, et al. Localized scleroderma in childhood is not just a skin disease. Arthritis Rheum 2005;52:2873–81.

[33] Blaszczyk M, Krolicki L, Krasu M, et al. Progressive facial hemiatrophy: central nervous system involvement and relationship with scleroderma en coup de sabre. J Rheumatol 2003;30(9):1997–2004.

[34] DeFelipe J, Segura T, Arellano JI, et al. Neuropathological findings in a patient with epilepsy and the Parry-Romberg syndrome. Epilepsia 2001;42:1198–203.

[35] Flores-Alvarado DE, Esquivel-Valerio JA, Garza-Elizondo M, et al. Linear scleroderma en coup de sabre and brain calcification: is there a pathogenic relationship? J Rheumatol 2003; 30:193–5.

[36] Holland KE, Steffes B, Nocton JJ, et al. Linear scleroderma en coup de sabre with associated neurologic abnormalities. Pediatrics 2006;117:132–6.

[37] Weber P, Ganser G, Frosch M, et al. Twenty-four hour intraesophageal pH monitoring in children and adolescents with scleroderma and mixed connective tissue disease. J Rheumatol 2000;27:2692–5.

[38] Guariso G, Conte S, Galeazzi F, et al. Esophageal involvement in juvenile localized scleroderma. Clin Exp Rheumatol 2007;25:786–9.

[39] Takehara K, Sato S. Localized scleroderma is an autoimmune disease. Rheumatology (Oxford) 2005;44:274–9.

[40] Ruffatti A, Peserico A, Glorioso S, et al. Anticentromere antibody in localized scleroderma. J Am Acad Dermatol 1986;15:637–42.

[41] Mimura Y, Ihn H, Jinnin M, et al. Rheumatoid factor isotypes in localized scleroderma. Clin Exp Dermatol 2005;30:405–8.

[42] Hayakawa I, Hasegawa M, Takehara K, et al. Anti-DNA topoisomerase IIα autoantibodies in localised scleroderma. Arthritis Rheum 2004;50:227–32.

[43] Grigolo B, Mazzetti I, Borzi RM, et al. Mapping of topoisomerase IIα epitopes recognized by autoantibodies in idiopathic pulmonary fibrosis. Clin Exp Immunol 1998;114:339–46.

[44] Sato S, Fujimoto M, Hasegawa M, et al. Antiphospholipid antibody in localised scleroderma. Ann Rheum Dis 2003;62:771–4.

[45] Vila P, Hernandez MC, Lopez-Fernandez MF, et al. Prevalence, follow-up and clinical significance of the anticardiolipin antibodies in normal subjects. Thromb Haemost 1994; 72:209–13.

[46] Martini G, Murray KJ, Howell KJ, et al. Juvenile-onset localized scleroderma activity detection by infrared thermography. Rheumatology (Oxford) 2002;41:1178–82.

[47] Wiebel L, Howell KJ, Visentin MT, et al. Laser Doppler flowmetry for assessing localized scleroderma in children. Arthritis Rheum 2007;56:3489–95.

[48] Zulian F, Meneghesso D, Grisan E, et al. A new computerized method for the assessment of skin lesions in localized scleroderma. Rheumatology (Oxford) 2007;46:856–60.

[49] Liu P, Uziel Y, Chuang S, et al. Localized scleroderma: imaging features. Pediatr Radiol 1994;24:207–9.

[50] Cunningham BB, Landells ID, Langman C, et al. Topical calcipotriene for morphea/linear scleroderma. J Am Acad Dermatol 1998;39:211–5.

[51] Dytoc M, Ting PT, Man J, et al. First case series on the use of imiquimod for morphoea Br J Dermatol 2005;153:815–20.

[52] Caca-Biljanovska NG, Vlckova-Laskoska MT, Dervendi DV, et al. Treatment of generalized morphea with oral 1,25-dihydroxyvitamin D3. Adv Exp Med Biol 1999;455:299–304.

[53] Hulshof MM, Bouwes BJN, Bergman W, et al. Double-blind, placebo-controlled study of oral calcitriol for the treatment of localized scleroderma and systemic scleroderma. J Am Acad Dermatol 2000;43:1017–23.

[54] Kerscher M, volkenandt M, Gruss C, et al. Low dose UVA phototherapy for treatment of localized scleroderma. J Am Acad Dermatol 1998;38:21–3.

[55] Kreuter A, Gambichler T, Avermaete A, et al. Combined treatment with calcipotriol ointment and low-dose ultraviolet A1 phototherapy in childhood morphea. Pediatr Dermatol 2001;18:241–5.

[56] Gurss CJ, von Kobyletzki G, Behrens-Williams SC, et al. Effects of low dose ultraviolet A-1 phototherapy on morphea. Photodermatol Photoimmunol Photomed 2001;17:149–55.

[57] De Rie MA, Bos JD. Photochemotherapy for systemic and localized scleroderma. J Am Acad Dermatol 2000;43:725–6.

[58] El-Mofty M, Mostafa W, Esmat S, et al. Suggested mechanisms of action of UVA phototherapy in morphea: a molecular study. Photodermatol Photoimmunol Photomed 2004;20:93–100.

[59] Kreuter A, Hyun J, Stucker M, et al. A randomized controlled study of low-dose UVA1, medium-dose UVA1, and narrowband UVB phototherapy in the treatment of localized scleroderma. J Am Acad Dermatol 2006;54:440–7.

[60] Staberg B, Wulf HC, Klemp P, et al. The carcinogenic effect of UVA irradiation. J Invest Dermatol 1983;81:517–9.

[61] Setlow RB, Grist E, Thompson K, et al. Wavelengths effective in induction of malignant melanoma. Proc Natl Acad Sci U S A 1993;90:6666–70.

[62] Seyger MM, van den Hoogen FH, de Boo T, et al. Low-dose methotrexate in the treatment of widespread morphea. J Am Acad Dermatol 1998;39:220–5.

[63] Uziel Y, Feldman BM, Krafchik BR, et al. Methotrexate and corticosteroid therapy for pediatric localized scleroderma. J Pediatr 2000;136:91–5.

[64] Kreuter A, Gambichler T, Breuckmann F, et al. Pulsed high-dose corticosteroids combined with low-dose methotrexate in severe localized scleroderma. Arch Dermatol 2005;141:847–52.

[65] Fitch PG, Retting P, Burnham JM, et al. Treatment of pediatric localized scleroderma with methotrexate. J Rheumatol 2006;33:609–14.

[66] Weibel L, Sampaio MC, Visentin MT, et al. Evaluation of methotrexate and corticosteroids for the treatment of localized scleroderma (morphea) in children. Br J Dermatol 2006;155:1013–20.

ELSEVIER
SAUNDERS

Rheum Dis Clin N Am
34 (2008) 257–265

RHEUMATIC
DISEASE CLINICS
OF NORTH AMERICA

Index

Note: Page numbers of article titles are in **boldface** type.

A

Abdominal discomfort, 228

c-Abelson, in fibrosis, 127–128

ACE gene polymorphisms, 26

Acro-osteolysis, 221–223

Activin-like kinases, 124

Adhesion molecules, 62, 67

Adrenomedullin, for pulmonary arterial hypertension, 194

Adrenoreceptors, in Raynaud's syndrome, 81–85

AIF1 gene polymorphisms, 22, 25

Allograft inflammatory factor-1, 22

Allopurinol, for vascular disease, 105

Alpha-adrenergic blockers, for vascular disease, 103

Angiogenesis, 45–47, **73–79**

Angiography, 99–100

Angioplasty, 106

Angiostatin, 76–77

Angiotensin II receptor antagonists
for fibrosis, 123
for vascular disease, 102

Angiotensin-converting enzyme, 26, 67

Angiotensin-converting enzyme inhibitors
for juvenile systemic sclerosis, 243
for vascular disease, 102

Aniline, in food oils, toxic oil syndrome due to, 207

Animal models, of scleroderma, 133–135

Ankle-brachial pressure index, 90

Anorectal dysfunction, 228–229

Anti-angiogenic factors, 73–79

Antibody(ies). *See also* Antinuclear antibodies.
cardiolipin, 248
CD20, 171
centromere, 2, 6–7, 32
discovery of, 1–2
endothelial, 62
histone, 247
in juvenile localized scleroderma, 247–248
Pm/Scl, 5, 8, 32
RNA polymerase, 3, 5–6, 10–11, 32
Scl 70 antigen (topoisomerase), 2–3, 5–6, 9–11, 32, 247
subsets of, 2–3
Th/To, 5, 7–8
titer of, 94–95
transforming growth factor, 150–151, 173
U1-RNP, 5, 8–9
U3-RNP, 6, 9, 11, 32

Antibody-dependent cellular cytotoxicity, 61–62

Anticardiolipin antibodies, 248

Anticentromere antibodies, 2, 6–7, 32

Antifibrotic therapy, for skin disease, 172–173

Antinuclear antibodies, 4
in juvenile localized scleroderma, 247–248
in limited scleroderma, 5
in pediatric patients, 242

Antioxidants, for vascular disease, 105

Antiplatelet agents, for vascular disease, 105–106

Anti-thymocyte globulin
for skin disease, 169–170
with stem cell transplantation
for fibrosis, 146–147, 149
for skin disease, 167–169

Apoptosis, endothelial, 47, 59–63

Arrhythmias, 186–187

Surgery, for vascular disease, 106

Sympathectomy, cervical, for vascular
     disease, 106

T

T cells
     cytotoxic, 61
     in vascular repair, 74

Tadalafil, for vascular disease, 104

TGFβ gene polymorphisms, 25, 27

Thalidomide, for scleromyxedema, 212–213

Thermography, 95, 98–99, 248

β-Thromboglobulin, 65

Thrombomodulin, 67

Th/To antibodies, 5, 7–8

Thyroid gland, fibrosis of, 231–232

Tissue plasminogen activator, for vascular
     disease, 106

Topoisomerase, antibodies to, 2–3, 5–6,
     9–11, 32, 247–248

Toxic oil syndrome, 207

Transforming growth factor beta, 27, 63,
     117
     antibodies to
          for skin disease, 173
          recombinant, for fibrosis,
               150–151
     as biomarker, 174
     in eosinophilic fasciitis, 207
     in fibrosis, 122–135

Transplant atherosclerosis, 43, 50

Transplantation, stem cell, 50
     for fibrosis, 145–150
     for skin disease, 167–169

Trichostatin, for fibrosis, 156–157

Tricuspid Annular Plane Systolic
     Excursion, 185

Tricuspid valve disease, 187

Trigeminal neuropathy, 232

L-Tryptophan, toxicity of, 207

Tumor necrosis factor-a, antibodies to,
     for skin disease, 171

Twin studies, 18–19

Tyrosine kinase inhibitors. *See also*
     Imatinib.
     for fibrosis, 153–155

U

Ulnar artery occlusion, 91

Ultrasound
     Doppler, 95–96
     in skin disease assessment, 174

Ultraviolet light therapy, for scleredema,
     215

Unilateral morphea, 245

U1-RNP antibodies, 5, 8–9

U3-RNP antibodies, 6, 9, 11, 32

Urokinase, 77

V

Valvular heart disease, 187

Vascular cell adhesion molecule, 62

Vascular disease. *See also* Raynaud's
     phenomenon.
     circulating markers of, 66–67
     pathophysiology of. *See*
          Pathophysiology.
     peripheral, **89–114**
     vascular repair in, **73–79**

Vascular endothelial cadherin, 45–48

Vascular endothelial growth factor, 26, 42,
     73–76

Vasoactive intestinal peptide, for
     pulmonary arterial hypertension, 193

Vasoconstriction, in Raynaud's syndrome,
     81–85

Vasodilators, for vascular disease, 103–105

Ventricle(s), left, dysfunction of, 184

Vibration, Raynaud's phenomenon and,
     84–85

Videomicroscopy, 98

Viruses, as triggers, 60–63

Vitamin D, 249

von Willebrand factor, 66–67

W

Warfarin, for vascular disease, 106

Weakness, 233

Wrist, avascular necrosis of, 223

X

Xerostomia, 224